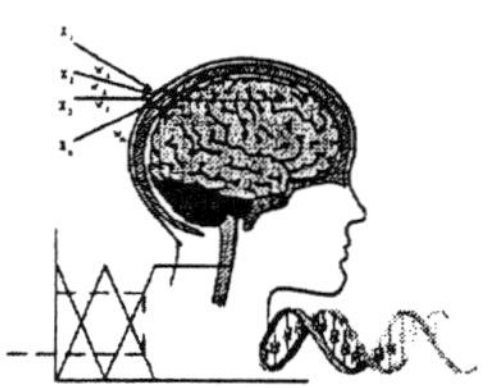

The CRC Press
International Series on Computational Intelligence

Series Editor
L.C. Jain, Ph.D., M.E., B.E., (Hons), Fellow I.E. (Australia)

L.C. Jain, R.P. Johnson, Y. Takefuji, and L.A. Zadeh
Knowledge-Based Intelligent Techniques in Industry

L.C. Jain and C.W. de Silva
Intelligent Adaptive Control: Industrial Applications

L.C. Jain and N.M. Martin
Fusion of Neural Networks, Fuzzy Systems, and Genetic Algorithms: Industrial Applications

H.N. Teodorescu, A. Kandel, and L.C. Jain
Fuzzy and Neuro-Fuzzy Systems in Medicine

C.L. Karr and L.M. Freeman
Industrial Applications of Genetic Algorithms

L.C. Jain and Beatrice Lazzerini
Knowledge-Based Intelligent Techniques in Character Recognition

L.C. Jain and V. Vemuri
Industrial Applications of Neural Networks

H.N. Teodorescu, A. Kandel, and L.C. Jain
Soft Computing in Human-Related Science

B. Lazzerini, D. Dumitrescu, L.C. Jain, and A. Dumitrescu
Evolutionary Computing and Applications

B. Lazzerini, D. Dumitrescu, and L.C. Jain
Fuzzy Sets and Their Application to Clustering and Training

L.C. Jain, U. Halici, I. Hayashi, S.B. Lee, and S. Tsutsui
Intelligent Biometric Techniques in Fingerprint and Face Recognition: Practical Applications

Z. Chen
Computational Intelligence for Decision Support

L.C. Jain
Evolution of Engineering and Information System and Their Applications

H.N. Teodorescu and A. Kandel
Dynamic Fuzzy Systems and Chaos Applications

L. Medsker and L.C. Jain
Recurrent Neural Networks: Design and Applications

SOFT COMPUTING
in
HUMAN-RELATED
SCIENCES

Edited by
Horia-Nicolai Teodorescu
Abraham Kandel
Lakhmi C. Jain

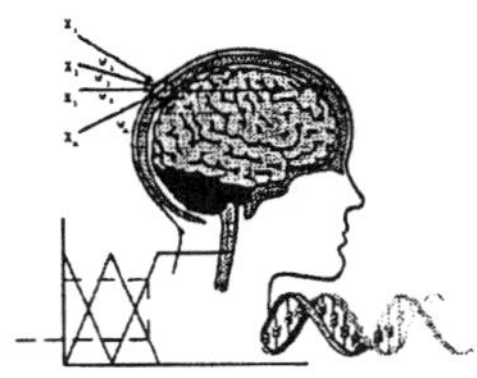

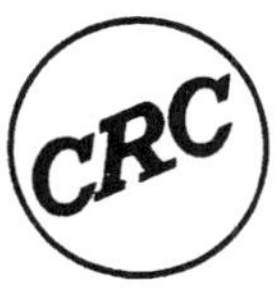

CRC Press

Boca Raton   London   New York   Washington, D.C.

Library of Congress Cataloging-in-Publication Data

Soft-computing in human-related sciences / Horia-Nicolai L.
    Teodorescu, Abraham Kandel, Lakhmi C. Jain (editors).
            p.   cm. -- (International series on computational
    intelligence)
        Includes bibliographical references and index.
        ISBN 0-8493-1635-9 (alk. paper)
        1. Medical informatics. 2. Soft computing. 3. Life sciences-
    -Data processing. I. Teodorescu, Horia-Nicolai. II. Kandel,
    Abraham. III. Jain, L. C. IV. Series.
    R858.S625 1999
    610′.285—dc21   99-11923
                                                                       CIP

Preface

There is a tendency to say that we live in the *post numerical computing and control* era, an era based on numerous emerging fields, many of them devoted to knowledge processing. Hard boundaries between such fields as fuzzy systems, neural networks, chaotic systems, and expert systems tend to vanish, and "intelligent systems" mixing these different approaches are replacing the classic, signal- and data-driven systems.

The present volume *Soft Computing in Human-related Sciences* is intended to demonstrate how new technologies derived from human reasoning and knowledge processing, such as neural networks, fuzzy logic, genetic algorithms, and virtual reality), can be applied to human-related sciences. There are several human-related sciences addressed in this volume: man-machine interaction, robotics (mainly anthropomorphic robots) and prosthetic devices, human-like information processing and control, medicine (including rehabilitation medicine), psychology (emotion representation and recognition), nutrition (health and social problems), medical information management, and the validation of training and education.

This volume we provides an up-to-date, extensive review of recent developments and trends for students and researchers in robotics, man-machine communication, cybernetics, medicine, psychology, biomedical engineering, system engineering, communication, control engineering, and other human-related sciences. Computer scientists, electrical engineers, and control engineers interested in the development of soft computing systems and their applications, as well as experts in the application of intelligent technologies, should find this volume a valuable resource in their research.

This volume is composed of three sections. The first section deals with the fundamentals of soft computing and intelligent systems, as well as issues in robotic and prosthetic systems. The second section is devoted to medical applications in the broader sense: information systems for medical use, intelligent diagnosis in maternal and fetal medicine, applications based on new tools such as wavelet neural systems, and signal processing and control in pattern recognition by human experts. The third section deals with the interpretation of emotion by computers, nutrition education and planning based on fuzzy techniques, and the assessment of competence after training.

In **Chapter 1**, *Fuzzy control methodology: basics and state of the art*, the authors provide a very complete introduction containing a review of the current research and the state of the art in the field of intelligent control and related applications. A thorough review of genetic methods is presented, and a comprehensive yet concise overview of fuzzy control and neural networks is provided. A focus of the chapter is the combination of neuro-fuzzy systems with genetic methods in order to realize a truly "intelligent" system. The main concepts in fuzzy systems (inference mechanisms for fuzzy controllers, defuzzification methods, functional fuzzy inference) are explained; moreover, several topics related to fuzzy control are reviewed. Learning, adaptation, and evolution for fuzzy controllers and several applications in image processing, diagnosis systems, and biomedical engineering are described.

In **Chapter 2**, *Learning stiffness characteristics of the human hand using a neuro-fuzzy system,* the authors investigate human hand stiffness and motor learning. A neuro-fuzzy system (ANFIS type) is used in modeling the stiffness characteristics of the human hand for different postures. The theoretical aspect of the model as well as the model itself, the simulation protocol and results are discussed. The methodology and results of this paper may be used in designing robotic manipulators and prosthetic devices; in addition, the results are useful in rehabilitation medicine.

In **Chapter 3**, *Fuzzy neural networks and their applications to learning sensory-motor coordination*, the author deals with fuzzy logic neurons, whose synaptic operators are modeled by triangular norms, and whose somatic operators are modeled by triangular co-norms. Applications to problems of sensory-motor mapping (more precisely eye-arm coordination) are discussed. A neural network is trained with sets of images of the arm-joint control value pairs. In particular, the imitation of human movements by robots is addressed. After learning, the network is able to control a robotic arm that imitates the movement of a master arm observed by a camera, achieving a form of vision-based telemanipulation. Such systems have applications in prosthetics, remote surgery, and industrial robotics.

In **Chapter 4**, *Fuzzy Reduction Control of Acceleration and Vibration of a Stretcher-Cart on an Ambulance,* the authors present the use of fuzzy logic control in the active control of vibrations and acceleration on on stretcher-carts in ambulances.

In **Chapter 5**, *Computational intelligence for medical information analysis and refinement*, the authors describe the design of an automated data analysis and decision support system - the Clinician's Workstation - for the clinical diagnostic environment. The system uses a neural network to automatically create and utilize disease-specific expert systems. The neural network used in the Clinician's Workstation has a specialized architecture which is presented in the paper.

In **Chapter 6**, *Intelligent diagnostic systems in maternal and fetal medicine*, a team of computer scientists and physicians present a thorough review of intelligent systems as used in the area of maternal and fetal medicine. The authors present a broad introduction to the related areas of prenatal diagnosis and perinatal surveillance, and they discuss technological advances that have affected these fields. A review of wavelet theory, fuzzy logic, neural networks, and feature extraction is given. Emphasis is placed on intelligent signal processing, since one of the goals of fetal medicine is to use noninvasive techniques to monitor the fetus. The authors describe several systems they have constructed for use in fetal medicine.

In **Chapter 7**, *Wavelet network with convex wavelets: Applications to nonlinear system modeling and feature extraction in vectorcardiography,* the authors present a family of systems combining wavelets, neural networks, and fuzzy concepts. The wavelet networks are used to solve several types of problems, including chaotic time series prediction and a major medical diagnosis problem, namely vectorcardiogram processing and interpretation. A thorough analysis of the wavelet networks and of the corresponding learning algorithms is performed. Appendices dealing with mathematical details complement the chapter.

In **Chapter 8**, *Features-oriented filtering of biological signals*, the authors present a new interpretation of signal processing and control as a task-oriented process. The methodology is based on a feature space representation of the signals, rather than a sample space representation. All subsequent operations are related to the feature space. The final aim is to perform human-like processing and to generate results that are more appropriate for human interpretation. Various techniques (principal component analysis, multilayer perceptron, radial basis function networks) are used in the development of the feature space processing systems. Applications in the field of biomedical engineering are used to demonstrate the methods.

In **Chapter 9**, *An emotion processing system based on fuzzy inference and subjective observations*, the authors propose an interesting tool for representing and processing mixed emotions, and for the interpretation of emotions by machines. Computer simulations and the results of emotional clustering and interpretation demonstrate the validity of the system. Although the authors base their approach on a detailed mathematical representation, the reader can skip the mathematical details without losing sight of the main ideas in the chapter. The research demonstrates tremendous potential in man-machine interaction and in virtual reality; moreover, it significantly contributes to the design of more human-friendly support systems and machines. The field of psychology will benefit from a new tool for emotion representation, and linguists will have the benefit of a more intelligent system for interpreting the semantics of natural languages.

In **Chapter 10**, *Fuzzy methods in nutrition planning and education and in clinical nutrition*, the authors deal with a softer interpretation of the recommended daily allowances for diets based on fuzzy sets and fuzzy logic. The authors present a complete methodology and several applications in nutrition control, nutrition planning, and nutrition education, using as examples large project orders by a major European health insurance company for its customers in Germany and by WHO for a developing country. In addition, various aspects related to nutrition education and economic and social issues are addressed.

In **Chapter 11**, *Designing experiments for medical diagnosis evaluation using membership functions*, competency evaluation of a junior specialists is dealt with, namely the professional evaluation for medical diagnosis in a clinical context. The authors introduce a fuzzy sets-based evaluation experiment design. The membership functions are built using the scaling methods of the Theory of Psychological Measurement. The basic tasks related to the scaling methods are analyzed, and conditions for extracting the membership functions are derived. The proposed experiment is designed to promote the acquisition of experience in medical diagnosis for the purpose of competency evaluation. The applications of the presented methodology range from training evaluation in various fields to the design of supervisory systems in hierarchical structures.

The contributors to this volume are computer scientists, engineers, and physicians. Almost all chapters are written by teams of physicians, biomedical engineers, computer scientists, and electrical engineers. This insures that both the medical audience and the engineering audience will find this volume interesting and useful.

The backgrounds of the contributors to this volume indicate a well-balanced, worldwide authorship: four chapters are contributed by scientists from the USA, four chapters by researchers from Europe, four chapters by researchers from Japan, two chapters by contributors from the Middle East, and one chapter has a contributor from Australia. (The sum of the contributors is larger than the number of chapters because many chapters have contributors from several different regions.)

It is a challenge to adequately present a team of contributors when so many are renowned experts in their fields. Furthermore, their vitae indicate that each one is now serving or has served as either a president or vice-president of an international society, as a chief editor or a vice-editor of an international journal, or both. Without any risk of exaggeration, we can summarize the many contributions of the authors of this volume by saying that the field of intelligent systems would be quite different today if it had not been for them.

All of the chapters were reviewed by five or more referees, which contributed significantly to the improvements in contents and style. Six out of eleven chapters were partly rewritten, while others were largely edited by the Editors to insure a uniform style. An Index of Terms supplements the volume, and the first editor added some remarks to two of the chapters.

This volume, in combination with the volume *Fuzzy and Neuro-Fuzzy Systems in Medicine,* H.N. Teodorescu, A. Kandel, L.C. Jain (Eds.), CRC Press, FL, 1998, is designed to offer comprehensive reading for a variety of classes. Courses related to intelligent technologies in colleges and departments of medicine, psychology, and biomedical engineering will have, for the first time, reading materials in their fields that are suitable for graduate students. In addition, engineering courses on neuro-fuzzy systems and other intelligent technologies may find that the two volumes provide good reading for their students as well.

October 1998

Horia-Nicolai Teodorescu
Abraham Kandel
Tampa, Florida

Lakhmi C. Jain
Adelaide, South Australia

About the Editors

Horia-Nicolai L. Teodorescu has served as a professor in several universities; he is currently teaching courses at the University of South Florida, Tampa, FL, U.S.A., Swiss National Institute of Technology, Lausanne, Switzerland, and Technical University of Iasi, Iasi, Romania. Dr. Teodorescu received an M.S. degree and a Doctoral degree in Electronics in 1975 and 1981, respectively. He is a founding director of the Center for Fuzzy Systems and Approximate Reasoning at Technical University of Iasi, Iasi, Romania, since 1990. He has been a professor at that university since 1990 as well. He was an invited or visiting professor in Japan in 1992, 1993, and 1994, in Switzerland in 1994, 1995, and 1996, and in Spain in 1993 and 1996.

Dr. Teodorescu has written about 250 papers, authored/co-authored, edited/co-edited more than 20 volumes, and holds 21 patents. He has won several gold and silver medals for his inventions at various invention exhibitions. He has authored many papers on biomedical engineering and the applications of fuzzy and neuro-fuzzy systems to medical engineering. 11 patents held by Dr. Teodorescu are in the field of biomedical engineering, and he has won several grants for research on the application of fuzzy systems to biomedicine. He is a Senior Member of the IEEE and holds several honorific titles, including "Eminent Scientist" from the Fuzzy Logic Systems Institute in Japan and the Honorary Medal of the Higher Economic School in Barcelona, Spain. He has been a *correspondent member* of the Romanian Academy since 1993.

Dr. Teodorescu is one of the Chief Editors of *Fuzzy Systems & A.I.– Reports and Letters, International Journal for Chaos Theory and Applications, Iasi Polytechnic Magazine,* and *Magazine for Fuzzy Systems,* as well as a Co-Director of *Fuzzy Economic Review.* He is a member of the editorial boards of *Fuzzy Sets and Systems, The Journal of Grey Systems, BUSEFAL – Bulletin for Studies and Exchange of Fuzziness and its Applications, Journal of Information Sciences of Moldavia, Review for Inventions, Romanian Journal of Information Science and Technology,* and *Journal of AEDEM.* He has served as a chairman of the scientific committees of several international conferences, and he has been a member of the scientific committees of more than 40 international conferences.

Address: Computer Science and Engineering Department, University of South Florida, ENB 118, 4202 East Fowler Avenue, Tampa, FL 33620, USA

Abraham Kandel received a B.Sc. from the Technion – Israel Institute of Technology and an M.S. from the University of California, both in Electrical Engineering, and a Ph.D. in Electrical Engineering and Computer Science from the University of New Mexico. Dr. Kandel, a Professor and the Endowed Eminent Scholar in Computer Science and Engineering, is the Chairman of the Department of Computer Science and Engineering at the University of South Florida. Previously, he was a Professor and Founding Chairman of the Computer Science Department of Florida State University, as well as the Director of the Institute of Expert Systems and Robotics at FSU and the Director of the State University System Center for Artificial Intelligence at FSU. He is Editor of *The Fuzzy Track – IEEE MICRO*, an Associate Editor of *IEEE Transactions of Systems, Man, and Cybernetics*, and a member of the editorial board of the international journals *Fuzzy Sets and Systems*, *Information Sciences*, *Expert Systems*, *Engineering Applications of Artificial Intelligence*, *The Journal of Grey Systems*, *Control Engineering Practice*, *Fuzzy Systems – Reports and Letters*, *IEEE Transactions on Fuzzy Systems*, a book series on *Studies in Fuzzy Decision and Control*, *Applied Computing Review Journal*, *Journal of Neural Network World*, *The Journal of Fuzzy Mathematics*, and *BUSEFAL – Bulletin for Studies and Exchange of Fuzziness and Its Applications*.

Dr. Kandel has published over 350 research papers for numerous professional publications in Computer Science and Engineering. He is also the author/co-author, editor/co-editor of 26 texts in Computer Science and Engineering. Dr. Kandel is a Fellow of the ACM, Fellow of the IEEE, Fellow of the New York Academy of Sciences, Fellow of AAAS, as well as a member of NAFIPS, IFSA, ASEE, and Sigma-Xi.

Dr. Kandel has been awarded the College of Engineering Outstanding Research Award, USF, 1993-94; Sigma-Xi Outstanding Faculty Researcher Award, 1995; The Theodore and Venette-Askounes Ashford Distinguished Scholar Award, USF, 1995; MOISIL International Foundation Gold Medal for Lifetime Achievements, 1996; and the Distinguished Researcher Award, USF, 1997.

Address: Computer Science and Engineering Department, University of South Florida, ENB 118, 4202 East Fowler Avenue, Tampa, FL 33620, USA

Lakhmi C. Jain is a founding director of the Knowledge-Based Intelligent Engineering Systems (KES) Centre, located in the Faculty of Information Technology at the University of South Australia. He is a fellow of the Institution of Engineers Australia. He has initiated a postgraduate research program in knowledge-based intelligent engineering systems. He is the Founding Editor-in-Chief of the *International Journal of Knowledge-Based Intelligent Engineering Systems* and serves as an Associate Editor of the *IEEE Transactions on Industrial Electronics*. Dr. Jain was the Technical Chair of the ETD2000 International Conference in 1995, Publications Chair of the Australian and New Zealand Conference on Intelligent Information Systems in 1996 and a Conference Chair of the International Conference on Knowledge-based Intelligent Electronic Systems in 1997 and 1998. He served as the Vice-President of the Electronics Association of South Australia in 1997. He is the Editor-in-Chief of the *International Book Series on Computational Intelligence*, CRC Press, USA. His interests focus on the development of novel techniques such as knowledge-based systems, artificial neural networks, fuzzy systems, genetic algorithms, and the application of these techniques.

Address: KES Center, Faculty of Information Technology, University of South Australia, Adelaide, Warrendi Road, The Levels, South Australia 5095

Contributors

Sezer Aksel is a Professor of Obstetrics and Gynecology. She is affiliated with the University of South Alabama, USA. Her field of interest is reproductive endocrinology and infertility.
Address: 100 Tower Dr. 703, Daphne Alabama, 36526, USA. Fax: +1 205 639 7433. E-mail: sezer@Dibbs.net

Volkan Atalay graduated from the Department of Electrical and Electronics Engineering, Middle East Technical University, Ankara, Turkey, in 1987. He received the degree of Master of Science from the same department. He pursued doctoral studies in Computer Science at the Universite Rene Descartes-Paris V, Paris, France, and obtained the Ph.D. in 1993. He was a visiting scholar at the New Jersey Institute of Technology, NJ, USA, for a year. He has been an Assistant Professor of Computer Engineering at METU since 1993. His research areas are computer vision, particularly texture analysis, document analysis, and applications of neural networks.
Address: Dept. of Computer Eng., Middle East Technical University, 06531, Ankara, Turkey. Phone: +90 312 210 5576, Fax: +90 312 210 1259. E-mail: volkan@ceng.metu.edu.tr

Meral Beksac graduated from Hacettepe University, Faculty of Medicine, Ankara, Turkey, in 1980. She received her degree in Internal Medicine in 1985 and in Hematology in 1991. Her fields of interest are hematological malignancies, tissue typing, umbilical cord blood transplantation, and morphological assessment of hematological images. She has been a Professor of Hematology since 1993 at Ankara University, Turkey.
Address: Dept. of Hematology, Ankara University, 06100, Ankara. Phone: +90 312 310 8606, Fax: +90 312 311 5474. E-mail: mbeksac@neuron.ato.org.tr

Sinan Beksac graduated from Hacettepe University, Faculty of Medicine, Ankara, Turkey in 1976. He received his degree in Obstetrics and Gynecology in 1980. He has been a Professor of Obstetrics and Gynecology since 1992 at

Hacettepe University. His fields of interest are prenatal diagnosis, perinatal surveillance, and intelligent diagnostic systems in maternal and fetal medicine. *Address: Division of Maternal and Fetal Medicine, Dept. of Obstetrics and Gynecology, Hacettepe University, 06100, Ankara, Turkey. Phone: +90 312 310 1011, Fax: +90 312 310 5552. E-mail: mbeksac@neuron.ato.org.tr*

Patrik Eklund received his Ph.D. in Mathematics at Abo Akademi University in 1986. Since 1995 he has been a Professor in Computer Science at Umea University. His research interests include foundations of computer science, AI, health informatics, distributed systems, and industrial information systems. He actively develops cooperative ventures with both industry and health care. *Address: Umea University, Department of Computing Science, Se-90187, Umeå, Sweden. Phone: +46 90 7869914, Fax +46 90 166126. E-mail: peklund@cs.umu.se, URL: http://www.cs.umu.se/~peklund*

Aydan M. Erkmen received her B.S. degree from Bogazici University, Department of Electrical Engineering, Istanbul, Turkey, in 1978 with a major in Mathematics. Her M.S. degree in 1981 was earned at Drexel University, Department of Electrical and Computer Engineering, Philadelphia, PA, USA. She pursued her Ph.D. studies at the School of Information Technology and Engineering, George Mason University, Fairfax, VA, USA. She is now an Associate Professor at the Middle East Technical University, Department of Electrical and Electronics Engineering, Ankara, Turkey. Her research interests include intelligent control and diagnostic systems with applications in bioengineering, robotics with an emphasis on grasping with anthropomorphic robot hands, and intelligent scheduling in automation. *Address: Dept. of Electrical and Electronics Eng., Middle East Technical University, 06531, Ankara, Turkey. Phone: +90 312 210 2325, Fax: +90 312 210 1261. E-mail: aydan@rorqual.cc.metu.edu.tr*

Toshio Fukuda graduated from Waseda University in 1971. He received the M.S. and D.E. from the University of Tokyo in 1973 and 1977, respectively. He also studied at the graduate school of Yale University from 1973 to 1975. In 1977 he joined the National Mechanical Engineering Laboratory and became a Visiting Research Fellow at the University of Stuttgart from 1979 to 1980. He joined the Science University of Tokyo in 1981 and then moved to Nagoya University in 1989. Currently he is a Professor at the Center for Cooperative Research in Advanced Science & Technology, Nagoya University, Japan. His research interests are in the fields of intelligent robotic systems, mechatronics, and micro robotics. He was made an IEEE Fellow in 1995 and was awarded the IEEE Eugene Mittlemann Award in 1997. He has been the Vice President of IEEE-IES (1990~), IFSA Vice President (1997~), IEEE Robotics and Automation Society President (1998~).

Address: Center for Cooperative Research in Advanced Science and Technology, Dept. of Mechano-Informatics and Systems & Dept. of Micro System Engineering, Nagoya University, Furo-cho, Chikusa-ku, Nagoya 464-01 JAPAN. Fax: +81 52 789 3909 / 3115. E-mail: fukuda@mein.nagoya-u.ac.jp

Andreas Hahn was born in 1962 and is a university lecturer. From 1989 to 1993 he was a researcher in the Nutritional Biochemistry Department at the University of Giessen. Since 1993 he has been the resident lecturer for Nutritional Physiology and Human Nutrition in the Department of Food Science at the University of Hannover. His special interests are the use of fuzzy logic in food science work, the assessment of alternative nutritional programs, questions regarding nutritional supplements, and interactions between nutrients and drugs.

Address: HD Dr. Andreas Hahn, Institut für Lebensmittelwissenschaft, Universität Hannover, Wunstorfer Str. 14, D-30453 Hannover, Germany, Phone: +49 511 762 5093, Fax: +49 511 762 4927. E-mail: a-w@freway.de

Ugur Halici graduated from the Department of Electrical and Electronics Engineering, Middle East Technical University, Ankara, Turkey. She received her M.S. degree in 1983 and her Ph.D. in 1988 from the same department. She has been a Professor of the Department of Electrical and Electronics Engineering, METU, since 1996. Her research interests include intelligent systems, computer vision, fingerprint recognition, and artificial neural networks.

Address: Computer Vision and Artificial Neural Networks Research Lab., Dept. of Electrical and Electronics Eng., Middle East Technical University, 06531, Ankara, Turkey. Phone: +90 312 210 2333, Fax: +90 312 210 1261. E-mail: halici@rorqual.cc.metu.edu.tr

Alexander Iliesh received his B.S. degree in Mechanical Engineering in 1987 and his M.S. in Biomedical Engineering in 1995, both from Tel-Aviv University, Israel. He is currently continuing his Ph.D. research at the Department of Applied Mathematics, the Weizmann Institute of Science, Rehovot, Israel. The focus of his current research work is the use of modular structures for learning and adaptation in motor control.

Address: Department of Applied Mathematics and Computer Science, Weizmann Institute of Science, Rehovot, Israel, 76283. Phone: +972 8 934 2651, Fax: +972 8 934 2945. E-mail: alexi@wisdom.weizmann.ac.il

Lena Kallin is a Ph.D. student in the Computing Science Department at Umea University, where she also earned her M.S. Her research interests include

medical informatics, hybrid neural networks and fuzzy logic systems, data mining, and knowledge discovery.
Address: Department of Computing Science, Umeå University, Se-90187, Umeå Sweden. Phone +46 90 786 68 33, Fax: +46 90 786 61 26. E-mail: Kallin@Cs.Umu.Se

Naoyuki Kubota graduated from Osaka Education University in 1992, received the M.E. from the Hokkaido University in 1994, and received the D.E. from Nagoya University in 1997. He is currently with the Department of Mechanical Engineering, Osaka Institute of Technology, Japan. He received the Best Paper Award of IECON'96 and the Best Paper Award of CIRA'97, among others. His main researches are computational intelligence, intelligent robotic systems, and intelligent manufacturing systems.
Address: Dept. of Mechanical Engineering, Osaka Institute of Technology, 5-16-1 Omiya, Asahi-ku, Osaka 535-8585, Japan. Phone: +81 6 954 4254, Fax: +81 6 957 2134, E-mail: kubota@med.oit.ac.jp

Kemal Leblebicioglu received the B.S. degree in Electrical and Electronics Engineering in 1979 and the M.S. and Ph.D. degrees in Mathematics in 1982 and 1988, respectively, all from the Middle East Technical University, Ankara, Turkey. From 1980 to 1988 he was with the Department of Mathematics at the METU as a graduate assistant. Since 1988 he has been on the faculty of the Department of Electrical and Electronics Engineering at METU, where he is currently an Associate Professor. His research interests include numerical methods for partial differential equations, inverse problems, optimization, optimal control theory, neural networks, neuro and fuzzy controllers, and image processing.
Address: Computer Vision and Artificial Neural Networks Research Lab., Dept. of Electrical and Electronics Eng., Middle East Technical University, 06531, Ankara, Turkey. Phone: +90 312 210 2358, Fax: +90 312 210 1261. E-mail: kleb@rorqual.cc.metu.edu.tr

Mikio Maeda received the S.B.E. in Radio Electronics in 1969 from Kumamoto Radio College, Kumamoto. He earned his Ph.D. in 1990 in System Science from Tokyo Institute of Technology, Tokyo, Japan. He joined the Department of Control Engineering at KIT in 1969 as an engineer. In 1989 he became a research assistant at the Computer Engineering Department. Since 1996 he has been an Associate Professor in Control Engineering Systems. His research work has concentrated on fuzzy expert systems, fuzzy control, medical information systems, and AI systems. He is a member of the Japan Society of Instrument and Control Engineers, the Japan Society for Fuzzy Theory and Systems, the Biomedical Fuzzy Systems Association, and the Japan Society of Mechanical Engineers.

Address: Dept. of Computer Engineering, Faculty of Engineering, Kyushu Institute of Technology, Sensuicho 1-1, Tobata, Kitakyushu, 804, Japan. Phone: +81 93 884 3249, Fax: +81 93 871 5835. E-mail: mmaeda@comp.kyutech.ac.jp.

Shuta Murakami received the B.E. degree in Control Engineering from the Kyushu Institute of Technology (KIT), Kitakyushu, in 1964 and the M.E. degree in 1966. He received his Ph.D. in 1969 in Control Engineering from Tokyo Institute of Technology, Tokyo, Japan. He joined the Department of Control Engineering at KIT in 1969 as a lecturer on Control. He has been a Professor in Control Systems since 1988. His research work has focused on fuzzy control, fuzzy modeling, and fuzzy decisions. He is a member of the SICE, Operations Research, and the International Fuzzy Systems Association.
Address: Dept. of Computer Engineering, Faculty of Engineering, Kyushu Institute of Technology, Sensuicho 1-1, Tobata, Kitakyushu, 804, Japan. Phone: +81 93 884 3249, Fax: +81 93 871 5835.
E-mail: murakami@comp.kyutech.ac.jp

Masahiro Nagamatu received his B.S. degree in Electronic Engineering from KIT in 1972. He received his M.S. and Ph.D. degrees in Engineering from Tohoku University, Japan, in 1974 and 1977, respectively. Since graduation he has been with the Department of Electrical, Electronic, and Computer Engineering at KIT. Currently, he is an Associate Professor. His primary research interests are discrete optimization algorithms.
Address: Department of Electrical Engineering, Faculty of Engineering, Kyushu Institute of Technology, Sensui, Tobata, Kitakyushu city, Fukuoka 804 Japan. Phone : +81 93 884 3257, Fax : +81 93 871 5835.
E-mail: nagamatsu@comp.kyutech.ac.jp

Takashi Samatsu received his Ph.D. degree in Computer Science and Systems Engineering from Kyushu Institute of Technology in 1998. He is currently with the Department of Electrical Engineering, Kyushu Tokai University, Japan. His primary areas of interest are in soft computing and system analysis.
Address: Department of Electrical Engineering, Kyushu Tokai University, 9-1-1 Toroku, Kumamoto 862-8652, Japan. Phone: +81 96 382 1141, Fax: +81 96 381 7956. E-mail: tsamatsu@ktmail.ktokai-u.ac.jp

Alejandro Sancho-Royo received his M.S. degree in Mathematics (1984) from the University of Sevilla, Spain, and his Ph.D. Degree in Sciences (1998) from the University of Granada, Spain. Since 1986 he has been at the School of Arts and Crafts of Granada, where he is Professor and Chair of the Department of Mathematics. He has participated in experimental education programs. He has been a Coordinator and Professor for Interior Design Expert Title in The

University of Almeria, Spain, (1994-1995) mainly in the courses "Ergonomics in Environmental Design" and "Habitat Psychosocial Aspects." His main research interests are in the methodology of psychosocial sciences, with a special emphasis in fuzzy sets and systems tools.

Address: Departamento de Matemáticas, Escuela de Artes Aplicadas, Gracia 2 y 4, 18190 Granada, Spain. Phone: +34 958 264462, Fax: +34 958 264500. E-mail: eaaoagr@arrakis.es

Gustaf Selén is a Ph.D. student at the Computer Science Department at Åbo Akademi University, Åbo, Finland, where he also earned his M.S. His research interests include medical informatics, data mining, and related software development.

Address: Department of Computer Science, Åbo Akademi University, SF-20520 Åbo, Finland. Phone: +358 2 215 40 71, Fax +358 2 215 47 32. E-mail gselen@abo.fi

Naruki Shirahama received the M.E. degree in Electronics from Kyushu Institute of Technology (KIT), Kitakyushu, Japan, in 1994. He has been working as a research assistant at Kitakyushu National College of Technology. His present research interests include applications of the subjective observation model. Mr. Shirahama is a member of the Japan Society for Fuzzy Theory and Systems (SOFT) and the Biomedical Fuzzy Systems Association (BMFSA).

Address: Department of Electrical Engineering, Kitakyushu National College of Technology, 5-20-1 Shii, Kokuraminamiku, Kitakyushu, Fukuoka 803-0985 Japan. Phone: +81 93 964 7340, Fax: +81 93 964 7242. E-mail: naruki@kct.ac.jp

Adrian Stoica is a senior member of the technical staff at the Jet Propulsion Laboratory at the California Institute of Technology. He received his M.S. engineering degree in Electronics from the Technical University of Iasi, Romania, in 1986, and his Ph.D. in Robotics from Victoria University, Melbourne, Australia, in 1996. His research focuses on intelligence, learning, and adaptation techniques for space robots and humanoids. He has published about 40 papers in the field. Dr. Stoica is currently conducting research on robotics and machine intelligence.

Address: Jet Propulsion Laboratory, California Institute of Technology, Pasadena, CA, 91109, USA. Phone: +818 354 2190, Fax: +818 393 1545. E-mail: adrian.stoica@jpl.nasa.gov

Eiji Uchino received his Ph.D. degree in Systems Engineering in 1988. He is presently a Professor at Yamaguchi University. His research interests include adaptive system modeling, intelligent signal and image processing, and human brain-based information-processing systems.

Address: Department of Physics, Biology, and Informatics, Yamaguchi University, 1677-1 Yoshida, Yamaguchi 753-8512, Japan. Phone/Fax: +81 839 33 5699, Fax: +81 839 33 5768. E-mail: uchino@sci.yamaguchi-u.ac.jp

Jose-Luis Verdegay received his M.S. degree in Mathematics (1975) and his Ph.D. degree in Sciences (1980) from the University of Granada, Spain. Since 1975 he has been at the University of Granada as a Full Professor and former Chair of the Department of Computer Science and Artificial Intelligence. Professor Verdegay has co-edited five books and is the author/co-author of numerous technical papers. He has been an advisor of seven Ph.D. theses and director of a number of national and international research projects. He has also served on the program committees of several major international conferences and has been President of the Spanish Association for Fuzzy Logic and Technologies. Dr. Verdegay is presently serving on various editorial boards of leading journals. His main research interests are in decision making problems in fuzzy environments, including optimization problems and genetic algorithms, group decision making, and decision support systems.

Address: Dept. Ciencias de la Computacion e Inteligencia Artificial, ETS Ingenieria Informatica, Universidad de Granada, 18071 Granada, Spain, Phone: +34 58244019, Fax: +34 58 243317. E-mail: verdegay@goliat.ugr.es

Bernd Wirsam (born 1944) was a university lecturer for Theoretical Physics and Quantum Chemistry at the University in Giessen until 1977. Special fields of interest are optimizations and fuzzy decision making, applied to industrial processes and nutrition. Together with Renate Albat, he founded the software company *"Albat+Wirsam"* (A+W) that won the "Innovative German Companies" award in 1995.

Address: ALBAT + WIRSAM Software-Vertriebs GmbH, Konrad-Adenauer-Str. 15, D-35440 Linden, Germany, Phone: +49 6403 9700, Fax: +49 6403 64390. E-mail: a-w@freeway.de

Takeshi Yamakawa received his Ph.D. degree in Electrochemistry from Tohoku University. He is a Professor in the Department of Computer Science and Control Engineering, Kyushu Institute of Technology, Iizuka, Japan. He is also the Chairman of a Japanese foundation, the Fuzzy Logic Systems Institute (FLSI), which he established to create an international collaboration on soft computing. He received the *Grigore Moisil* Gold Medal in 1994 for his contribution to engineering application of fuzzy systems. He acted as an organizing/program committee member for over 60 international conferences and serves as an associate editor for over 10 international journals in the field of soft computing.

Address: Department of Computer Science and Control Engineering, Kyushu Institute of Technology, 680-4 Kawazu, Iizuka, Fukuoka 820-0044, Japan, Phone: +81 948 29 7712, Fax: +81 948 29 7742.
E-mail: yamakawa@ces.kyutech.ac.jp

Torao Yanaru received the M.S. degree in Electrical Engineering from KIT in 1967, and the Ph.D. degree in Engineering in 1982. He has worked as a Professor in the Department of Electrical Engineering, Faculty of Engineering at KIT. He worked as an Associate Professor in the Information Scientific Center at KIT from 1975 to 1988. He worked as an Associate Professor in the Department of Artificial Intelligence Engineering at KIT from 1989 to 1991. His present research interests include development of an emotion processing system based on the theory of subjective observation models. Dr. Yanaru is a member of BMFSA, SOFT, and many other societies.

Address: Department of Electric Engineering, Faculty of Engineering, Kyushu Institute of Technology, Sensui, Tobata, Kitakyushu city, Fukuoka 806 Japan. Phone and Fax: +81 93 884 3245. E-mail: yanaru@comp.kyutech.ac.jp

Acknowledgments

The Editors thank the contributors for their commitment, hard work, and patience during the preparation of the chapters. Without the considerable efforts of the authors and of the reviewers, this volume could not have come to fulfillment.

The Editors thank Ms. Dawn Mesa, Editor of the volume, Ms. Josephine Gilmore, Editor, Ms. Suzanne Lassandro, Production Manager, and Ms. Mimi Williams from CRC Press, and Ms. Mary Parrish, Senior Word Processor, Computer Science and Engineering Department, University of South Florida, for their kind support, professional advice, and commitment to the project during the preparation of this volume.

The Editors are grateful to all the reviewers of the chapters in this volume, namely (in alphabetic order) Dragos Arotaritei (Romanian Academy, Computer Science Institute), James Black (University of South Florida, Tampa, USA), Mircea Chelaru (Duke University), Scott Dick (University of South Florida, Tampa, USA), A.M. Fanelli (University of Bari, Italy), Noboru Iwata (University of Kitakyushu and University of South Florida), R.K. Jain (University of South Australia, Adelaide, Australia), Naoki Kugihara (Kyushu Institute of Technology), Doron Leca (Tel Aviv, Israel), B. Lazzerini (University of Pisa), Daniel Mlynek (Swiss Federal Institute of Technology, Lausanne), Daniel Moses (University of South Florida, Tampa, USA), Wladimir Rodriguez (University of South Florida, Tampa), Alexander Rothstein (Technical University of Vilnnita, Ukraine), Adam Schenker (University of South Florida, Tampa, USA), Sorina Zahan (University of Cluj, Romania).

October 1998

Horia-Nicolai Teodorescu
Abraham Kandel
Tampa, Florida

Lakhmi C. Jain
Adelaide, South Australia

Contents

Chapter 6.

Intelligent diagnostic systems in maternal and fetal medicine
Sinan Beksac, Aydan J. Erkmen, Sezer Aksel, Ugur Halici, Kemal Leblebicioglu, Meral Beksac, Volkan Atalay, and Lakhmi C. Jain **137**

Part 3. Applications in Psychology, Nutrition, and Professional Evaluation

Chapter 9.

An emotion-processing system based on fuzzy inference and subjective observations
Naruki Shirahama, Torao Yanaru, and Masahiro Nagamatsu **293**

Chapter 10.
Fuzzy methods in nutrition planning and education and in clinical nutrition
Bernd Wirsam and Andreas Hahn **335**

Chapter 11.
Designing experiments for medical diagnosis evaluation using membership functions
José Luis Verdegay and Alejandro Sancho-Royo **351**

Part 1.

Robotics,

Prostheses,

Control

Chapter 1

Fuzzy control methodology: basics and state of the art

Toshio Fukuda and Naoyuki Kubota

1. Introduction

Recently, fuzzy systems have been applied to such fields as knowledge engineering, computer science, mechatronics and robotics. In addition, various inference methods have been proposed to deal with human language, imprecise information, complicated problems and nonlinear mapping [3-6, 9]. In general, a fuzzy system has no learning mechanism, and therefore, fuzzy neural networks and network-based fuzzy systems have been developed [3, 4, 6]. Furthermore, genetic algorithms have also been applied to tune fuzzy rules [3, 4, 6].

On the other hand, various methodologies concerning intelligence have been successfully developed, and their implementation was made possible by the progresses in computation capabilities. Artificial intelligence (AI) is used to describe and build an intelligent agent, which perceives its environment by sensors, makes decisions and takes action [1]. McCulloch and Pitts suggested that suitably defined networks could learn [2], and furthermore, Newell and Simon developed [1] the General Problem Solver. Afterward, knowledge-based systems, including expert systems, were developed [1].

Many developments in artificial intelligence are related to human language and to the information representation specific to humans. Human language enables the symbolic processing of information. The information is done and the classification is performed by dropping meaningless information, that is, by focusing on attributes that include most information. In addition, the task planning is also performed by logically dividing a complex task into several simple subtasks. All these operations, in conjunction with the symbolic processing of information, have resulted in success in AI.

Furthermore, the recent research thrusts concerning intelligence include brain science, soft computing, artificial life, and computational intelligence [1-16]. It is very difficult to distinguish one research field from the others; we simply describe the aim of each research field. Brain science aims to understand the biochemical and physical mechanism of the human brain, and to construct a highly interconnected neural network like the human brain [1-4]. Soft computing, which was proposed by Zadeh, is a new concept for information processing, whose objective is to realize a new approach for analyzing and creating human-like, flexible information processing such as sensing, understanding, learning, recognizing and thinking [5, 6]. Artificial life (A-life) means life created by humans rather than nature [7]. A-life has three types of approaches: 1) a wetware system from the molecular level, 2) a software system from the cellular level and 3) a hardware system from the organism level [7]. Bezdek discussed intelligence from a triple level point of view: artificial, biological, and computational [3, 4, 8]. In the strictest sense, computational intelligence (CI) depends on numerical data and does not rely on knowledge [3, 8]. Furthermore, Eberhart defined CI as a methodology involving computing [4]. Based on the above discussion, we can summarize that CI aims to realize intelligence from the viewpoints of biology, evolution and self-organization. CI tries to realize intelligence by internal description, while classical AI tries to construct intelligence by external (explicit) description. Therefore, information and knowledge in a CI system should be learned or acquired by the system itself.

These research fields use neural networks (NN), fuzzy system (FS) and genetic algorithms (GA) [2-16]. Each technique plays a specific role in intelligent systems. Neural networks have been applied for nonlinear mapping of objective problems. FS has been applied for representing human linguistic rules. GA has been applied for solving optimization problems. However, no single technique is ideal for realizing all features of intelligence. Therefore, we should integrate and combine some techniques to offset the disadvantages of each technique by the advantages of the others.

1.1. Fuzzy computing and neural computing

Artificial neural networks and fuzzy logic are based on the mechanisms of the human brain (Figure 1). The human brain processes information super-quickly and super-accurately thanks to its network structure. McCulloch and Pitts [2] proposed in 1943 that a suitably defined network could learn. After that, the rediscovery of the back-propagation algorithm by Rumelhart popularized artificial NNs [2]. The artificial NN simulates the biological brain and can be trained to recognize patterns.

The basic attributes of NN are the architecture and the functional properties, including dynamic properties (neurodynamics.) In a limited sense, the neurodynamics play the role of nonlinear mapping from input to output (see Figure 1). An NN is composed of many interconnected neurons, each having inputs, outputs, synaptic strength, and activation. The learning algorithm is, in general, determined by the type of problem involved. The learning algorithms for adjusting weights of synaptic strength are classified into supervised learning with target responses, unsupervised learning without target responses, and reinforcement learning with only success or failure reported. In general, when supervised learning is used, a multilayer NN is trained by a back propagation algorithm based on the error function between the output response and the target response. However, the back propagation algorithm, which is a gradient method, is often trapped in local minima. In addition, the learning capability of NNs depends on the structure of the NN and the initial weights of the synaptic strength. Therefore, the optimization of the structure and the synaptic strength is very important for obtaining the desired target responses.

Other types of artificial NNs include the Hopfield network, the Boltzmann Machine, Adaptive Resonance Theory and Self-Organizing Maps [2, 9, 15, 16]. The Hopfield network is regarded as an autoassociative fully connected network which has symmetrically weighted links [2]. The Boltzmann Machine is based on the simulated annealing according to Metropolis dynamics [2]. The Adaptive Resonance Theory model, which was developed by Grossberg and Carpenter, is an unsupervised NN based on competitive learning [9, 15]. The Self-Organizing Map, which was proposed by Kohonen, is a clustering algorithm creating a map of relationships among input patterns [9, 16].

While an NN simulates physiological features of the human brain, fuzzy theory simulates psychological features of the human brain. Fuzzy theory provides us linguistic representations such as 'slow' and 'fast'. Fuzzy theory [5, 6, 9] uses truth degrees, which are represented as grades of a membership function (see Figure 1). Fuzzy logic is a powerful tool for non-probabilistic and ill-defined structures.

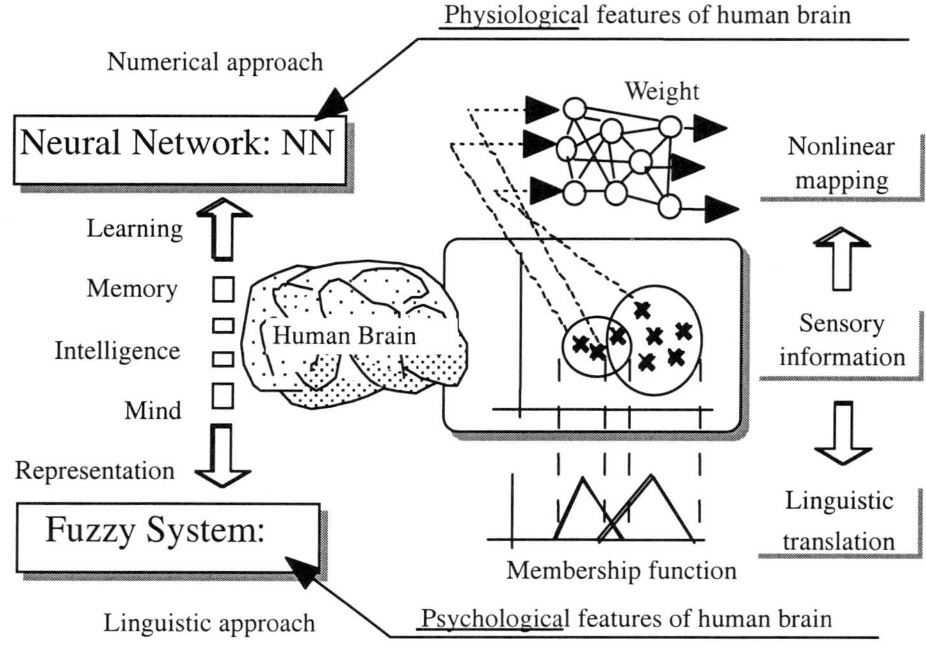

Figure 1. Neural network and fuzzy system simulating the mechanism of the human brain.

A fuzzy inference system is based on the concepts of fuzzy set theory, fuzzy if-then rules, and fuzzy inference. Fuzzy inference derives conclusions from a set of fuzzy if-then rules. A fuzzy inference system implements a mapping from its input space to output space by a number of fuzzy if-then rules. The most widely used fuzzy inference systems are Mamdani fuzzy models and Takagi-Sugeno fuzzy models, which are used as fuzzy controllers. The main features of the fuzzy controller are the local action of the control and the interpolation (aggregation) of local control laws. In the fuzzy controller, the state space of the system is divided into several regions as membership functions, which are antecedents (conditions). The output (consequence) for the system control is designed as singletons or membership functions [5, 6]. Next, the fuzzy rules are interpolated as a global controller. In order to tune the fuzzy rules, the delta rule is often applied [6, 25].

1.2. Evolutionary computing

Evolutionary computing (EC) works by simulating evolution on a computer [11]. From an historical point of view, the evolutionary optimization methods are divided into three main categories: genetic algorithms (GA), evolutionary programming (EP) and evolution strategy (ES) [3, 4, 10-14]. These methods are fundamentally iterative generation and alteration processes operating on a set of candidate solutions, which form a population. The entire population evolves toward better candidate solutions via the selection operation and genetic operators such as crossover and mutation. The selection operator decides which candidate solutions move on into the next generation, which limits the search space. The crossover and mutation operators generate new candidate solutions from the search space. There is no unique classification of the EC methods in the literature. In this chapter, we classify the EC methods into *genetic algorithms* (GA) and *evolutionary algorithms* (EA), based on the representation level (Figure 2).

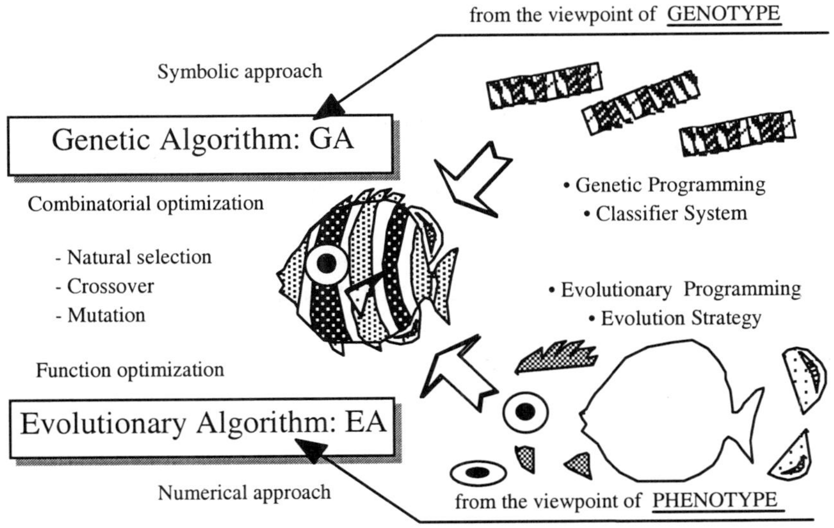

Figure 2. Evolutionary computation: genetic algorithm and evolutionary algorithm.

GAs operate from the genotype viewpoint, using simple symbolic operations. GAs are often applied to combinatorial optimization problems such as knapsack problems, traveling salesman problems and job shop scheduling problems [10-14]. It is experimentally known that GAs can obtain near or approximately optimal solutions with low computational cost. Other GAs are genetic programming and classifier systems. Genetic programming, which was proposed by Koza [12, 13], can deal with the tree structure, and has been applied for generating computer programs. The classifier system, which is called GA-based machine learning, can learn syntactically simple string production rules to guide its performance in an arbitrary environment.

On the other hand, EAs operate from the phenotype viewpoint, using numerical operations, in addition to symbolic operations, such as mutation and crossover. EAs, including EP and ES, have been used to solve numerical optimization problems such as function optimization problems and weight optimization of neural networks [11]. The important feature of EAs is self-adaptation. Self-adaptive mutation is a particularly useful operation, as it can self-tune the search range according to historical success records [11]. In EAs, tournament selection and deterministic selection are often used as the selection scheme.

In addition, GAs provide the evolution mechanism for population dynamics, robot society and A-life [7]. From the viewpoint of simulated evolution, GAs can maintain genetic diversity in a population, enabling it to adapt to a dynamic environment. Therefore, GAs are often called adaptive systems. However, GAs eliminate worse individuals from the population according to an evaluation of the current environment only. As a result, it is difficult to adapt the population to a significant change of the environment. Therefore, GAs often require methods to maintain genetic diversity in a population to cope with the dynamically changing environment.

1.3. Emerging synthesis for computational intelligence

To realize a highly intelligent system, a synthesis of various techniques is required. Figure 3 shows the synthesis of NN, FS, and GA. Each technique plays a specific role in intelligent systems. The main characteristics of NN are to recognize patterns and to classify input, and to adapt themselves to dynamic environments by learning. However, the mapping structure of NN is a black box, making it difficult to understand. Fuzzy systems, on the other hand, can cope with human knowledge and can perform inference, but FSs do not fundamentally have a learning mechanism.

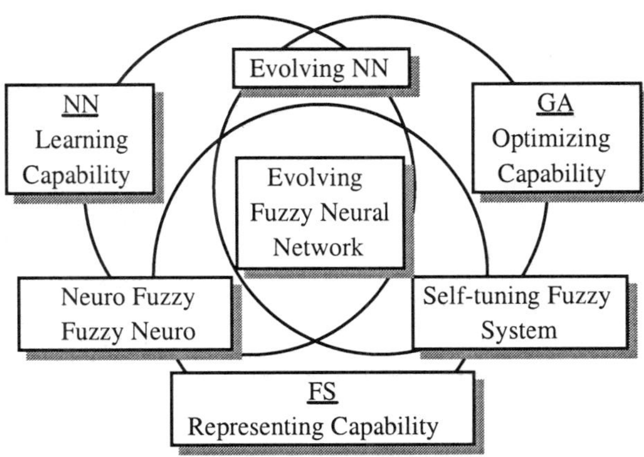

Figure 3. Synthesis of NN, Fuzzy, and GA.

Neuro-fuzzy computing overcomes these disadvantages of NN and FS [6]. In general, the neural network part is used for learning, while the fuzzy logic part is used for representing knowledge. Learning is performed through incremental learning, the back propagation method and the delta rule, based on error functions. GA can also tune NN and FS. However, evolution can be defined as resultant or accidental change, since the GA cannot predict and estimate the effect of the change. To summarize, an intelligent system can quickly adapt to a dynamic environment by NN and FS with the back propagation method and the delta rule, and furthermore, the structure of an intelligent system can globally evolve by using GA. The adaptation and evolution capabilities allow us building systems that are more intelligent. As mentioned before, the intelligence arises from the linkage of perception, decision making and action.

2. Inference mechanisms for fuzzy controller

Fuzzy control does not require mathematical models for the controlled system, while classical control theory requires a mathematical model expressing the controlled system. If the system is complex, the mathematical modeling becomes difficult. The fuzzy controller uses a linguistic representation of a human expert knowledge to automatically control a system.

The fuzzy controller is composed of four main modules: fuzzification, rule-base, inference mechanism, and defuzzification. The fuzzification is a mapping from a crisp input space to fuzzy sets represented as membership functions. The rule-base is generally described as a set of production rules (fuzzy if-then rule): *if* [conditions], *then* [consequences]. The rule base is generally designed by using a human expert's knowledge about the controlled system. We show an example of an if-then rule for collision avoidance in a mobile robot (see Figure 4),

if [the left is very dangerous] and [the front is dangerous],
then [turn right].

This linguistic expression describes the relationship between the condition and the consequence. Figure 5 shows the fuzzy sets for the degree of danger in the collision avoidance problem. The linguistic variable 'distance' means the distance from the obstacles. Each membership function describes a fuzzy set corresponding to a linguistic expression (label). In general, the fuzzy if-then rule is described as follows,

if x_1 is $A_{i,1}$ and x_2 is $A_{i,2}$ and ... and x_n is $A_{i,n}$, then y is B_i,

where $A_{i,j}$ is a membership function for the j-th input of the i-th rule, and B_i is a membership function for the output of the i-th rule.

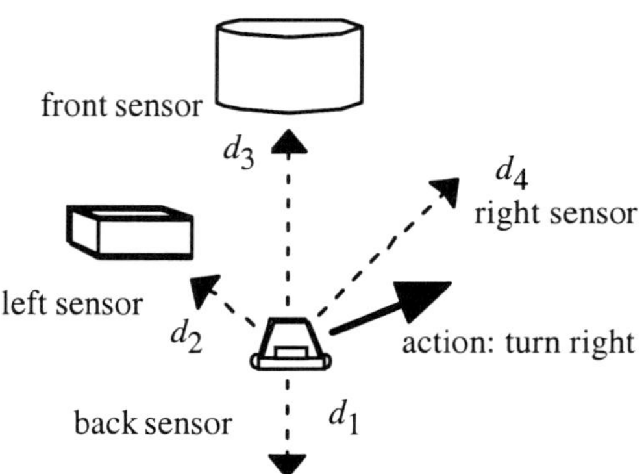

Figure 4. Collision avoidance problem for a mobile robot.

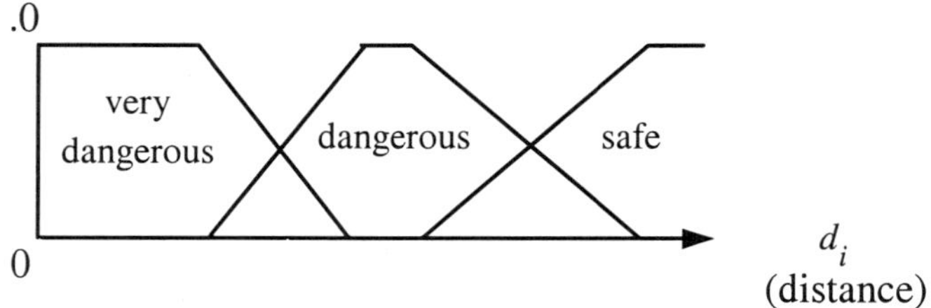

Figure 5. Membership functions for linguistic values:
"very dangerous", "dangerous", and "safe".

The most commonly used linguistic variables in the fuzzy controller are state variables, state error, and differential and integral of state error Furthermore, the consequence is often described as a singleton or function.

The inference mechanism derives a resulting output from fuzzy if-then rules using crisp input values. When the consequences of fuzzy rules are fuzzy sets, the resulting output is also a fuzzy set. Since we need crisp output values for real-world control, the result must be translated into a crisp output value. The defuzzification is used for this translation. Various inference mechanisms and defuzzification methods have been proposed [6, 47]. In the following subsections, we introduce some inference and defuzzification methods for the fuzzy controller.

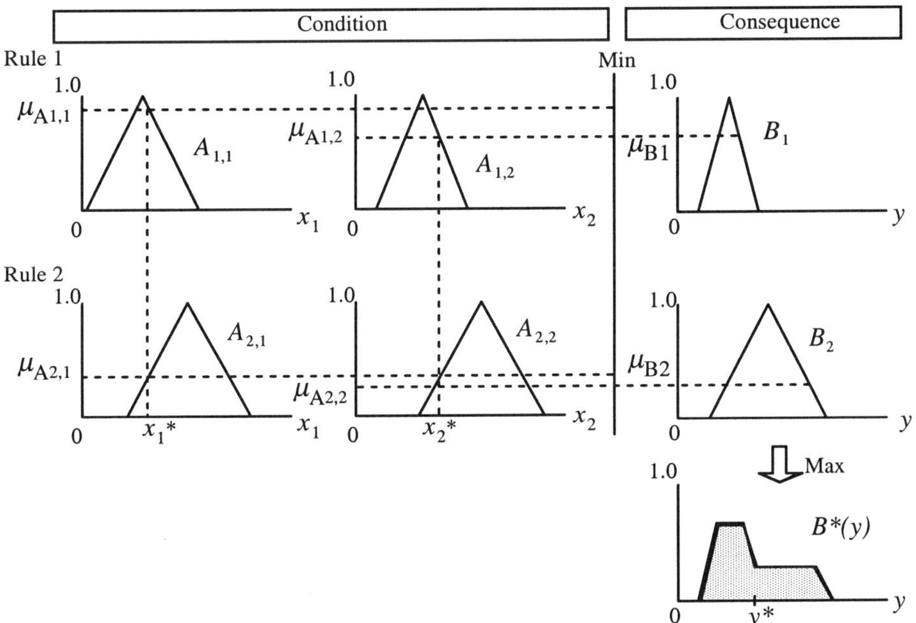

Figure 6. Inference procedure of the min-max-gravity method.

2.1. Min-max-gravity method

The min-max-gravity method, which was proposed by Mamdani, is widely used in control systems. We show an inference procedure of the min-max-gravity method where x_1 and x_2 are input variables and y is an output variable (Figure 6). We present the procedure of the min-max-gravity method when two crisp inputs x_1^* and x_2^* are given.

Step 1:   Calculate the membership degrees of $\mu_{A_{i,1}}(x_1{}^*)$ and $\mu_{A_{i,2}}(x_2{}^*)$ of the *i*-th rule ($i = 1,2$),

Step 2:   Calculate the consequence of the *i*-th rule by *min* t-norm for the rule premise and implication,

$$\mu_{B_i}{}^*(y) = (\mu_{A_{i,1}}(x_1{}^*) \wedge \mu_{A_{i,2}}(x_2{}^*)) \wedge \mu_{B_i}(y) \tag{1}$$

Step 3:   Calculate the resulting output by using *max* the co-norm (corresponding to the *min* t-norm),

$$\mu_B{}^*(y) = \mu_{B1}{}^*(y) \vee \mu_{B2}{}^*(y) \tag{2}$$

Step 4:   Calculate the center of gravity of the fuzzy set $B^*(y)$,

$$y^* = \frac{\int B^*(y)\,y\,dy}{\int B^*(y)\,dy} \tag{3}$$

The crisp output y^* is calculated by the defuzzification formula (3) in Step 4. This defuzzification method is called center of gravity (COG). Various defuzzification methods have been proposed, such as the max-criterion method, bisector of area (BOA), mean of maximum (MOM), smallest of maximum (SOM), and largest of maximum (LOM) method [6].

2.2. Product-sum-gravity method

In the product-sum-gravity method, *min* and *max* operators of the *min-max*-gravity method are replaced with the product and sum operators. We show an inference procedure based on the product-sum-gravity method (Figure 7).

Step 1:   Calculate the membership degrees of $\mu_{A_{i,1}}(x_1{}^*)$ and $\mu_{A_{i,2}}(x_2{}^*)$ of the *i*-th rule ($i = 1, 2$).

Step 2: Calculate the rule premise and implication by using the product t-norm operator,

$$\mu_{B_i}{}^*(y) = \mu_{A_{i,1}}(x_1{}^*) \times \mu_{A_{i,2}}(x_2{}^*) \times \mu_{B_i}(y) \tag{4}$$

Step 3:   Calculate the resulting output by summing,

$$\mu_B{}^*(y) = \mu_{B1}{}^*(y) + \mu_{B2}{}^*(y) \tag{5}$$

Step 4:   Calculate the center of gravity of the fuzzy set $B^*(y)$ using Equation (3),

$$y^* = \frac{\int B^*(y)\,y\,dy}{\int B^*(y)\,dy}$$

The crisp output y^* is calculated by defuzzification in Step 4.

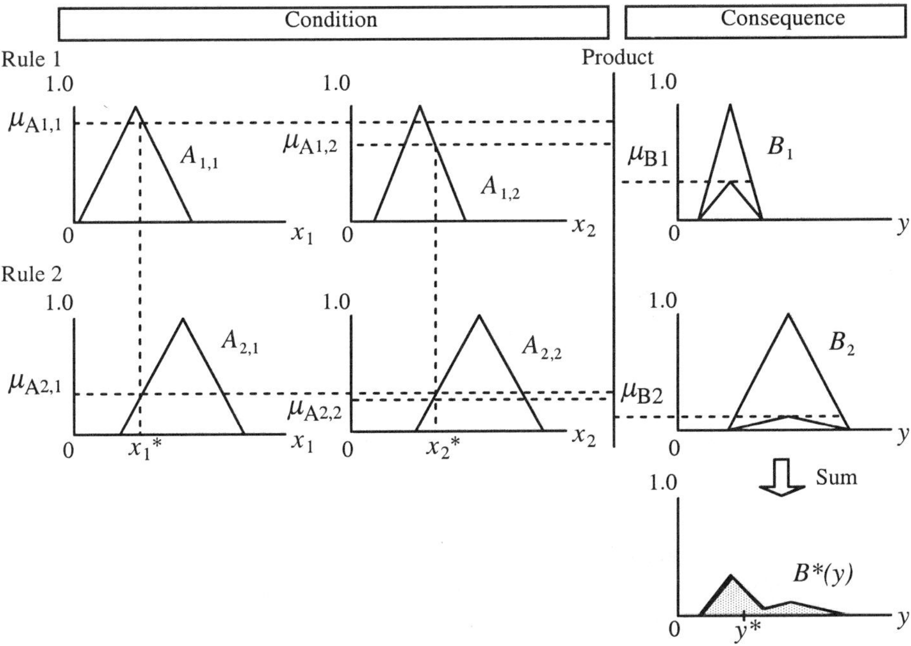

Figure 7. Inference procedure of the product-sum-gravity method.

2.3. Functional fuzzy inference method

The functional fuzzy inference method, also known as the Sugeno fuzzy model or TSK Fuzzy model, uses a numerical function in the consequence. A polynomial function is often used for simplifying the consequence. In general, a fuzzy if-then rule using the functional fuzzy inference method is described with the form

If x_i is $A_{i,1}$ and x_2 is $A_{i,2}$ and ... and x_n is $A_{i,n}$, then y is $f_i(x_1, \cdots, x_n)$

where $A_{i,j}$ is a membership function for the j-th input of the i-th rule, and $f_i(x_1,\cdots,x_n)$ is a function for the output of the i-th rule. A commonly used function is as follows:

$$f_i(x_1, \cdots, x_n) = a_0 + a_1 x_1 + \cdots + a_n x_n \tag{6}$$

where a_0, a_1, $\cdots$, and a_n are coefficients. We show below an inference procedure of the functional fuzzy inference method.

Step 1: Calculate the membership degrees of $\mu_{A_{i,j}}(x_j{}^*)$ of the j-th input of the i-th rule ($i = 1,\cdots, r$)

Step 2: Calculate the firing strength of the i-th rule by product

$$\mu_i = \prod_{j=1}^{n} \mu_{A_i, j}(x_j{}^*) \tag{7}$$

Step 3: Calculate the resulting output by the weighted average, based on the firing strength

$$y^* = \frac{\displaystyle\sum_{i=1}^{r} \mu_i \cdot f_i(x_1, \cdots, x_n)}{\displaystyle\sum_{i=1}^{r} \mu_i} \tag{8}$$

This method is regarded as a special case of the product-sum-gravity method. Moreover, the min operator can be used instead of product in Step 2. In addition, the functional fuzzy inference method can use PID control rules for a fuzzy set corresponding to the divided state space.

2.4. Simplified fuzzy inference method

The min-max-gravity method and product-sum-gravity method use fuzzy sets in the consequences, but calculating the center of gravity is computationally intensive. Therefore, the simplified fuzzy inference method has been proposed to reduce computational time. The simplified fuzzy inference method uses a singleton instead of a fuzzy set in the consequence. In general, a fuzzy if-then rule using the simplified fuzzy inference method is of the form

$$\text{if } x_i \text{ is } A_{i,1} \text{ and } x_2 \text{ is } A_{i,2} \text{ and ... and } x_n \text{ is } A_{i,n}, \text{ then } y \text{ is } w_I,$$

where $A_{i,j}$ is a membership function for the j-th input of the i-th rule, and w_i is a singleton for the output of the i-th rule. We show the procedure of the simplified fuzzy inference method as follows:

Step 1: Calculate the membership degrees of $\mu_{Ai,j}(x_j{}^*)$ of the j-th input of the i-th rule ($i = 1, \cdots, r$).

Step 2: Calculate the firing strength of the i-th rule by product using Equation (7).

$$\mu_i = \prod_{j=1}^{n} \mu_{Ai,\,j}(x_j{}^*)$$

Step 3: Calculate the resulting output by weighted average based on the firing strength,

$$y^* = \frac{\displaystyle\sum_{i=1}^{r} \mu_i \cdot w_i}{\displaystyle\sum_{i=1}^{r} \mu_i} \tag{9}$$

This method is also regarded as a special case of the product-sum-gravity method. Moreover, this method can be regarded as a special case of the functional fuzzy inference method when the consequence is constant in the functional fuzzy inference method.

2.5. Tsukamoto fuzzy model

The Tsukamoto fuzzy model uses a fuzzy set with a monotonic membership function in the consequence. Therefore, the resulting output of each rule takes a crisp value based on the firing strength. We show an example of the Tsukamoto fuzzy model below (Figure 8).

Step 1: Calculate the membership degrees of $\mu_{Ai,j}(x_j{}^*)$ the j-th input of the i-th rule ($i = 1, \ldots, r$).

Step 2: Calculate the firing strength of the i-th rule by using the *min* t-norm for the rule premise

$$\mu_i(y) = \mu_{Ai,1}(x_1{}^*) \wedge \mu_{Ai,2}(x_2{}^*) \wedge \cdots \wedge \mu_{Ai,n}(x_n{}^*) \tag{10}$$

Step 3: Calculate the output corresponding to the firing strength

$$w_i = \mu_{Bi}{}^{-1}(\mu_i(y)) \tag{11}$$

Step 4: Calculate the output by weighted average of the firing strength using Equation (9)

$$y^* = \frac{\displaystyle\sum_{i=1}^{r} \mu_i \cdot w_i}{\displaystyle\sum_{i=1}^{r} \mu_i}$$

In this fuzzy model, the antecedent membership functions $A_{i,j}$ are not required to be monotonic.

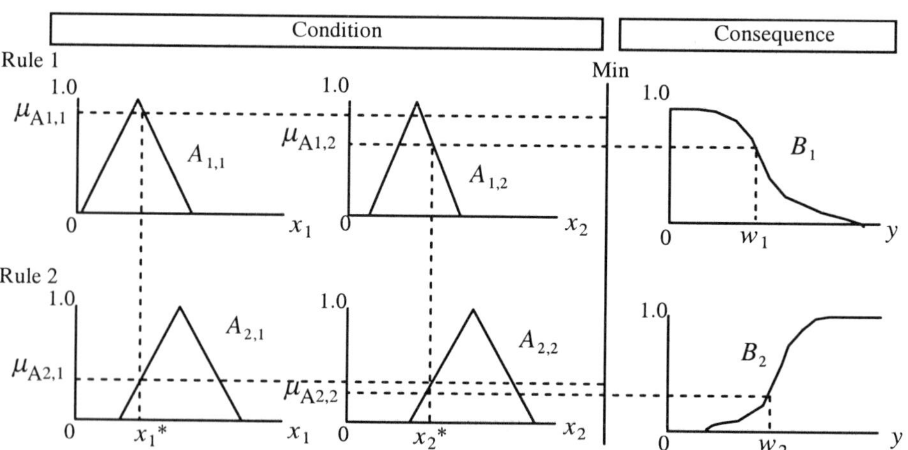

Figure 8. Inference procedure of the Tsukamoto fuzzy model.

3. Learning, adaptation, and evolution for fuzzy controller

This section considers a fuzzy controller as an intelligent system from the viewpoints of learning, adaptation, and evolution. Human beings have evolved and formed ecosystems in various environments by adapting to their dynamic environments, by searching for a livable environment, and by rebuilding their environments. Living things are hierarchical systems and interact at various levels, such as organs, cells, and genes. Living things evolve by the change of genetic information and continuous natural selection by competition between individuals or species. In addition, living things can adapt to their dynamic environments during a single lifetime. It is generally said that '*adaptation*' is change over a short time and '*evolution*' is change over a long time. In this chapter, the meaning of adaptation and evolution is more restrictive, namely,

- Adaptation is to improve an individual through interaction with environment. Adaptation performance is determined under the evaluation criterion in the context of environmental factors (Figure 9.a).

$$Evaluation = f_{criterion}(form \circ environment) \tag{12}$$

- Evolution is to globally change the form of a population and to maintain diversity of form. Evolution performance is determined based on the form only (Figure 9.b).

$$Evaluation = f_{criterion}(form) \tag{13}$$

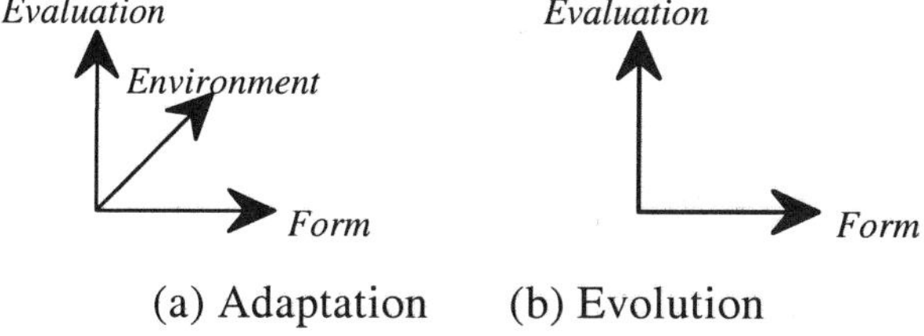

Figure 9. Evaluations for adaptation and evolution.

For example, it is often said that a form evolves when a simple form changes into a more complex one. Here, the form includes figure, pattern, function, and organization. Adaptation emphasizes improvement, while evolution emphasizes change. Implicitly, both adaptation and evolution are related to the concept of time, but they do not depend on the scale of time.

The driving force for adaptation and evolution is mainly learning and inheritance (Figure 10). Learning is a process of gaining knowledge or skill. Adaptation includes improvement by learning and simple adjustment. In general, the adaptation of the system to a dynamic environment is performed by means of a learning mechanism, and this learning process is fundamentally regarded as a necessary change based on error functions. On the other hand, inheritance is a process of receiving characteristics from the previous form. In nature, mutation occasionally changes genetic information as transmitting errors, and as a result, the phenotype of a living thing also changes. Consequently, evolution can be regarded as resultant or accidental change. Therefore, evolutionary change can change the global form. Consequently, evolutionary methods are often used for the global search of forms. In the following subsections, we introduce a learning mechanism and an evolution mechanism for fuzzy controllers.

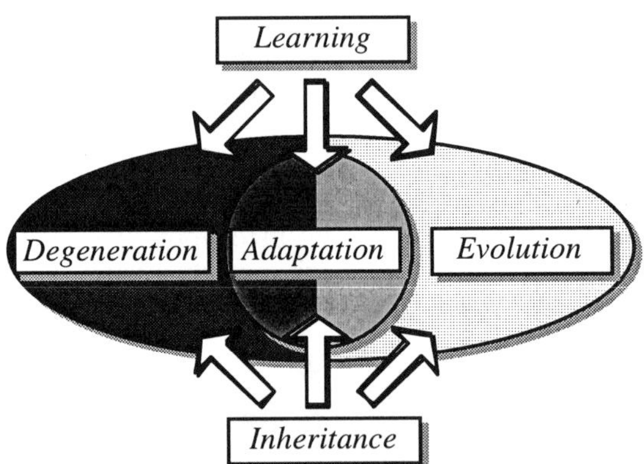

Figure 10. Evolution and adaptation by learning and inheritance.

3.1. Learning for a fuzzy controller

Learning methodologies includes learning by discovery, learning by observation, and reinforcement learning through interaction with the environment. In the case of the human beings, knowledge can be acquired by children from parents by transmitting information by teaching and showing.

The linguistic information processing enables the easy transfer of knowledge to offspring. Symbolic information processing is especially easy to understand.

The rule base for a fuzzy controller can be designed by human expert knowledge, an operator's control actions, fuzzy modeling, and learning based on experience [6, 47]. Here we focus on the simplified fuzzy inference system. When a set of input-output data is given, the simplified fuzzy inference system can be trained by the delta rule [47].

We consider a set of fuzzy if-then rules using the simplified fuzzy inference method as follows:

$$\textit{If } x_i \textit{ is } A_{i,1} \textit{ and } x_2 \textit{ is } A_{i,2} \textit{ and ... and } x_n \textit{ is } A_{i,n}, \textit{ then } y \textit{ is } w_I,$$

where $A_{i,j}$ is a membership function for the j-th input of the i-th rule, and w_i is a singleton for the output of the i-th rule. One can use various types of membership functions such as triangular membership function, trapezoidal membership function, and gaussian membership function. First, we consider a triangular membership function (Figure 11). A triangular membership function is generally described as

$$\mu_{Ai,j}(x_j) = \begin{cases} 1 - \dfrac{|x_j - a_{i,j}|}{b_{i,j}} & |x_j - a_{i,j}| \le b_{i,j} \\ 0 & \textit{otherwise} \end{cases} \tag{14}$$

where $a_{i,j}$ and $b_{i,j}$ are the central value and the width of the membership function $A_{i,j}$. Consequently, the firing strength is calculated by

$$\mu_i = \prod_{j=1}^{n} \mu_{Ai,j}(x_j) = \prod_{j=1}^{n}\left(1 - \dfrac{|a_{i,j} - x_j|}{b_i}\right) \tag{15}$$

By using Equation (9), we obtain the resulting output.

$$y^* = \dfrac{\displaystyle\sum_{i=1}^{r} \mu_i \cdot w_i}{\displaystyle\sum_{i=1}^{r} \mu_i} \tag{9}$$

When y^* is the target output of the controlled system, the error function is defined as

$$E = \frac{1}{2}(y^* - y)^2 \tag{16}$$

To construct a fuzzy controller using the relationship between input values and output values, we must minimize the error function E. When the condition parts (membership functions) are fixed, we can easily train the output w_k of the k-th rule according to the delta rule based on the error function. The derivative of E is as follows:

$$\frac{\partial E}{\partial w_k} = \frac{\partial E}{\partial y}\frac{\partial y}{\partial w_k} = -\left(y^* - \frac{\sum \mu_i \cdot w_i}{\sum \mu_i}\right)\frac{\mu_k}{\sum \mu_i} \tag{17}$$

Consequently, we can update the output of the consequence of the k-th rule by,

$$w_k(t+1) = w_k(t) - \tau \cdot \frac{\partial E}{\partial w_k}$$

$$= w_k(t) + \tau \cdot \left(y^* - \frac{\sum \mu_i \cdot w_i}{\sum \mu_i}\right)\frac{\mu_k}{\sum \mu_i} \tag{18}$$

where τ is the learning rate satisfying $0 < \tau < 1.0$ and t is the learning iteration. Other frequently used types of membership functions are trapezoidal membership functions and Gaussian membership functions (Figure 12). A Gaussian membership function is generally described as

$$\mu_{Ai,j}(x_j) = \exp\left(-\frac{(x_j - a_{i,j})^2}{b_{i,j}}\right) \tag{19}$$

where $a_{i,j}$ and $b_{i,j}$ are the central value and the width of the membership function $A_{i,j}$. In any type of membership function, the outputs of fuzzy rules can be trained by the delta rule, since the output is dependent on the firing strength of each rule for a given input.

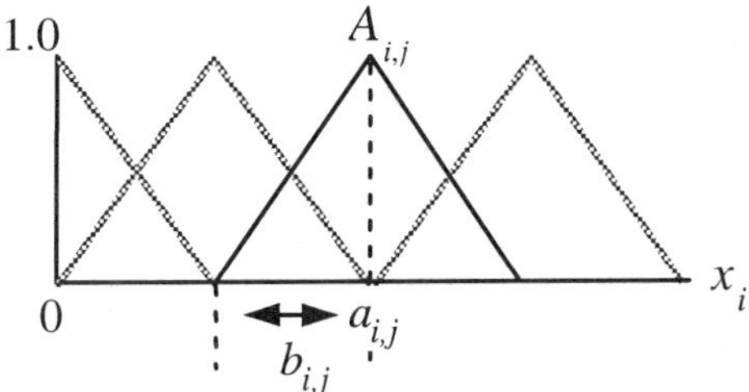

Figure 11. An example of triangular membership function.

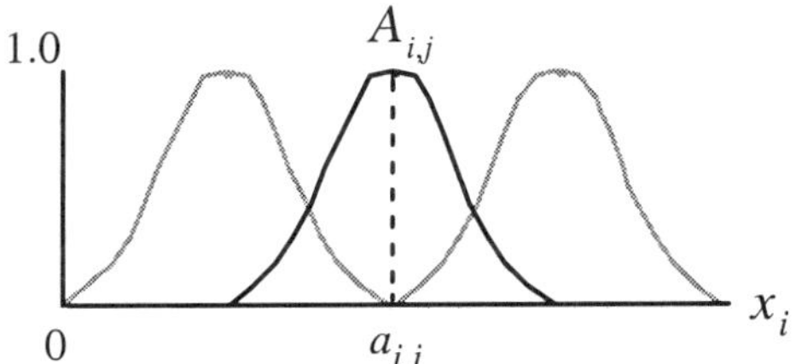

Figure 12. An example of Gaussian membership function.

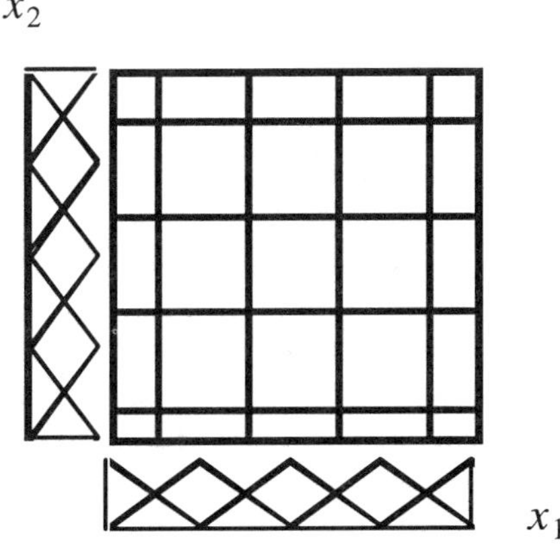

Figure 13. Input space partition for two input variables.

In designing a fuzzy controller, one needs to determine the structure of the inference system. The structure of the inference system includes input dimensionality (the number of input variables), output dimensionality (the number of output variables), the number of fuzzy sets for each input and output, the shape of membership functions, and the number of fuzzy rules. The input and output dimensions are determined beforehand by the objective control problem. The fuzzy rules to be tuned are dependent on the inference mechanism. Therefore, first of all, the inference method should be determined. Next, we determine fuzzy sets for each input variable of a fuzzy rule. The simplest method for representing fuzzy rules is to make partitions covering all the input space. Figure 13 shows the input space partition of two input variables, x_1 and x_2, where there are five fuzzy sets for each input. Each region partitioned by the membership functions corresponds to a fuzzy rule. In this case, the number of fuzzy rules is 25. The outputs of the fuzzy rules can easily be tuned by the delta rule.

In addition, the partition of the input space can be trained by the delta rule [6, 17]. However, it is difficult to determine the number of fuzzy sets and the shape of membership functions before learning. Therefore, a fuzzy controller requires a structure optimization mechanism.

3.2. Evolution of a fuzzy controller

The previous subsection described the simplest learning mechanism for fuzzy controllers. This method is often called a fuzzy neural network based upon the back propagation method [19, 20]. In addition, various self-tuning methods have been proposed such as a fuzzy learning controller with radial basis functions [21, 22], a fuzzy logic controller using GAs for determining the shapes of membership functions and fuzzy rules [23, 25, 27, 28, 29], and incremental learning based on the error function [26]. These methods can often learn faster than NNs. However, the learning ability and approximation accuracy of each method are related to the number and shape of membership functions.

A fuzzy inference system composed of many membership functions and fuzzy rules has high learning ability, but there are some redundant fuzzy rules. Basically, the number of fuzzy rules is the n-th power of the number of membership functions for each input variable, when the number of input variables is n, in order to completely cover the input space. Consequently, the number of rules increases exponentially with the number of input variables. We must pay attention to determine the structure of the membership functions, but to determine the structure before learning is very difficult. Therefore, this subsection introduces a self-tuning method of the fuzzy controller based on the evolutionary computation, to cope with this difficult problem.

3.2.1. Representation of a candidate solution

GAs have been applied for combinatorial optimization problems, while the EAs have been applied for numerical optimization, as mentioned before. Here we consider the optimization problem of a fuzzy controller as a numerical and combinatorial optimization problem. The decision variables refer to the shape of the membership functions, the combination of membership functions, and the fuzzy rules. The maximal number of fuzzy rules, and the numbers of input and output variables, are r, n, and o, respectively. We use a Gaussian membership function given by Equation (19),

$$\mu_{Ai,j}(x_j) = \exp\left(-\frac{(x_j - a_{i,j})^2}{b_{i,j}} \right)$$

where $a_{i,j}$ and $b_{i,j}$ are the central value and the width of the membership function $A_{i,j}$ for the j-th input of the i-th rule.

We use the following fuzzy if-then rule:

if x_i is $A_{i,1}$ and ... and x_n is $A_{i,n}$, then y_1 is $w_{i,1}$, ..., y_o is $w_{i,o}$

where $w_{i,k}$ is a singleton for the k-th output of the i-th rule. The decision variables are $a_{i,j}$, $b_{i,j}$ and $w_{i,k}$. Furthermore, we should determine the combination of input variables of the condition part of each fuzzy rule. Based on these optimization parameters, a set of fuzzy rules as a candidate solution is represented in Figure 14. The combination of fuzzy rules is determined by the validity of each rule (r_{valid}), and the combination of membership functions is determined by the validity of each membership function (m_{valid}). By changing these validity parameters, we can obtain the optimal combination, which reduces the number of fuzzy rules and membership functions while maintaining inference performance. The string length of a set of fuzzy rules is $(n*3+o+1)*r$. In addition, the continuous decision variables (represented as real numbers), can be transformed into discrete binary coding. The binary coding can reduce the search space to an arbitrary precision. A population is composed of candidate solutions, and evolves toward optimal fuzzy if-then rules through the genetic operators and selection. Next, we consider genetic operators of crossover and mutation for the search.

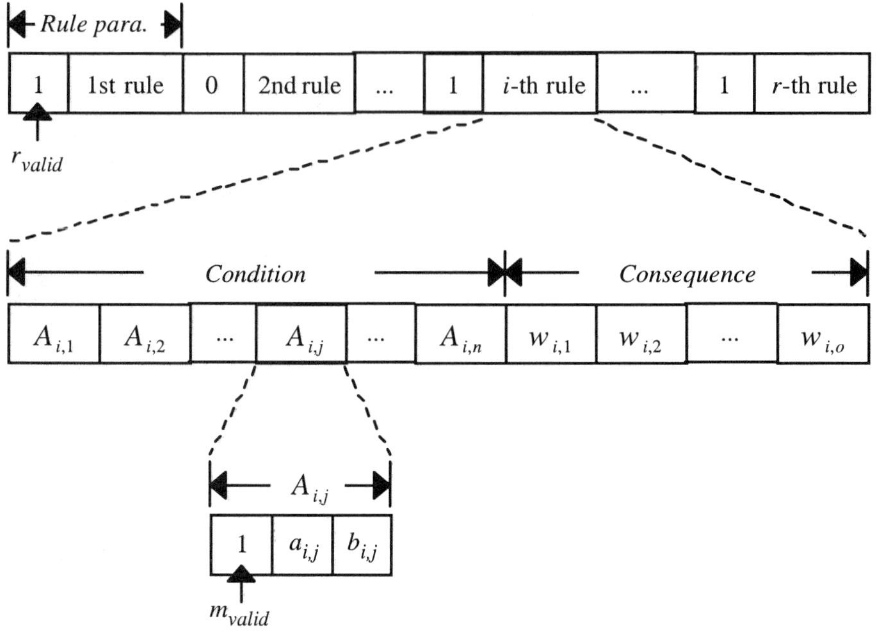

Figure 14. Representation of fuzzy rules.

3.2.2. Genetic operators

Genetic operators change some candidate solutions, such as the fuzzy rules. The crossover changes the combination of fuzzy rules and membership functions between two candidate solutions. Figure 15 shows an example of a one-point crossover. Membership functions for x_i in each rule are depicted, but other membership functions are also exchanged between two candidate solutions. Other crossover operators such as multi-point crossover and uniform crossover are often applied to produce exchanges between candidate solutions [10, 11].

In this problem, two types of combinatorial mutation operations can be used for the search. The first is to change the validity parameters for the fuzzy rules and the membership functions. This simple mutation is shown in Figure 16. The validity of the second rule is changed from 1 to 0. The second type is to exchange membership functions between the fuzzy rules in a candidate solution. We refer to these operators as an exchanging mutation. Figure 17 shows an example of exchanging mutation. In this figure, $A_{2,1}$ and $A_{3,1}$ are exchanged in the fuzzy rules. Thus, crossover and mutation operators can change the global and local combinations of fuzzy rules, respectively.

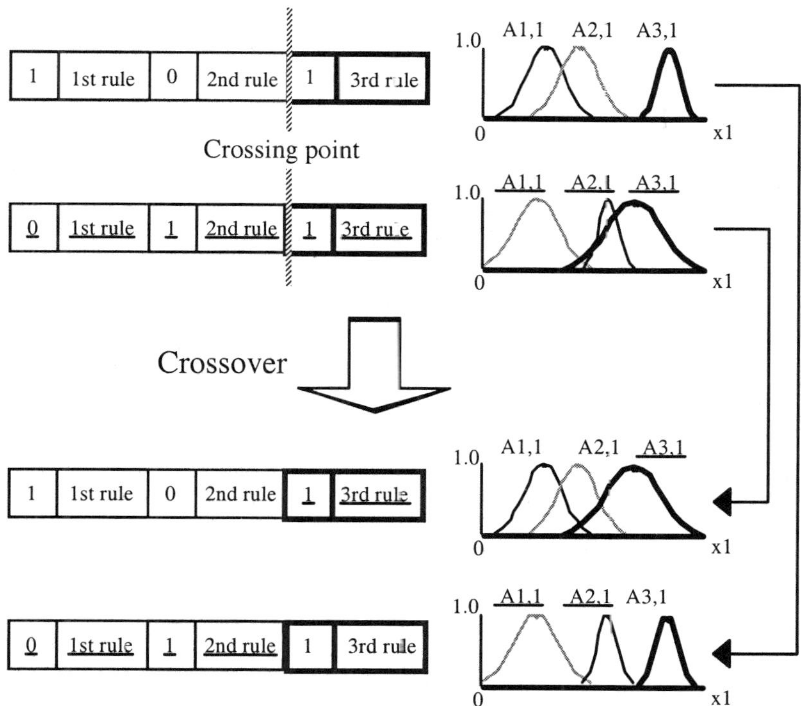

Figure 15. A one-point crossover operation: the third rules are exchanged (membership functions for x_i in each rule).

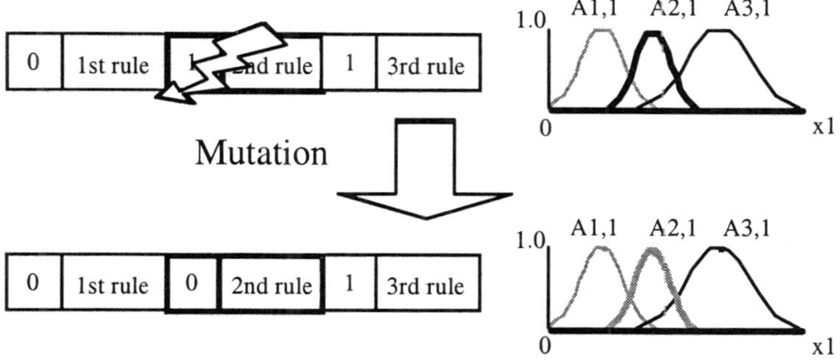

Figure 16. A simple mutation: the validity of the second rule is changed.

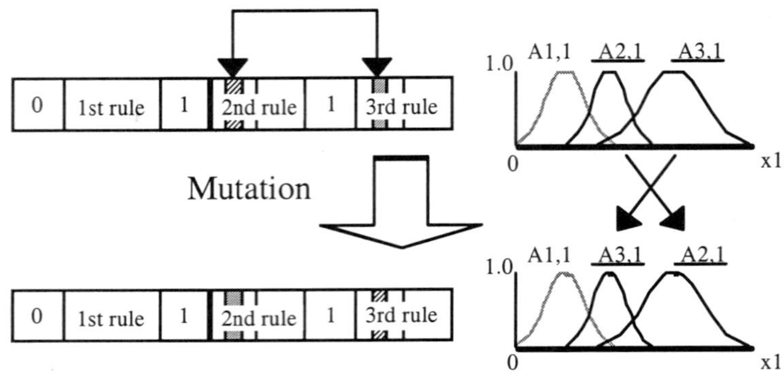

Figure 17. An exchanging mutation: membership functions are exchanged.

Next, numerical mutation is used for optimizing parameters for the membership functions and output variables. Various types of numerical mutation operators have been proposed [11]. One is normal random value based mutation as follows:

$$a_{i,j}(t+1) = a_{i,j}(t) + N(0,\sigma^2) \tag{20}$$

where t is the generation (iteration times) and σ^2 is the variance. This is the most basic numerical mutation, but the search range is fixed *a priori*. To overcome this problem, self-adaptive mutation has been proposed [11]. The self-adaptive mutation changes the variance according to the historical fitness record. As Rechenberg suggested [11],

The ratio of successful mutations to all mutations should be 1/5. If this ratio is greater than 1/5, increase the variance; if it is less, decrease the variance.

This ratio has been often discussed in previous studies. The self-adaptive mutation can self-adaptively change the searching range according to the success ratio based on the landscape of the fitness function. While self-adaptive mutation refers to its own fitness record, adaptive mutation refers to the average, maximum, and minimum of fitness values of the candidate solutions. In other words, adaptive mutation changes the searching range relative to the fitness values of the population. However, sometimes this mutation is also called a self-adaptive mutation. The widely used adaptive mutation is as follows:

$$a_{i,j}(t+1) = a_{i,j}(t) + N\left(0, \alpha_{i,j} \times \frac{f - \min f}{\max f - \min f} + \beta_{i,j}\right) \tag{21}$$

where f is the fitness value of a candidate solution, and $\alpha_{i,j}$ and $\beta_{i,j}$ are the coefficient and offset, respectively. The search range of the adaptive mutation operator is scaled according to the distribution of fitness values at the iteration times t. Consequently, adaptive mutation can scale the search range according to the evolution of the population. To summarize, the numerical mutation operations can be conceptually classified into three types: 1) numerical mutation without using fitness values, 2) self-adaptive mutation based on the fitness record of a candidate solution, and 3) adaptive mutation based on relative evaluation with other candidate solutions.

3.2.3. Fitness function and selection mechanism

The objective is to find a fuzzy controller minimizing the error function between the target outputs and the inference results, and reducing redundant fuzzy rules and the number of membership functions. The fitness function (f) consists of the error function (E), the number of the membership functions (M_{NUM}) and the number of fuzzy rules (R_{NUM}) as follows:

$$f = W_E \cdot E + W_M \cdot M_{NUM} + W_R \cdot R_{NUM} \tag{22}$$

$$M_{NUM} = \sum_{i=1}^{r} \sum_{j=1}^{n} m_{valid\_i,j} \tag{23}$$

$$R_{NUM} = \sum_{i=1}^{r} r_{valid\_i} \tag{24}$$

where $m_{valid\_i,j}$ is the validity of the membership function for the j-th input of the i-th rule, r_{valid_i} is the validity of the i-th rule, and W_E, W_M, and W_R are coefficients. Consequently, this problem results in a multi-objective optimization problem.

The selection operator generates a new population for the next generation. The basic selection methods are the roulette wheel selection and elitist selection [10]. Roulette wheel selection selects an individual l with the probability (p_l) as follows:

$$p_l = \frac{f_l}{\displaystyle\sum_{i=1}^{s} f_i} \tag{25}$$

where s is the population size. Accordingly, an individual with a higher fitness value can reproduce more offspring. Elitist selection passes the best individual into the next generation without considering the fitness value. Therefore, the hybrid method of roulette wheel selection and elitist selection is often used. Other selection methods are tournament selection, expected value selection, and ranking selection [10].

3.2.4. Evolutionary process with learning

The evolution of candidate solutions is dependent on the combination of genetic operators and the selection mechanism. A general procedure (pseudo code) of GA for a fuzzy controller is as follows:

> *begin*
>   *Initialization*
>   *repeat*
>   *Crossover*
>   *Mutation*
>   *Selection*
>   *until Termination condition = True*
> *end.*

Initialization randomly generates candidate solutions with uniform random distribution. Next, the crossover operator exchanges the combination of fuzzy rules and membership functions, and the mutation operator changes the validity parameters and adds normal random value to the decision variables. Here, we can apply any crossover and mutation operators, but we should be careful with self-adaptive mutation. When the crossover globally changes the combination of fuzzy rules, the previous fitness record of a candidate solution is meaningless. Consequently, we should not use global crossover operators with the self-adaptive mutation. In addition, we can easily incorporate other operators such as virus infection operators [28].

The evolutionary tuning of fuzzy controller is time consuming, because GAs represent a stochastic search method. Therefore, we can incorporate human knowledge and the learning mechanism such as the delta rule. The procedure of GA with the delta rule is shown in Figure 17. We can introduce human knowledge into fuzzy rules in the initialization. When the human knowledge is not complete, GA can correct or tune the fuzzy rules based on the human knowledge. Furthermore, the learning can be introduced in three stages of fuzzy controller evolutionary process. First, after initialization, the fuzzy rules can be trained by learning. In this stage, the structure of fuzzy rules is not optimized, and thus, the number of iterations and the learning rate should be relatively small and high, respectively. Next, we consider learning during the evolution. As the genetic operators might break good candidate solutions, only the best several candidate solutions should be trained through learning. This learning can be regarded as a hill climbing-like operator. Here we must consider the searching ratio between GA and delta rule. The fuzzy rules can be effectively trained by the learning, when the combination of membership functions is determined. However, the combination can be easily changed by crossovers during the evolution by GA. Consequently, to reduce the computation cost, we should take into account the searching ratio between learning and evolution according to the state of the fuzzy rules. After tuning by GA, the final learning is performed as a fine tuning of fuzzy rules with a small learning rate.

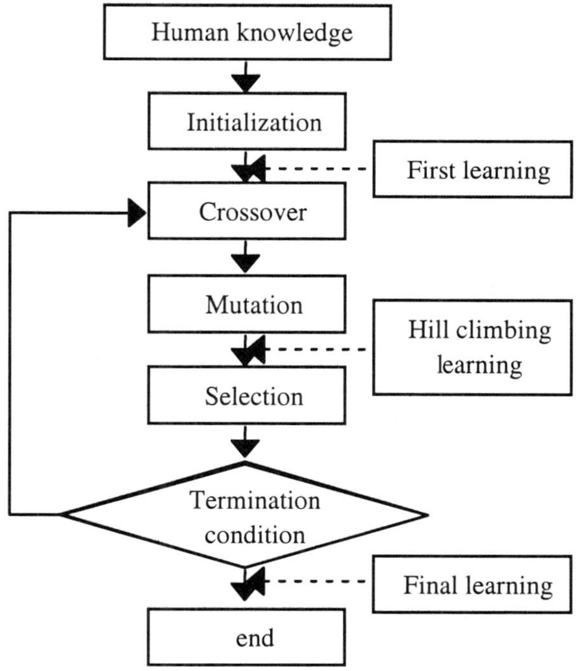

Figure 18. Procedure of GA with learning mechanism.

4. Application of fuzzy controllers to biomedical engineering

Fuzzy inference systems have been applied to image processing, diagnosis, classification problems, control problems, and decision support systems in biomedical engineering [30-45]. This section introduces recent applications of fuzzy systems to biomedical engineering.

4.1. Fuzzy image processing in biomedical engineering

Image processing is very important in biomedical engineering. Fuzzy systems are used for image processing tasks such as edge detection, image enhancement, and image segmentation in x-ray images, megavoltage images, and magnetic resonance images [30-35]. First, we introduce the studies in human brain image processing.

Structure identification or extraction of the human brain in magnetic resonance images is an important issue in neurology and radiology, as the structure of the human brain is very complex. Hata et al. applied fuzzy inference systems for 3D magnetic resonance human brain image segmentation [30, 31]. In this study, the fuzzy if-then rules are generated according to the expert knowledge of position, boundary surface, and intensity. Chang et al. designed a fuzzy rule-based system incorporating knowledge of spatial relationships between brain structures for labeling human brain components in magnetic resonance images [32].

On the other hand, Runkler and Bezdek proposed a segmentation algorithm based on fuzzy c-elliptotypes clustering and applied fuzzy clustering based on fractal features to the digital mammograms [33]. Tizhoosh et al. implemented four fuzzy methods for the enhancement of megavoltage images; minimization of fuzziness, equalization based on fuzzy expected value, fuzzy histogram hyperbolization, and fuzzy rule-based approach [34]. In addition, the analysis of vessel morphology is also a popular subject in medical image processing. Tolias et al. proposed an unsupervised fuzzy algorithm for vessel tracking and applied this tracking algorithm to detect the ocular fundus vessels [42].

4.2. Fuzzy diagnosis system in biomedical engineering

Fuzzy diagnosis systems have been applied in biomedical engineering [36-41]. The design of a fuzzy diagnosis system is mainly dependent on expert knowledge. Skilled clinicians can linguistically express practical knowledge using if-then rules. The criteria for the design of a fuzzy diagnosis system are the accuracy of the diagnosis, transparency of the decision process, and computational requirements [40].

Babinec and Novotny developed a fuzzy expert system supporting multicriteria decision making for exercise therapy prescription [37]. Orr et al. proposed a fuzzy logic extension to standard statistical modeling and applied a fuzzy additive risk model to estimate the mortality risk of cardiac surgery [36].

In addition, Hirota et al. have proposed a fuzzy diagnostic logic to find the surgical site infection based on the method of the differential count of white blood cells due to Stab and Lymph [38]. Furthermore, Arita has applied fuzzy theory to fields such as ultrasonographic diagnosis and diagnosis of diabetes mellitus [39].

4.3. Related applications

There are fuzzy controls for prosthesis and bioprocess, etc., as well as other applications to biomedical engineering [43, 44, 45]. Linkens et al. have developed a hierarchical fuzzy-based support system for anesthesia monitoring and control [43].

In addition, fuzzy control systems are used in plant controls. Horiuchi et al. proposed an on-line control system combining the phase identification mechanism with fuzzy inference and applied it to the phase control of fed-batch cultures for α-Amylase production [44]. Furthermore, Horiuchi et al. applied the culture phase identification by fuzzy set theory to effective b-Galactosidase production by recombinant Escherichia coli [45].

5. Summary

This chapter presented the basics of fuzzy inference systems and fuzzy controllers, and discussed learning, adaptation, and evolution for fuzzy controllers. Furthermore, this chapter presented recent applications of fuzzy systems to biomedical engineering.

The fundamental methodology is based on the concepts of brain science and intelligent systems including neural networks, fuzzy theory, and genetic algorithms. An intelligent system requires a learning ability for adaptation to a dynamic environment, and an evolutionary mechanism for structure optimization. The performance of intelligent systems depends on the available knowledge and information from both human beings and the environment. The intelligence of a system emerges from the information processing abilities structured as a whole [46].

Acknowledgment

The authors are grateful to Professor H.N. Teodorescu and Professor L.C. Jain for their very constructive comments, which have improved the presentation of this chapter.

References and Further Reading

[1]   Russell, S.J. and Norvig, P., (1995), *Artificial Intelligence*, Prentice-Hall, Inc.

[2]   Anderson, J.A. and Rosenfeld, E., (1988), *Neurocomputing - Foundations of Research*, The MIT Press.

[3]   Zurada, J.M., Marks II, R.J., and Robinson, C.J., (1994), *Computational Intelligence - Imitating Life*, IEEE Press.

[4]   Palaniswami, M., Attikiouzel, Y., Marks II, R.J., Fogel, D., and Fukuda, T., (1995), *Computational Intelligence - A Dynamic System Perspective*, IEEE Press.

[5]   Zadeh, L.A., (1965), *Fuzzy Sets, Information, and Control*, Vol. 8, pp. 338-353.

[6]   Jang, J-S.R., Sun, C-T., and Mizutani, E., (1997), *Neuro-Fuzzy and Soft Computing*, New Jersey: Prentice-Hall, Inc.

[7]   Langton, C.G., (1995), *Artificial Life – An Overview*, The MIT Press.

[8]   Marks II, R.J., (1993), Intelligence: computational versus artificial, *IEEE Transactions in Neural Networks*, Vol. 4, No. 5, pp. 737-739.

[9]   Kartalopoulos, S.V., (1996), *Understanding Neural Networks and Fuzzy Logic*, IEEE Press.

[10]   Goldberg, D.E., (1989), *Genetic Algorithms in Search, Optimization, and Machine Learning*, Addison Welsey.

[11]   Fogel, D.B., (1995), *Evolutionary Computation*, IEEE Press.

[12]   Koza, J., (1992), *Genetic Programming*, Massachusetts: The MIT Press.

[13]   Koza, J., (1994), *Genetic Programming II*, Massachusetts: The MIT Press.

[14]   Holland, J., (1975), *Adaptation in Natural and Artificial Systems*, Ann Arbor, MI: University of Michigan Press.

[15] Carpenter, G.A. and Grossberg, S., (1988), The art of adaptive pattern recognition by a self-organizing neural network, *Computer*, Vol. 21, pp. 77-88.

[16] Kohonen, T., (1984), *Self-Organization and Associative Memory*, Springer-Verlag, Berlin.

[17] Shi, Y., Mizumoto, M., Yubazaki, N., and Otani, M., (1996), A learning algorithm for tuning fuzzy rules based on the gradient method, *Proceedings of the Fifth IEEE International Conference on Fuzzy Systems*, New Orleans, LA, pp. 55-61.

[18] Fukuda, T., Shiotani, S., and Arai, F., (1992), A New Neuron Model for Additional Learning, *Proceedings of 1992 International Joint Conference on Neural Networks*, pp. 938-943.

[19] Horikawa, S., Furuhashi, T., and Uchikawa, Y., (1992), On fuzzy modeling using fuzzy neural networks with the back-propagation algorithm, *IEEE Transactions on Neural Networks*, Vol. 3, No. 5, pp. 801-806.

[20] Higgins, C.M. and Goodman, R.M., (1992), Learning fuzzy rule-based neural networks for function approximation, *Proceedings of International Joint Conference on Neural Networks*, Vol. 1, pp. 251-256.

[21] Katayama, R., Kajitani, Y., Kuwata, K., and Nishida, Y., (1993), Self generating radial basis function as neuro-fuzzy model and its application to nonlinear prediction of chaotic time series, *IEEE International Conference on Fuzzy Systems*, pp. 407-414.

[22] Linkens, D.A. and Nie, J., (1993), Fuzzified RBF network-based learning control: structure and self-construction, *IEEE International Conference on Neural Networks*, pp. 1016-1021.

[23] Whitley, D., Strakweather, T., and Bogart, T., (1990), Genetic algorithms and neural networks: optimizing connection and connectivity, *Parallel Computing*, 14, pp. 347-361.

[24] Nomura, H., Hayashi, I., and Wakami, N., (1991), A Self-Tuning Method of Fuzzy Control by Decent Method, *Proceedings of 4th IFSA Congress, Engineering*, pp. 155-158.

[25] Lee, M.A. and Takagi, H., (1993), Integrating Design Stages of Fuzzy Systems Using Genetic Algorithms, *Proceedings of Second IEEE International Conference on Fuzzy Systems*, pp. 612-617.

[26] Shimojima, K., Fukuda, T., and Hasegawa, Y., (1995), RBF-fuzzy system with GA Based unsupervised/supervised learning method, *Proceedings of International Joint Conference on 4th Fuzz-IEEE / 2nd IFES*, pp. 253-258.

[27] Shimojima, K., Kubota, N., and Fukuda, T., (1996), RBF fuzzy controller with virus-evolutionary genetic algorithm, *Proceedings of the International Conference on Neural Networks*, pp. 1040-1043.

[28] Shimojima, K., Kubota, N., and Fukuda, T., (1997), Virus-evolutionary genetic algorithm for fuzzy controller optimization, studies in fuzziness, Vol. 8, *Genetic Algorithms and Soft Computing*, Physica-Verlag, A Springer-Verlag Company, pp. 369-388.

[29] Kubota, N., Arakawa, T., Fukuda, T., and Shimojima, K., (1997), Fuzzy manufacturing scheduling by virus-evolutionary genetic algorithm in self-organizing manufacturing system, *Proceedings of the Sixth IEEE International Conference on Fuzzy Systems*, pp. 1283-1288.

[30] Hata, Y., Kobashi, S., Kamiura, N., and Ishikawa, M., (1997), Fuzzy logic approach to 3D magnetic resonance image segmentation, information processing in medical imaging, *Lecture Notes in Computer Science*, Vol. 1230, pp. 387-392.

[31] Kobashi, S., Kamiura, N., Hata, Y., and Ishikawa, M., (1997), Automatic robust threshold finding aided by fuzzy information granulation, *Proceedings of IEEE 1997 International Conference on Image Processing*, Vol. 1, pp. 711-714.

[32] Chang, C.-W., Hillman, R., Ying, H., Kent, T., and Yen, J., (1996), A fuzzy rule-based system for labeling the structures in 3D human brain magnetic resonance images, *Proceedings of the Fifth IEEE International Conference on Fuzzy Systems*, pp. 1973-1982.

[33] Runkler, T.A. and Bezdek, J.C., (1997), Image segmentation using fuzzy clustering with fractal features, *Proceedings of The Sixth IEEE International Conference on Fuzzy Systems*, pp. 1393-1398.

[34] Tizhoosh, H.R., Krell, G., and Michaelis, B., (1997), *On Fuzzy Enhancement of Megavoltage Images in Radiation Therapy*, Proceedings of the Sixth IEEE International Conference on Fuzzy Systems, pp. 1399-1404.

[35] Waschek, T., Levegrun, S., Schlegel, W., Kampen, M., and Cabill, R.E., (1996), Target volume definition for three dimensional radiotherapy of cancer patients with a fuzzy rule based system, *Proceedings of the Fifth IEEE International Conference on Fuzzy Systems*, pp. 1718-1725.

[36] Orr, R.K., (1996), Estimating mortality risk of cardiac surgery using a fuzzy additive model, *Proceedings of the Fifth IEEE International Conference on Fuzzy Systems*, pp. 1983-1988.

[37] Babinec, F. and Novotny, J., (1997), Fuzzy logic approach to exercise therapy prescription in type 1 diabetics, *Seventh IFSA World Congress*, Vol. 4, pp. 401-405.

[38] Hirota, H., Arita, S., Hori, Y., Sakaguchi, S., Maniwa, Y., Tanimura, H., Mizumoto, M., Li, Z., and Nagasawa, R., (1997), Diagnostic system for surgical site infection based on differential counts of WBC using fuzzy inference, *Seventh IFSA World Congress*, Vol. 4, pp. 417-422.

Chapter 2

Learning eye-arm coordination using neural and fuzzy neural techniques

Adrian Stoica

Developing models for motor control, learning, and sensory-motor coordination is of equal interest to researchers studying human motor behavior and to engineers aiming at robots with capabilities closer to human performance, such as anthropomorphic or humanoid robots. This chapter proposes an approach to the transfer of motor skills to such robots, in which the robot's capability to control its limbs starts with the learning of motor coordination using self-directed exploration. Once it has control over its limbs, the robot could imitate the movements of an instructor or execute movements described verbally or in a succession of coordinates in Cartesian or joint spaces. The approach described in this chapter uses learning by imitation (or teaching by demonstration, as seen from the human perspective). This method of learning is considered promising, because it is human-friendly and efficient in illustrating postures hard to capture in linguistic descriptions or quantified in programming instructions. The model of eye-arm sensory-motor coordination described here is characterized by a system of equations, numerically solved using neural networks. Two models of neurons are explored: a classic neuron with a sigmoidal characteristic and a fuzzy (logic) neuron defined using triangular norms, used when the model of sensory-motor coordination was characterized by fuzzy relational equations. The interest in fuzzy neural models originates in the search for a unique structural element for a *nervous system* able to learn from both visual examples and linguistic descriptions of the movement. Both neural models successfully learned the functional mapping that associates images of the instructor arm with joint-commands necessary for positioning the robot arm in a similar posture. However, the fuzzy neural model has shown increased transparency. The experiments illustrate how the neural-guided robot is able to imitate 2D and 3D arm movements of a human and of another robot.

1. Introduction

1.1. Models of motor control and skill learning and their use in studies of human motor behavior, bioengineering, and robotics

Models of motor control, learning, and sensory-motor coordination have been developed at the confluence of technology-push – application-pull forces, as illustrated in Figure 1.

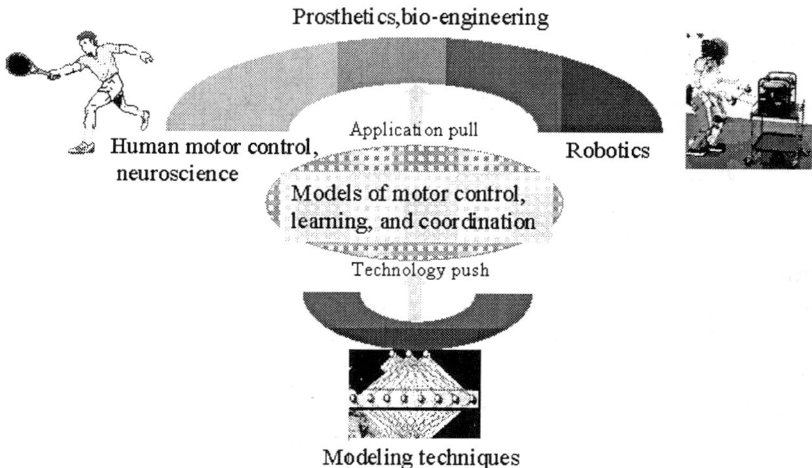

Figure 1. Models: result of applications pull – technology push.

Computer scientists, mathematicians, engineers, and other specialists are pushing modeling tools to help create better models of motor learning and control; these tools are often in the form of computational structures such as neural networks, fuzzy systems, etc. At one end of the spectrum of the application, users are researchers interested in human-oriented studies, such as human motor learning and control, vision, sensory-motor coordination, and neuro-control. At the other end of the spectrum are engineers interested in building efficient robots; when the robots are anthropomorphic and need to move like the humans, the source of inspiration is in models of human motor control. Somewhere in between these two categories of users are bioengineers and researchers developing prosthetic devices, with the role of using technology to correct or ameliorate human disabilities.

1.2. Humanoid robots as personal assistants

Robots that look like humans, move, and have a general human-like behavior are no longer fiction-only characters. More than a decade of research on humanoids led to an impressive demonstration in 1997 of the Japanese Honda P2 humanoid robot, a robot that can autonomously walk, go up and down stairs, push a cart, etc. [1]. Honda's demonstration comes as a technology proof, showing that it is possible now to build self-contained (with power and computing on-board) humanoid robot bodies and ensure simple motor controls. Further work is needed in developing appropriate perceptual skills, motor skills for useful activities, basic levels of intelligence, etc. Humanoids belong to the larger category of service robots. It is predicted that service robotics will outstrip industrial robotics sometime early in the 21st century [2]. Humanoids will probably have an important role as personal assistants in household activities, elderly care, or assistance of the disabled. There are more than four million partially or fully disabled individuals in the U.S. alone [3]. Humanoids could be ideal in replacing humans in dangerous activities such as fire fighting, operations in nuclear-contaminated regions, or in space missions [4, 5].

1.3. Organization of the chapter

The chapter is organized as follows. Section 2 presents some aspects of learning of motor skills by anthropomorphic and humanoid robots. Section 3 addresses neural and fuzzy-neural modeling for motor learning, control, and sensory-motor coordination. It presents modeling by fuzzy relational equations and methods of model identification that are equivalent to the resolution of these equations. This resolution can be numerically approached as learning in a layered structure of fuzzy neurons. Section 4 presents an implementation of these models to real robots and 2D/3D experiments in learning the eye-arm coordination that allowed the robots to imitate the arm movement of human and robot teachers.

An extension forcing overall body imitation is possible if the body is covered with appropriately placed sensors. Imitation and capturing of elements of human movement is of great interest not only to robotics engineers but also to computer-assisted movie and game makers. For such users, Sarcos (Salt Lake City, Utah) has developed the SenSuit™ (illustrated in Figure 3) that enables real-time teleoperator control of robotic figures and computer generated icons [13].

Real imitation, however, is when the robot itself watches and moves freely to reproduce human movements. This chapter presents initial work in this area, describing how an anthropomorphic robot arm learns to imitate the movements of a teacher. See [14] for a more detailed presentation of the subject. The robot learner and the teacher (a human or an identical anthropomorphic robot) stay next to each other, and the eye of the learning robot watches the movement of the teacher. Figure 4 shows the robot imitating the 3D movement of an identical robot; the camera through which the learner robot gets the video input is mounted at the approximate position of an eye of a 1.80 m tall human. Figure 13 in Section 4.2 will show the robot imitating a human teacher in a set-up where the robot has a *bird's eye view* of the scene.

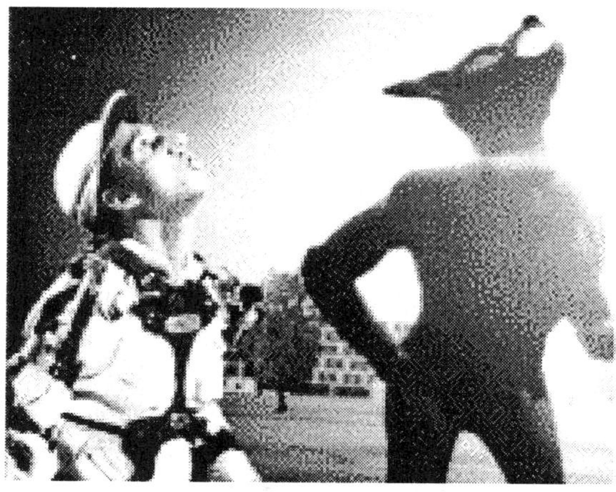

Figure 3. Operator in Sarcos' SenSuit controls a virtual anthropomorphic creature. (Copyright Sarcos Inc, reprinted with permission.)

Other researchers worldwide are working on different aspects of imitation. For example, researchers at Tokyo University developed a human skull-shaped robot imitating the facial expression of a human teacher. In several other centers, the analysis and understanding of human gestures has recently received considerable interest from the perspective of developing a next generation of human-friendly computer interfaces.

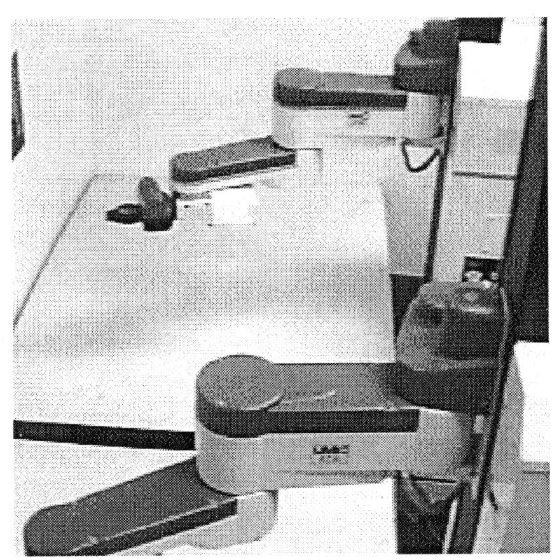

Figure 4. A learner arm imitates a teacher arm.

Learning by imitation appears promising for making humanoid robots move like humans. However, many other important aspects need to be addressed when aiming for such an endeavor.

2.3. Learning to walk

Biped motion control must contend with the serious problem of maintaining stability. One can, however, alleviate the need for a very stable design by initially supporting the robot on a *walker*, such as a circular ring at waist level used to maintain stability, on which the robot's hands lean on, and which is pushed along when the robot walks. Force sensors would then provide feedback, and the control of the robot could be adaptively changed. Thus, the robot could learn to walk while trying to minimize the force applied to the walker (seen as an optimization problem); when finally no force is put on the walker, the robot will be able to maintain by itself a stable biped motion. This approach would lessen the possibility of an expensive robot accidentally losing stability and falling, possibly damaging itself.

Once learned, *the knowledge of how to move* could be captured from the first learning robot in a generation and directly transferred (downloaded) to new, similar robots.

3. Neural and fuzzy neural modeling

3.1. Neural networks, fuzzy logic, and neuro-fuzzy hybrids

Human-like robotic movement requires models for motor generators, motor control, and sensory-motor coordination that find inspiration in models characterizing the movement of humans. The models described in this chapter use concepts of fuzzy logic and neural networks, briefly reviewed in the following paragraphs.

For the purpose of this chapter, a classic neuron is an elementary computational unit that performs a transformation from a multidimensional input space to a unidimensional output space. In a loose analogy with biological neurons, the inputs are modulated by weighting factors at the *synaptic* level and then summed together at the *somatic* level; finally, a sigmoidal transformation is applied to the weighted sum. The output is expressed by the formula

$$o = \frac{1}{1 + \exp(-ay)} \tag{1}$$

$$y = \sum_i w_i \cdot x_i + b \tag{2}$$

In the above equations, x_i denote the inputs, w_i the weights, y is the somatic activation, o is neuron output, a is a factor characterizing the slope of the neuron characteristic, and b is a bias term. Networks of neurons can have various topologies in which the signal can flow from network inputs to outputs in a feedforward only manner, or can have feedback at various points. A popular topology is multilayer; all neurons in a layer share the same inputs, which could be network inputs or outputs of a previous layer. In the more general case, learning consists of determining the topology, the weights w, and sometimes the somatic parameter a, such that the inputs and outputs are in a certain relationship. However, learning often consists of determining only the weights and biases, the other factors being fixed.

Fuzzy set theory, introduced by Zadeh in 1965 [15], provides a rich extension framework to the modeling formalism employed in a variety of disciplines, including Eye engineering and social sciences. The term fuzzy logic (FL) is generically used for a variety of mechanisms, including mechanisms for approximate reasoning as applied, for example, in knowledge-based systems.

Fuzzy models have proved their usefulness in a variety of applications, see for example [16] and [17] for a review. These two techniques (FL and NN) complement each other. This may be exploited in structures that combine their individual strengths: the transparent knowledge embodied in fuzzy systems and the learning ability of NN. Combinations of elements of fuzzy logic and neural networks were initiated in the seventies, with a first model of fuzzy neuron (FN) and a fuzzy neural network (FNN) being introduced in [18]. For reviews of work in this area, the reader is referred to [19-22].

3.2. The relational approach to system modeling

The definitions used in this section are due to Zadeh [14, 23], with some formulations taken from [24, 25].

Fuzzy relations. Recall that a fuzzy relation R from a set X to a set Y is a fuzzy subset of the Cartesian product $X{\times}Y$ ($X{\times}Y$ is the collection of all ordered pairs (x,y) of elements $x{\in}X$ and $y{\in}Y$). R is characterized by the membership function $\mu_R(x,y)$, and is expressed by

$$R = \left\{ \left((x, y), \mu_R(x, y)\right) \mid (x, y) \in X \times Y \right\} \tag{3}$$

A fuzzy relation (FR) can be seen as a mapping between two fuzzy sets described in terms of values of their membership function in points of their definition domains. Alternatively, a fuzzy relation can be seen as a mapping of fuzzy sets represented in terms of values of membership to some reference fuzzy sets defined on the universe of discourse. The mapping of sampled membership functions is referred here as *distributed*, while the mapping of labels is referred to as *compact*.

Composition of fuzzy relations. *MAX-MIN* **composition.** If Q is a relation from X to Y and R is a relation from Y to Z, then the composition of Q and R is a fuzzy relation denoted by $Q \circ R$ and defined pointwise by

$$\mu_{QoR}(x, z) = \bigvee_{y}(\mu_Q(x, y) \wedge \mu_R(y, z)) \tag{4}$$

where $\vee$ and $\wedge$ denote, respectively, *MAX* and *MIN*. More specifically, Equation (4) defines the *MAX-MIN composition*. The following assumes a finite universe of discourse, and *MAX* and *MIN* appear directly in the equations. The composition between a fuzzy set A and the fuzzy relation R, $R{:}X \rightarrow Y$, defines the *image* of fuzzy set A into the space Y (5), where $i = 1,...,m$ and $j = 1,...,n$

$$B(y_j) = (A \circ R)(x_i, y_j) = \bigvee_{i=1}^{m}(A(x_i) \wedge R(x_i, y_j)) \tag{5}$$

The *MAX-MIN* composition of fuzzy relations Q and R, defined on finite universes $Q:X \to Y$, $R:Y \to Z$, is given by

$$P(x_i, z_k) = (Q \circ R)(x_i, z_k) = \bigvee_{i=1}^{m} (Q(x_i, y_j) \wedge R(y_j, z_k)) \qquad (6)$$

MAX-MIN fuzzy relational equations. Let A and B be fuzzy sets, R a fuzzy relation, and $\circ$ a composition (not necessarily *MAX-MIN*). An equation of type $A \circ R = B$ is a *fuzzy relational equation* (FRE). A FRE can be addressed in the sense of solving for R, when A and B are known, or for A, if R and B are known (in which case it is called the inverse problem). Equation (5) describes a *MAX-MIN* FRE. The equation of type $Q \circ R = P$, with Q, P, R fuzzy relations, is called a *composite FRE*. As fuzzy relational matrices for Q and P are composed of rows, which correspond to fuzzy sets, one can consider that Equation (6) describes a system of equations of type (5); therefore, it is also called a system of FRE. The resolution of FRE was first addressed by Sanchez [26], who provided a methodology for solving *MAX-MIN* FRE, formulating conditions and analyzing theoretical aspects of obtaining a greatest (or maximal) solution. For a detailed presentation of results on *MAX-MIN* FRE, the reader is referred to [25].

Approximate solutions. If all the equations have a solution and their intersection is nonempty, then the system has a solution, and the presented methods of resolution can be applied. Practical situations may fail to meet the solvability conditions, in which case the system of FRE does not have (exact) solutions. In such a case, the problem of solvability can be approached in a passive way or in active ways [27]. The passive approach is related to the determination of a measure of solvability of the FRE, reflected in an index of solvability. One active approach is to look at modifications of fuzzy sets or to eliminate the equations that impede the existence of an exact solution. Another active approach is to try to fulfill the constraints to the highest possible degree, i.e., finding the best approximate solution [27, 28]. Most commonly, the approximation is sought in relation to the optimization of some index factor, which most often is the fuzzy Hamming distance (a sum of absolute errors) or the Euclidean distance between desired outputs and images obtained by composition with the fuzzy relation. Numerical methods are the most common way to determine approximate solutions for FRE. The problem of numerical resolution for approximate solutions was first addressed in [29], where a modified Newton method was proposed. Before genetic algorithms were attempted [30, 31], all numerical methods for finding a solution were gradient-based techniques [31]. Pedrycz [32] extended the *MAX-MIN* composition allowing *MIN* to be replaced by any operator from the class of triangular norms [33].

Triangular norms. [34]. A function T: $[0,1] \times [0,1] \to [0,1]$ is called a triangular norm (t-norm for short) if it satisfies the following conditions:

- associativity: $T(x, T(y,z)) = T(T(x,y), z)$,
- commutativity: $T(x,y) = T(y,x)$,
- monotonicity: $T(x,y) \leq T(x,z)$, whenever $y \leq z$, and
- boundary condition $T(x,1) = x$.

A function S: $[0,1] \times [0,1] \to [0,1]$ is called a triangular co-norm (t-co-norm or s-norm for short) if it satisfies the conditions of associativity, commutativity, monotonicity, and the boundary condition $S(x,0) = x$. S and T are corresponding (or pairs), if they comply with De Morgan's laws.

N-ary extensions. The n-ary extensions for T and S are defined recursively [25], for example,

$$\overset{m+1}{\underset{i=1}{T}}(x_1, x_2, ..., x_m) = \begin{cases} m = 1: & T(x_1, x_2) \\ m \geq 2: & T(x_{m+1}, \overset{m}{\underset{i=1}{T}}(x_1, x_2, ..., x_m)) \end{cases} \tag{7}$$

In a similar way, $\overset{m+1}{\underset{i=1}{S}}$ is defined.

Examples of t-norms. Table 1 presents 12 operators [34, 35].

S-T composition. Let A be a fuzzy set defined in X ($X = \{x_1, x_2, ..., x_m\}$), and R a fuzzy relation between X and Y. The S-T composition of a fuzzy set A and a fuzzy relation R is the fuzzy set B defined in Y ($Y = \{y_1, y_2, ..., y_n\}$), whose membership function is given by

$$B(y_j) = (A \circ_{t,s} R)(x_i, y_j) = \overset{m}{\underset{i=1}{S}}(A(x_i) \, T \, R(x_i, y_j)) \tag{8}$$

Let $Q: X \to Y$ and $R: Y \to Z$ be fuzzy relations. The S-T composition of Q and R is the fuzzy relation denoted $Q \circ_{t,s} R$ between X and Z, defined by

$$(Q \circ_{t,s} R)(x_i, z_k) = \overset{m}{\underset{i=1}{S}}(Q(x_i, y_j) \, T \, R(y_j, z_k)) \tag{9}$$

(The indices in $\circ_{ts}$ show that the operation is defined by means of a specific couple of t-norm and s-co-norm.)

Table 1. Triangular norms and co-norms.

T − norms

S − norms

$$T^1(x, y) = MIN(x, y)$$

$$S^1(x, y) = MAX(x, y)$$

$$T^2(x, y) = x \cdot y$$

$$S^2(x, y) = x + y - xy$$

$$T^3(x, y) = MAX(x + y - 1, 0)$$

$$S^3(x, y) = MIN(x + y, 1)$$

$$T^4(x, y) = \frac{xy}{x + y - xy}$$

$$S^4(x, y) = \frac{x + y - 2xy}{1 - xy}$$

$$T^5(x, y) = \begin{cases} x & if(y = 1) \\ y & if(x = 1) \\ 0 & else \end{cases}$$

$$S^5(x, y) = \begin{cases} x & if(y = 0) \\ y & if(x = 0) \\ 1 & else \end{cases}$$

$$T^6(x, y) = \frac{\lambda xy}{1 - (1 - \lambda)(x + y - xy)}$$

$$S^6(x, y) = \frac{\lambda(x + y) + xy(1 - 2\lambda)}{\lambda + xy(1 - \lambda)}$$

$$T^7(x, y) = MAX(1 - ((1 - x)^p + (1 - y)^p)^{\frac{1}{p}}, 0)$$

$$S^7(x, y) = MIN((x^p + y^p)^{\frac{1}{p}}, 1)$$

$$T^8(x, y) = \frac{1}{1 + ((\frac{1}{x} - 1)^\lambda + (\frac{1}{y} - 1)^\lambda)^{\frac{1}{\lambda}}}$$

$$S^8(x, y) = \frac{1}{1 + ((\frac{1}{x} - 1)^{-\lambda} + (\frac{1}{y} - 1)^{-\lambda})^{-\frac{1}{\lambda}}}$$

$$T^9(x, y) = \frac{xy}{MAX(x, y, \lambda)}$$

$$S^9(x, y) = 1 - \frac{(1 - x)(1 - y)}{MAX(1 - x, 1 - y, \lambda)}$$

$$T^{10}(x, y) = MAX\left(\frac{x + y - 1 + \lambda xy}{1 + \lambda}, 0\right)$$

$$S^{10}(x, y) = MIN(x + y + \lambda xy, 1)$$

$$T^{11}(x, y) = MAX((1 + \lambda)(x + y - 1) - \lambda xy, 0)$$

$$S^{11}(x, y) = MIN(x + y + \lambda xy, 1)$$

$$T^{12}(x, y) = \log_s\left(1 + \frac{(s^x - 1)(s^y - 1)}{s - 1}\right)$$

$$S^{12}(x, y) = 1 - \log_s\left(1 + \frac{(s^{1-x} - 1)(s^{1-y} - 1)}{s - 1}\right)$$

The *S-T* composition was introduced by Pedrycz in [32] and [36]. It received little attention in its general form (most studies being concerned with the particular cases max-t and max-min), but it resurfaced in the context of fuzzy neurons in [37, 38].

Resolution of *S-T* FRE. Conditions of solvability and an algorithm for determining a solution for one FRE given by Equation (8) were presented in [36]. For a solution of (8) to exist, it is necessary that

$$\forall k \in K, \quad B(y_k) \le \mathop{S}_{j \in J} (A(x_j)) \tag{10}$$

where $J = \{1,...,n\}$, $K = \{1,...,p\}$. The condition is sufficient provided that S and T are continuous. For the general form of a system of FRE (9), the resolution problem is open.

The relational approach to system modeling. In the relational approach to system modeling, information processing in a distributed fuzzy system is characterized by a composition of the input with a fuzzy relational equation that describes the system. Thus, processing can be considered to be performed by a network of distributed processors, each calculating the output in a particular point of the output domain. These processors can be neurons as in [39, 40].

3.3. Fuzzy logic neurons and numerical resolution of fuzzy relational equations

Fuzzy logics. A fuzzy logic is defined by a set of rules for determining the complement, intersection, and union of fuzzy sets. Zadeh's fuzzy logic is defined using *MIN* and *MAX* operators for intersection and union. A more general case is that of fuzzy logic based on triangular norms T and S, as defined, for example, in [41]. Such fuzzy logics are defined based on intersection and complement only, considering complementary t-norms. The complement A^c of a fuzzy set A is defined *by $A^c (x) = 1 - A(x)$,* the intersection $A\ T\ B$ of fuzzy sets A and B is defined *by $(A\ T\ B)(x) = T(A(x), B(x))$,* and the union $A\ S\ B$ of fuzzy sets A and B is defined *by $(A\ S\ B)(x) = S(A(x),B(x))$.* In the following, the specification of a certain fuzzy logic is semantically equivalent to the specification of an associated composition. For example, "applying the *MAX-MIN* composition" is equivalent to "working under the *MAX-MIN* logic."

Fuzzy logic neurons. Fuzzy logic can be used for defining logic neurons. Fuzzy logic neurons were introduced [42] using fuzzy logic operators to model synaptic and somatic activities. For example, a *MAX-MIN* fuzzy neuron (or simply *MAX-MIN* neuron) was defined based on Zadeh's fuzzy logic, i.e., using *MAX* as the union of activities at the somatic level, and *MIN* as the intersection or joint effect of inputs and synaptic states [43].

Pedrycz [43] has shown that a layer of *MAX-MIN* neurons implements the *MAX-MIN* composition and can be considered as the underlying structure of a fuzzy system in its relational definition (i.e., $X \circ R = Y$, where X are input fuzzy sets and Y are output fuzzy sets, R is a fuzzy relation between input and output, and $\circ$ is the *MAX-MIN* composition).

The following discussion refers to fuzzy neurons in the sense of Gupta [44] and Pedrycz and Rocha [45] (Pedrycz uses several neuron models, the one mentioned here being his OR neuron).

S-T fuzzy neurons and layers of S-T fuzzy neurons. Consider a neuron as an information processing element, having a number of inputs $\mathbf{x} = [x_1, x_2, ..., x_m]$ and a single output y. The inputs affect the neuron via synapses, which modulate the inputs with the values of the weights $w = [w_1, w_2, ..., w_m]$. The modulation can be modeled by a t-norm operation,

$$t_i = T(x_i, y_i) \tag{11}$$

$$y = \overset{m}{\underset{i=1}{S}}(t_i) \tag{12}$$

The effect of the modulated inputs as perceived by the neuron consists of a set of excitations t_i. All these t_i, $i = 1,2,...,m$, are somatic input contributions to the neuron, and the output is obtained by their aggregation. The aggregation can be performed by an *s*-norm operation. Equations (11) and (12) define an *S-T fuzzy neuron* (*S-T* FN), which is illustrated in Figure 5.

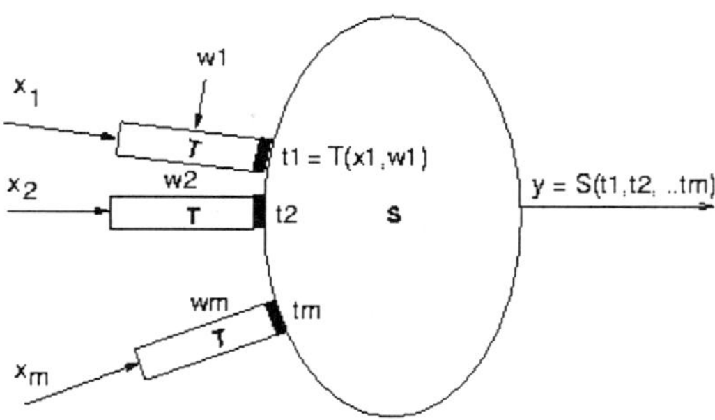

Figure 5. *S-T* fuzzy neuron.

Consider n similar neurons, each receiving inputs x via the set of *weights* $W = [w_1, w_2, ..., w_n]$. The equations for the j-th neuron, at instant k are

$$t_{i,j}^k = T\left(x_{k,i}, w_{i,j}\right) \qquad (13)$$

$$y_{k,j} = \mathop{S}_{i=1}^{m} (t_{i,j}^k) \qquad (14)$$

Considering that inputs at discrete moments of time $1,2,..., p$ are rows in a matrix $X = [x_1, x_2,...,x_p]$ and the same for outputs $Y = [y_1, y_2,...,y_p]$, then the detailed form of this batch processing is

$$Y = (X \circ W)(y_{kj}) = \mathop{S}_{i=1}^{m} (T(X(k,i), W(i,j)) \qquad (15)$$

which is the formal description of *S-T* composition of fuzzy relations.

Thus, a layer of fuzzy neurons performs the *S-T* composition (Figure 6). Presented with I-O pairs, learning in such a network is finally equivalent to the identification of a fuzzy model.

Fundamental fuzzy neurons (FFN). The equations for fuzzy neural processing written in terms of T and S operators are general, and for numerical calculations, it is necessary to select a particular pair of triangular norm/conorm to replace T and S in the formulas. In order to benefit from the great number of topologies and learning rules developed for classic neurons, fuzzy neurons need to respect some conditions, such as

- The neural model should permit gradient descent. Functions defined with thresholding by *MIN* or *MAX* are poor choices for gradient descent-like methods.
- The functions should be parametric. Parameterization offers modeling flexibility, as pointed out in [24, 25, 45].
- The selected t-norm (s-norm) should cover the *MIN* (*MAX*) case.

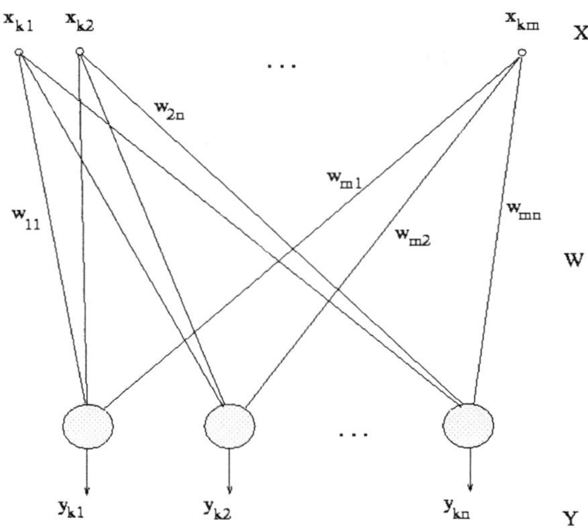

Figure 6. A layer of *S-T* neurons implements the *S-T* composition.

A comparison of the 12 operators presented in Table 1 shows that only T^8 and T^{12} satisfy the imposed requirements. It is possible to create new t-norms (for example, as shown in [46]), some of which may also satisfy the conditions imposed here. T^{12} has the advantage of covering the operators used in probabilistic reasoning, product/probabilistic sum (T^2/S^2), which is a limit case for (T^{12}_s / S^{12}_s) when $s \to 1$. The disadvantage is that in order to cover the case $s = 1$ (the point in which T^{12} is defined equal to T^2), one must switch between functions T^{12} and T^2.

A *fundamental fuzzy neuron* (FFN) is an *S-T* fuzzy neuron for which the *S* and *T* operators are the fundamental t-norms [47] (called fundamental in [34]) given by Equations (16), (17), for $0 < s < \infty$. A network of FFN forms a fundamental fuzzy neural network (FFNN).

$$
T_s(x, y) = \begin{cases}
MIN(x, y) & if\,(s = 0) \\
x \cdot y & if\,(s = 1) \\
\log_s\!\left(1 + \dfrac{\left(s^x - 1\right)\cdot\left(s^y - 1\right)}{s - 1}\right) & if\,((0 < s < \infty),\, s \neq 1) \\
MIN(1, x + y) & if\,(s = \infty)
\end{cases} \tag{16}
$$

$$S_s(x,y) = \begin{cases} MAX(x,y) & if \quad (s=0) \\ x+y-x\cdot y & if \quad (s=1) \\ 1-\log_s\left(1+\dfrac{\left(s^{1-x}-1\right)\cdot\left(s^{1-y}-1\right)}{s-1}\right) & if \quad ((0<s<\infty), s\neq 1) \\ MIN(1,x+y) & if \quad (s=\infty) \end{cases} \tag{17}$$

Due to the definition condition, the class of fuzzy neurons is restricted to $0 < s < \infty$, for which T_S, and S_S are continuous (as shown in [34]).

The characteristic function of a FFN with m inputs is expressed by

$$y = 1 - \log_{s_S}\left(1+\frac{\left(s_S^{1-t_1}-1\right)\cdot\left(s_S^{1-t_2}-1\right)\cdots\left(s_S^{1-t_m}-1\right)}{(s_S-1)^{(m-1)}}\right) \tag{18}$$

where each t_i represents the synaptic contribution of input x_i modulated by the weight w_i,

$$t_i = \log_{ST}\left(1+\frac{\left(s_T^{x_i}-1\right)\cdot\left(s_T^{w_i}-1\right)}{(s_T-1)}\right) \tag{19}$$

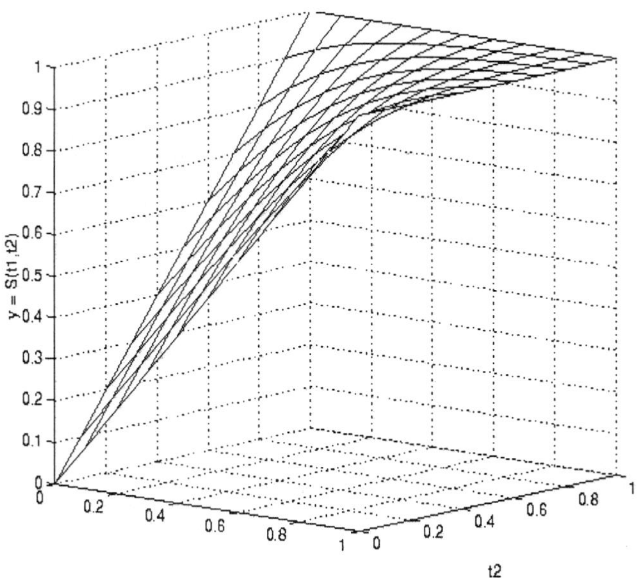

Figure 7. Characteristic of a fundamental s-norm fuzzy neuron.

The characteristic function for a *S-T* neuron with two inputs is presented in Figure 7. This illustrates the function $y = S_{100} (t_1, t_2)$, where t_1 and t_2 are the inputs after the synaptic composition.

Equations for learning and adaptation in FFN (numerical resolution of a system of FRE) are detailed in [14].

4. Experiments in learning eye-arm coordination

4.1. A model for eye-arm coordination

Motor skills can be broadly divided into two large categories: planning skills, i.e., the know-how expertise, and motor control skills, i.e., the ability acquired after performing a movement many times. Accordingly, the mapping between process characteristics and actions can be divided in a mapping between process characteristics and desired actions (determining the planning skills), and the mapping between desired and performed actions (corresponding to motor control skills), as in Figure 8.

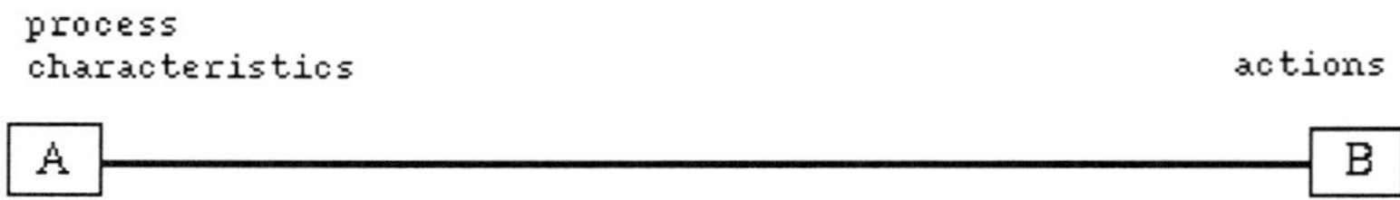

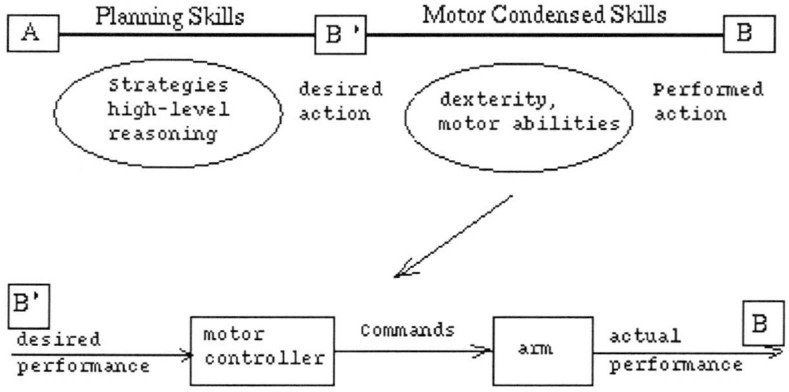

Figure 8. Planning skills and motor control skills.

The former motor skills are related to strategies at a higher level, while the latter refer to dexterity and motor abilities. In the case of arm coordination, the mapping between desired and actual performance is subject to a representation in which a motor controller maps the desired performance into commands, and the arm plays the role of the controlled plant, mapping commands to actual performance. The motor controller also performs a transformation from a sensory coordinate system to a motor coordinate system.

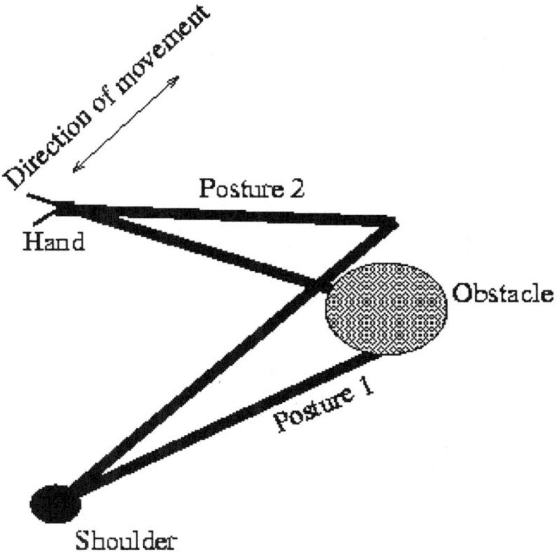

Figure 9. Two arm postures for the same hand position.

To be able to place its arm in a desired position, the robot needs to have a model of its eye-arm coordination. Traditionally, visuo-motor coordination in robotics addressed eye-hand coordination. For redundant manipulators (including here the human arm and anthropomorphic robot arms), the associated inverse kinematics problem is underconstrained, admitting more than one solution. In the context of acquiring motor skills by imitation, when the task requires specific postures or is imposed by obstacles in the environment, eye-hand coordination is insufficient. This is illustrated in the 3D situation in Figure 9, where Posture (1) given by an eye-hand model is unacceptable due to an obstacle, while Posture (2), shown by an instructor, provides a feasible alternative. The eye-arm coordination adds to other models of coordination, as shown in Figure 10.

We discuss a model of eye-arm coordination, schematically illustrated in Figure 11. During the learning of the visuo-motor model, the visual inputs could be from the robot's own arm, from the arm to follow, or from another teaching arm (these variations are discussed in detail later in this chapter). During the imitation of human arm movements, the visual inputs are images of the human arm. The model (W) reflects the mapping between visual inputs (X) and joint motor commands (Y). The inputs (X) to the model are low-resolution images originating in the images obtained from video cameras. The outputs (Y) are associated with shoulder and elbow joint angles as in Figure 12.

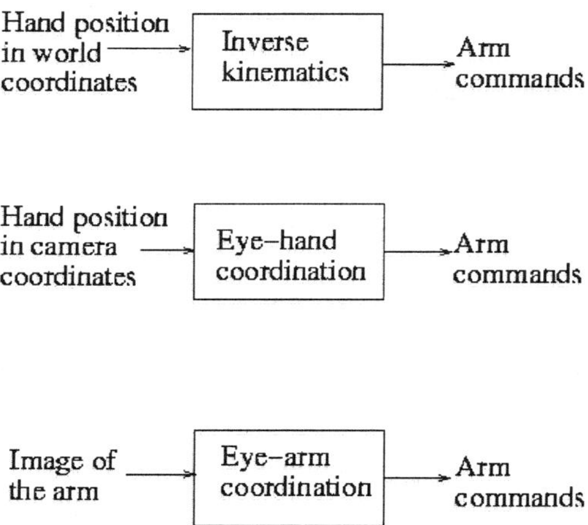

Figure 10. Models of arm coordination.

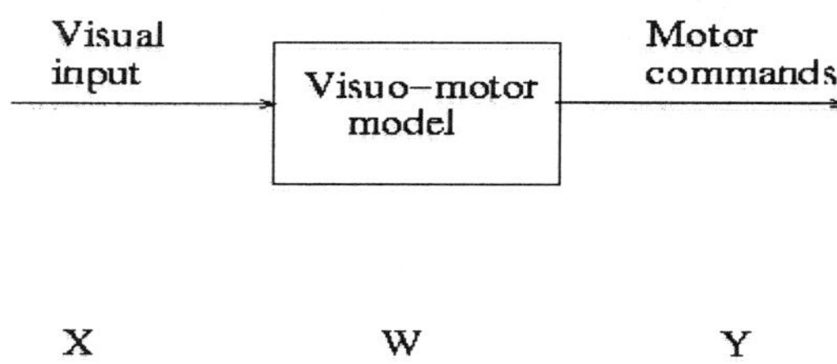

Figure 11. A model of visuo-motor coordination.

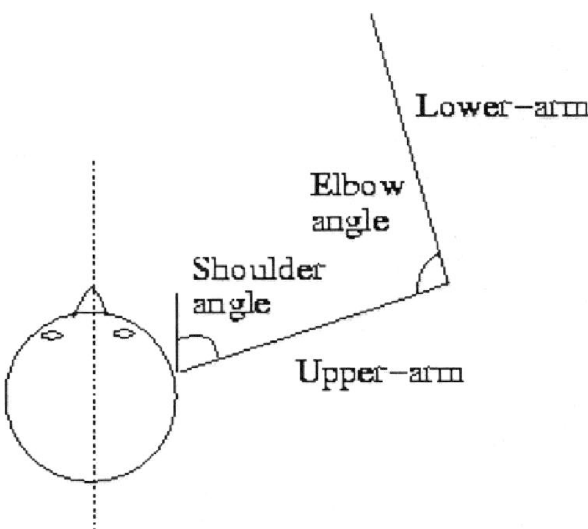

Figure 12. Arm skeleton showing shoulder and elbow angles.

Model identification from training examples consists of finding W, for given X and Y pairs.

4.2. Data acquisition for model identification: technique and experimental setup

In order to identify a model, it is necessary to obtain input-output data characterizing it. In this case, one needs to associate visual inputs to motor control outputs, which would position the arm in a posture similar to the visual input (showing the teacher arm). In most problems, the associations are between actions and determined perceptions through the same system. Here the robot must give controls to its own arm to place it in the position that it sees for the teacher's arm. To surpass this problem, in the technique adopted here for collecting training examples, *the human (teacher) imitates the robot.* The robot randomly flails its arm, and for each position of the arm, the human places his/her arm in a similar posture and gives a validation signal. Thus, the robot receives the information on how the human arm looks when it is in a posture similar to that of his arm, resulting as an effect of controls Y. Whenever it needs to achieve a posture like X, the robot will have to provide the commands Y.

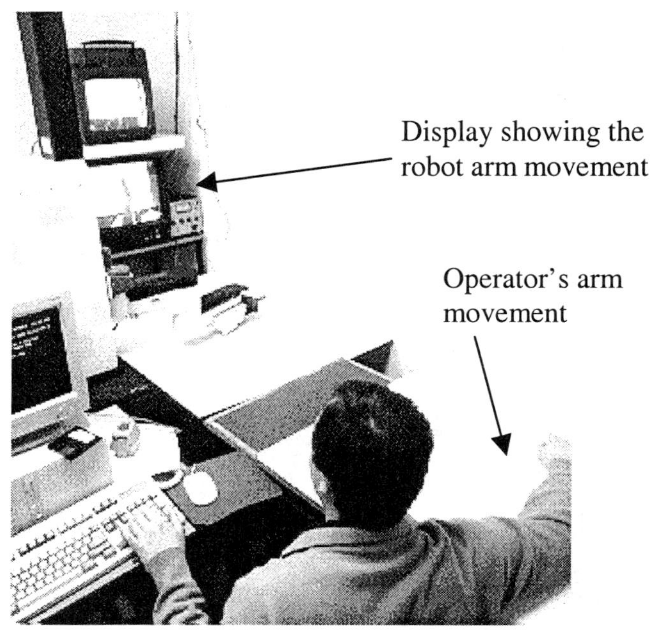

Figure 13. Anthropomorphic robot arm imitates arm movement of a human instructor.

A first type of experiment involved a robot imitating human arm movements performed in a horizontal plane. In its horizontal performance, the robot is anthropomorphic (see Figure 13).

The second type of experiments targeted how the approach extends to 3D performance. Two identical looking robots (RTX-type) were used, one learning to imitate the other (shown before in Figure 4). The human operator controls the teacher robot via a computer. This time the camera was placed at the approximate position of the human eye, gazing at an oblique angle to the teacher arm, as illustrated in the drawing in Figure 14.

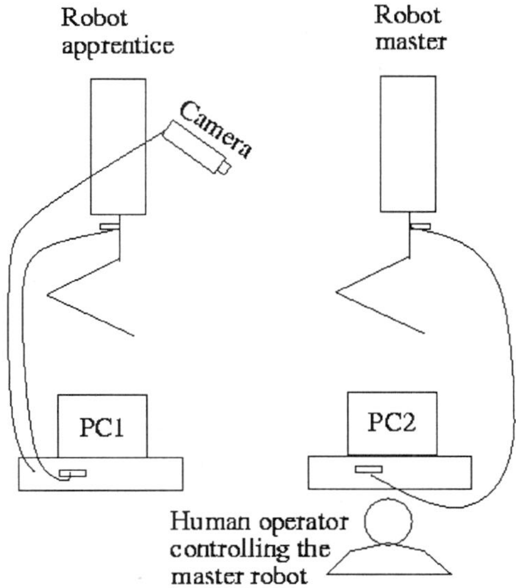

Figure 14. Set-up for 3D learning.

The image-command pairs were selected to (almost) uniformly cover the workspace. A total of 97 image-command pairs was collected and separated into a training set (88 pairs) and a test set (9 pairs), the number of pairs in the test being about 10% of the training set.

4.3. Neural and fuzzy-neural models for visuo-motor mapping

Both models (neural and fuzzy-neural) use only one neuron per joint (one neuron for the shoulder and one neuron for the elbow, for the 2D case in Figure 15). Inputs (X) were coming from a 192 pixel (12×16) low-resolution image, obtained by averaging regions of 16×16 neighboring pixels (Figure 16). Their intensity values were in the interval [0,1], with 256 gray levels. Similarly, the outputs Y were normalized to [0,1], which is the required definition domain for the fuzzy neural model.

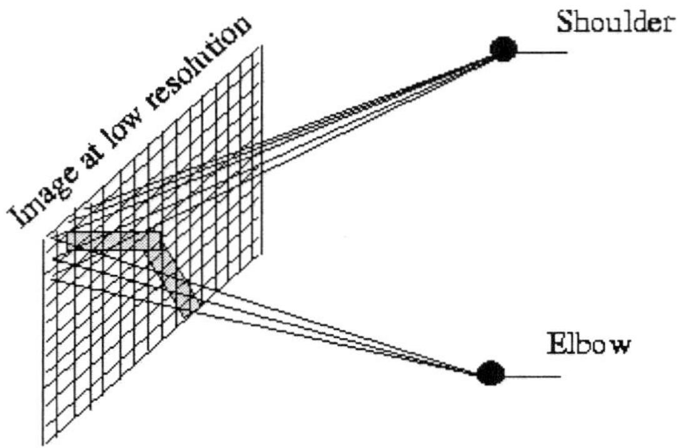

Figure 15. Shoulder and elbow neurons that map images to joint commands.

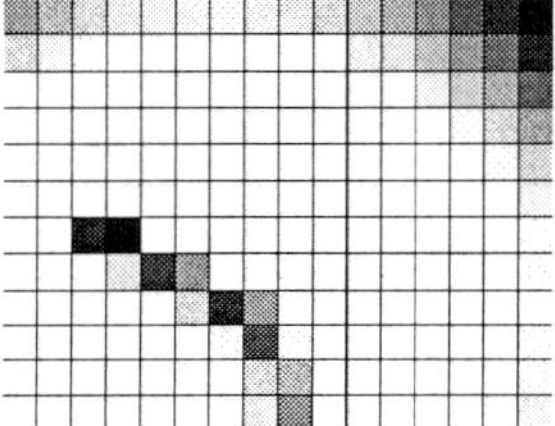

Figure 16. Low resolution image.

The classic neuron model employed in the tests was characterized by Equations (1) and (2). The training set was used for batch learning by gradient-descent with momentum and an adaptive learning rate. The performance of the neural model (evaluated on the test set and on the quality of imitation in a performance illustrated in the following) was considered good.

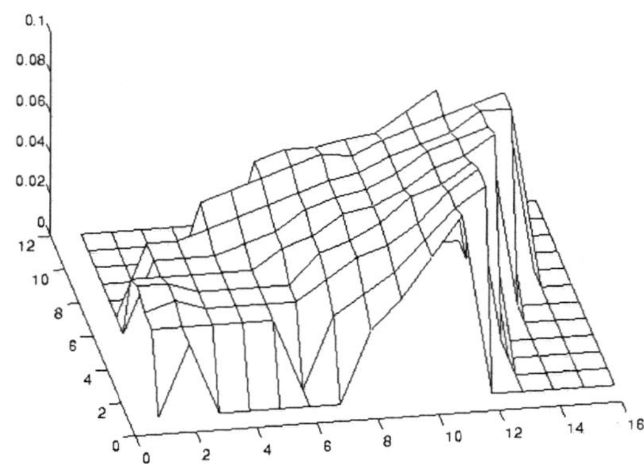

Figure 17. 3D representation of the weights of the shoulder neuron.

The fundamental fuzzy neural model characterized by Equations (18) and (19) was also tested. For the case $s = 0$, an analytical method similar to systems of *MAX-MIN* FRE was used to determine the weights, while for $s > 0$ a gradient-based technique was used [14]. The fuzzy neural model also has shown good learning performance. In addition, the weights of the fuzzy neuron model exhibit a *rule in the weights* representation, offering in this case transparency to the model. The weights act as a filter on input images. Higher values of the shoulder joint commands, which make the arm move to the right, are reflected in higher weights on the right. For the elbow, higher commands for extending the arm reflect in higher values along the radial direction.

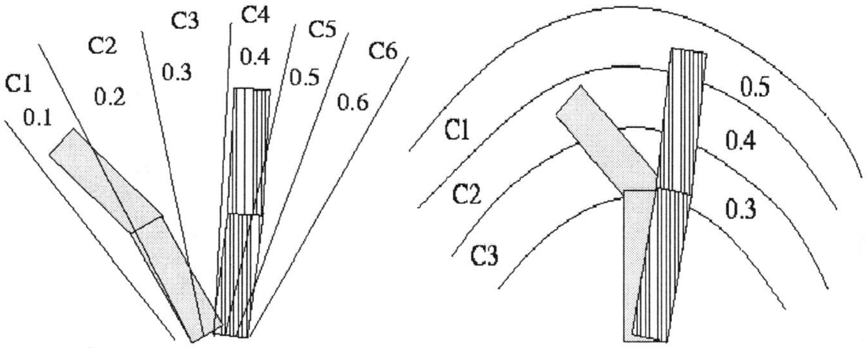

Figure 18. Schematic interpretation of the meaning in the weights.

For the shoulder, each class of the same gray level is disposed along a radial direction, the levels decreasing as the angle at the shoulder joint varies from right to left. For the elbow, the classes are circular, with higher values of the weights placed at greater distance from the shoulder joint and at the rightmost extremity. This can be seen in the simplified drawings of Figure 18, where classes C_i in input space have associated the numerical outputs indicated and an ordering exists of input classes along output values.

Thus, on this particular example, fuzzy neural models using t-norm based activation functions presented advantages over models using neurons based on sum-product-sigmoid operations. Namely,

• The weight space was directly interpretable by humans. The weights organized as filters took the shape of a right-left downhill slope for the shoulder neuron and a semicircular stadium shape for the elbow neurons. This organization, which for *MAX-MIN* neurons is independent of the color of the arm, lighting, and is little dependent on clothing folds, allows a model learned with one arm to be used with other arms of similar dimensions.

- Fuzzy neurons supported incremental learning well. This comes as a direct consequence that learning can be based on analytical methods of solving associated FRE.

- Fuzzy neural models have shown increased robustness to structured noise. The filters enable the robot to be highly insensitive to other objects in the image.

It should be noted, however, that in general the classical neural-only model has shown a greater approximation power. This is likely due to the fact that fuzzy neural models were limited to solutions in the [0,1] interval, while the weights of classic neurons can take any real value; moreover, the fuzzy models presented in this chapter used only excitatory inputs.

4.4. Robot imitating the movement of the teaching arm

The robot used the neural models determined by training to imitate (track) the movements of the teacher arm. The qualitative evaluation consisted of subjective assessments of the closeness of the posture of the robot arm to the posture of the human master arm. A series of images during imitation are shown in Figure 19.

When the training set included data from several different looking human arms, the model generalized and became robust to variation in the appearance of the teacher arm [14].

5. Discussion and conclusions

The work described in this chapter is only a first attempt to learn motor skills by imitation. The technique proposed here for obtaining training examples is general and can be applied to learning other types of movement. The fuzzy neural models are simple and have limited power. The neural models used in this chapter require that the vision system always "sees" the teacher's shoulder in a specified region of the space (at the bottom of the image). To obtain a robust system tolerant of position and rotation variations, one could expand the described system by introducing preprocessing models that perform appropriate compensating image transformation. A similar preprocessing is also needed to ensure scale invariance and other desirable features.

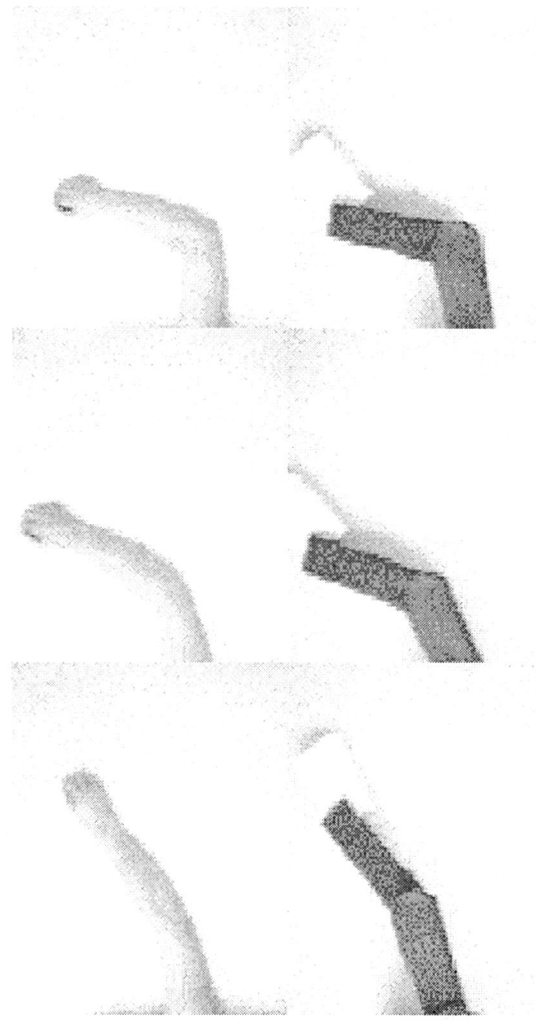

Figure 19. Robot moving after the human arm.

When imitation becomes possible in real world environments, the issue of correlating the motor behavior to the task to which it relates needs to be addressed. For example, a robot may imitate human arm movement quite well in hammering a nail with the small exception of hitting one millimeter away from the nail or hitting the nail at a low speed. It is necessary to have some *understanding* of the purpose of the movement. Imitation has the important role of providing a rough example of a movement. However, to enable task-related motor skill learning, one needs more sophisticated models than those for the simple perceptual skill addressed here.

Acknowledgment
This chapter describes research performed at Victoria University of Technology (VUT), Melbourne, Australia. I wish to thank Profs. Len Herron and Mike Wingate of VUT for their wise guidance during the Ph.D. research described here. I am grateful to Prof. Dan Butnariu of University of Haifa, Israel, for offering me insights into fuzzy theory, in particular on constructions based on triangular-norms. Finally, I thank Prof. Horia-Nicolai Teodorescu of Technical University of Iasi, Romania, for being my first academic mentor, for introducing me to fuzzy systems in the mid 80s, and for inviting me to write this chapter.

REFERENCES

[1] Honda's P2, http://www.honda.co.jp/home/hpr/e_news/robot/.

[2] Engelberger, J., Service robots arise, *International Federation of Robotics Newsletter*, 18:1, 1995.

[3] *** The assault on disabilities (Special Issue), *IEEE Spectrum*, Oct., 31:10, 1994.

[4] Merlyn, P.R., *Toward a Humanoid Robot: Artificial Intelligence and the Confluence of Technologies*, SRI Consulting, Business Intelligence Program, Report D96-2031, Menlo Park, CA, October 1996.

[5] Stoica, A., *Anthropomorphic Systems*, JPL Report D-14842, Jet Propulsion Laboratory, California Institute of Technology, Pasadena, CA, 1997.

[6] Nagell, K., Olguin, R.S., and Tomasello, M., Processes of social learning in the tool use of chimpanzees (pan troglodytes) and human children (homo sapiens), *Journal of Comparative Psychology*, 107 (2): 174-186, 1993.

[7] Mel, B., A connectionist model may shed light on neural mechanisms for visually guided reaching, *Journal of Cognitive Neuroscience*, 3 (3): 274-292, 1991.

[8] Kuperstein, M., INFANT neural controller for adaptive sensory-motor coordination, *Neural Networks*, 4: 131-145, 1991.

[9] Sheridan, T.B., *Telerobotics, Automation, and Human Supervisory Control*, MIT Press, Cambridge, MA, 1992.

[10] Pomerleau, D.A., *Neural Network Perception for Mobile Robot Navigation*, Kluwer Academics Company, Boston, MA, 1993.

[11] Lane, S.H., Handelman, D.A., and Gelfand, J.J., Can robots learn like people do?, *SPIE* (1294): 296-309, 1990.

[12] DART: http://tommy.jsc.nasa.gov/~li/dartfitt.html.

[13] SARCOS: http://www.sarcos.com.

[14] Stoica, A., *Motion Learning by Robot Apprentices: A Fuzzy Neural Approach*, Ph.D. Thesis, Victoria University, Melbourne, Australia, 1995.

[15] Zadeh, L.A., Fuzzy sets, *Information and Control*, 8: 338-353, 1965.

[16] Yager, R.R. and Filev, D., (Eds.), *Essentials of Fuzzy Modeling and Control*, John Wiley & Sons, New York, NY, 1994.

[17] Yager, R.R. and Zadeh, L.A., (Eds.), *Fuzzy Sets, Neural Networks, and Soft Computing*, Van Nostrand Reinhold, New York, NY, 1994.

[18] Lee, S.C. and Lee, E.T., Fuzzy neural networks, *Mathematical Biosciences*, 23: 151-177, 1975.

[19] Takagi, H., Fusion technology of fuzzy theory and neural networks - survey and future directions, *Proceedings of the International Conference on Fuzzy Logic and Neural Networks*, Iizuka, Japan, 13-26, 1990.

[20] Hellendorn, H., Neural-fuzzy: basics and industrial applications, *Proceedings of 2nd European Congress on Intelligent Techniques and Soft Computing*, Aachen, Sept. 20-23, 1: 131-134, 1994.

[21] Jang, J.S.R., Neuro-fuzzy modeling and control, *Proceedings of the IEEE*, March, 378-406, 1995.

[22] Nauck, D., Klawonn, F., and Kruse, R., *Foundations of Neuro-Fuzzy Systems*, John Wiley & Sons, New York, NY, 1997.

[23] Zadeh, L.A., Outline of a new approach to the analysis of complex systems and decision processes, *IEEE Transactions on Systems, Man, and Cybernetics*, SMC-3 (1): 28-44, 1973.

[24] Zimmermann, H-J., *Fuzzy Set Theory*, Kluwer Academics, Boston, MA, 1991.

[25] Nola, A., Sessa, S., Pedrycz, W., and Sanchez, E., *Fuzzy Relation Equations and Their Applications to Knowledge Engineering*, Kluwer Academic Publishers, Boston, MA, 1989.

[26] Sanchez, E., Resolution of composite fuzzy relation equations, *Information and Control*, 30: 38-48, 1976.

[27] Pedrycz, W., Processing in relational structures: fuzzy relational equations, *Fuzzy Sets and Systems*, 40: 77-106, 1991.

[28] Klir, G.J. and Yuan, B., Approximate solutions of systems of fuzzy relation equations, *Proceedings of the IEEE Conference on Fuzzy Logic, World Congress on Computational Intelligence*, Orlando, FL, 1452-1457, 1994.

[29] Pedrycz, W., Numerical and applicational aspects of fuzzy relational equations, *Fuzzy Sets and Systems*, 11: 1-18, 1983.

[30] Sanchez, E., Fuzzy genetic algorithms in soft computing environment, *Proceedings of the Fifth IFSA Congress*, Seoul, Korea, 44-50, 1993.

[31] Pedrycz, W., GAREL: A hybrid genetic learning in fuzzy relational equations, *Proceedings of the IEEE Conference on Fuzzy Logic, World Congress on Computational Intelligence*, Orlando, FL, 1354-1358, 1994.

[32] Pedrycz, W., Fuzzy relational equations with generalized connectives and their applications, *Fuzzy Sets and Systems*, 10: 185-201, 1983.

[33] Menger, K., Statistical metrics, *Proceedings of the National Academy of Sciences U.S.A.*, 28: 535-537, 1942.

[34] Butnariu, D. and Klement, E.P., *Triangular Norm-Based Measures and Games with Fuzzy Coalitions,* Kluwer Academics, Dordrecht, The Netherlands, 1993.

[35] Gupta, M.M. and Qi, J., Theory of t-norms and fuzzy inference methods, *Fuzzy Sets and Systems*, 40: 431-450, 1991.

[36] Bour, L. and Lamotte, M., Equations des relations floues avec la composition conorme-norme triangulaires, *BUSEFAL*, 34: 86-94, 1988.

[37] Pedrycz, W., Fuzzy neural networks with reference neurons as pattern classifiers, *IEEE Transactions on Neural Networks*, 3 (5): 770-775, 1992.

[38] Pedrycz, W., Lam, P.C.F., and Rocha, A.F., Distributed fuzzy system modeling, *IEEE Transactions on Systems, Man, and Cybernetics*, 25 (5): 769-780, 1995.

[39] Keller, J.M. and Tahani, H., Implementation of conjunctive and disjunctive fuzzy logic rules with neural networks, *International Journal of Approximate Reasoning*, 6: 221-240, 1992.

[40] Keller, J.M. and Krishnapuram, R., Evidence aggregation networks for fuzzy logic inference, *IEEE Transactions on Neural Networks*, 3 (5): 761-769, 1992.

[41] Butnariu, D., Klement, E.P., and Zafrani, S., On triangular norm-based propositional fuzzy logics, *Fuzzy Sets and Systems*, 69: 241-255, 1995.

[42] Gupta, M.M., Fuzzy logics and neural networks, *Proceedings of Tenth International Conference on Multiple Criteria Decision Making (TAIPEI'92)*, Taipei, Taiwan, 19-24, 1992.

[43] Pedrycz, W., Relational structures in fuzzy sets and neurocomputation, *Proceedings of the International Conference on Fuzzy Logic and Neural Networks*, Iizuka, Japan, 235-238, 1990.

[44] Gupta, M.M., Fuzzy neural computing system, *Proceedings of IMACS/SICE International Symposium on Robotics, Mechatronics, and Manufacturing Systems '92*, Kobe, Japan, 141-146, 1992.

[45] Pedrycz, W. and Rocha, A.F., Fuzzy-set based models of neurons and knowledge-based networks, *IEEE Transactions on Fuzzy Systems*, 1 (4): 254-266, 1993.

[46] Kaufmann, A. and Gupta, M.M., *Fuzzy Mathematical Models in Engineering and Management Science*, North-Holland, New York, 1988.

[47] Frank, M.J., On the simultaneous associativity of $F(x,y)$ and $x+y-F(x,y)$, *Aequationes Math.*, 19: 194-226, 1979.

Chapter 3

Learning stiffness characteristics of the human hand using a neuro-fuzzy system

Alexander Iliesh and Abraham Kandel

Motor control of the human hand or of robotic manipulators is one of many interesting issues concerning motor learning. One possible way to achieve this is by using stiffness as a control parameter. We built a system capable of learning and then successfully approximated the postural stiffness function of the human hand over a horizontal workspace. The adaptive model built is based on a hybrid neuro-fuzzy system, called ANFIS. This system incorporates a fuzzy inference system based on the Takagi-Sugeno-Kang method, together with a neural-network with learning capacities. The learning achieved has been used for fine-tuning the membership functions of the input. Simulations carried out demonstrate the effectiveness of the hybrid system for posture stiffness approximation of the human arm.

1. Introduction

The term "learning" may be defined as the ability to acquire additional knowledge or skill through study, with or without the supervision of a teacher, or by other means, such as past experience. Motor learning is intended to improve motor response to the changing environment, but it requires that the learner receive feedback to improve his next action. Learning methods make it possible to learn motor tasks like attending to objects in space, walking, swimming, or writing. Hand stiffness was found to be an important factor that can be used to control interaction with an environment, such as a tool, a tennis racket, a control joystick with or without force-feedback, or even a pen during writing.

The purpose of the research described in this chapter was to build a fuzzy system capable of learning to approximate and predicting the stiffness of the human hand during posture on a horizontal workspace. Such a system may also be used for learning and control of robotic manipulators, given a well-defined training data set.

1.1. Stiffness characteristics of the human hand during posture

While interacting with various environments, visco-elastic properties of the arm are regulated differently, according to the task. In order to investigate human multi-joint arm control mechanics, arm mechanical impedance at the hand has been characterized [12, 40, 51]. Impedance control [3] does not specify desired forces or positions, but rather a desired dynamic relationship between force and position, i.e., mechanical stiffness or "impedance." It is simple and robust to parameter uncertainty and imprecision of the environment, and it can be directly applied to redundant manipulators.

Previous research on the human arm movement [12] aimed to measure and characterize the field of elastic forces associated with hand posture in the horizontal plane. This research suggested that the reaching path of the human hand is planned and implemented by a hierarchical system. The upper layers of the brain deal with planning the desired movement of the hand, whereas the lower networks implement the motion by using the visco-elastic properties of the muscles. Motor adaptation to unexpected loads is one means that may be acquired by learning and control systems to supervise hand movement. Hence, various researchers have conducted experiments to determine characteristics of the postural stiffness field [11, 13, 47]. These experiments were conducted under varying arm configurations as well as under the influence of external forces called preloads, acting on the hand with different ranges of size and direction.

The arm stiffness at the hand during posture, on a horizontal plan, can be expressed mathematically by a characteristic matrix termed the stiffness matrix. This matrix describes the "spring-like" properties of the muscles by setting the relation between resisting forces, considered to be elastic, and imposed displacement perturbations. It can be represented as an ellipse having three parameters: area, shape (the ratio between the two main axes), and orientation (the angle between the main axis of the ellipse and the x-axis used in the reference frame of coordinates). The area of the ellipse is proportional to the size of the stiffness matrix. The shape designates the directions in which the arm stiffness is greater or less. The direction of the ellipse relates to the direction of the principal axis of stiffness, along which the resistance to external forces is maximum. The length of the main axis is linearly related to the maximum stiffness, whereas the length of the secondary axis is linearly related to the minimum stiffness.

Since the controllability and variability of the stiffness field at the hand during posture were important for various kind of interaction tasks, previous work has focused on the geometrical characteristics of the stiffness ellipse in the horizontal plane under different conditions of co-contraction and external force regulation [13, 14]. The experimental results support the hypothesis that humans can regulate arm stiffness characteristics to some extent, which enables achieving a variety of manipulation tasks.

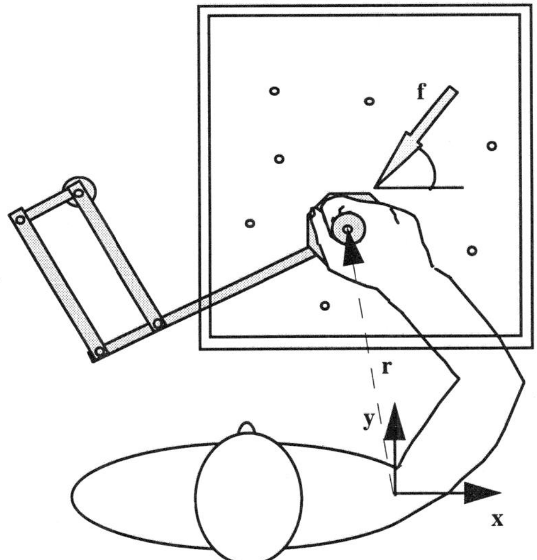

Figure 1. Typical experimental setup: the manipulandum and the reference coordinate system, including the radial distance (r) between the hand and the shoulder. Also shown is a typical preload (f) and its direction (ϕ).

Our model is based on characteristics extracted from experimental results [11, 13] that are used as input to a learning system. Figure 1 shows a characteristic experimental setup for measuring human stiffness. The experiment and its results, which were described in detail in the literature [11, 12, 13, 47], are discussed here briefly. A human subject grasped the instrumented handle of a two-link manipulandum and performed specified point-to-point planar arm trajectories. The subject was asked to hold the handle of a manipulandum at a fixed position in the horizontal plane. The initial position of the hand was set at an initial point termed the "target point", denoted by given coordinates (x_0, y_0). The hand was brought to the target, while holding the handle of the manipulator. During the experiment many small perturbations (in the range of several millimeters) were induced to the handle by the two torque motors of the manipulandum, in random directions and with changing amplitudes, as set by the computer used as controller. The elastic restoring forces, which developed instantaneously at the tip of the hand, were measured with great accuracy by force sensors mounted on the manipulandum. The measurements were done at zero velocity, without any contribution from the inertial or viscous properties of the musculoskeletal system. Hence, the restoring forces were considered to be an elastic response, resulting from the "spring-like" properties of the muscles. The response to a spontaneous movement may take several hundred milliseconds depending on the complexity of the response and the degree of precision required for the task [24]. In our case, the response was expected in up to 800 msec [40]. Since the measurements were taken after a shorter period of time, the measured restoring forces were expected to be due to muscle response only, without voluntary intervention. The experiment was held with different targets and changing preloads. A preload consisted of a certain force, actuated by the manipulator in a prechosen direction, to which the subject had to oppose and achieve posture before starting the perturbation stage.

The results of such an experiment make it possible, by using a model as described elsewhere [12, 47], to calculate a set of scalar variables that can be described as the hand-stiffness (or the end-effector). The stiffness can be expressed mathematically by using a characteristic matrix named the stiffness matrix. The matrix describes the "spring-like" properties of the muscles by setting the relation between the restoring forces (F_x, F_y), considered elastic, and the displacements (dx, dy) imposed by the manipulandum.

That can be described as follows:

$$F_x = -k_{xx}\, dx - k_{xy}\, dy \tag{1}$$

$$F_y = -k_{yx}\, dx - k_{yy}\, dy$$

or in vector notation

$$\underline{F} = -K\, d\,\underline{x} \tag{2}$$

where

$$\underline{F} = [F_x \quad F_y\,]^{\mathrm{T}} \tag{3}$$

$$d\underline{x} = \begin{bmatrix} dx & dy \end{bmatrix}^T \qquad (4)$$

$$\underline{K} = \begin{bmatrix} k_{xx} & k_{xy} \\ k_{yx} & k_{yy} \end{bmatrix}$$

The matrix K is called the stiffness matrix of the hand. It expresses the elastic behavior of the hand during posture, because of the action of the arm muscles. Here it is written in Cartesian coordinates, but it may also be expressed in the configuration space, in term of joint coordinates.

Graphically, it is possible to characterize the stiffness matrix as an ellipse (Figure 2a) having three parameters: area, shape (the ratio between the two main axes), and orientation (the angle between the main axis of the ellipse and the x-axis used in the reference frame of coordinates). The area of the ellipse is proportional to the size of the stiffness. The shape designates directional stiffness, which is actually the ability to oppose external forces coming from different directions. The orientation of the ellipse indicates the principal axis of stiffness, along which the resistance to external forces is maximum. The length of the main axis is linearly related to the maximum stiffness (K_{max}), whereas the length of the secondary axis is linearly related to the minimum stiffness (K_{min}).

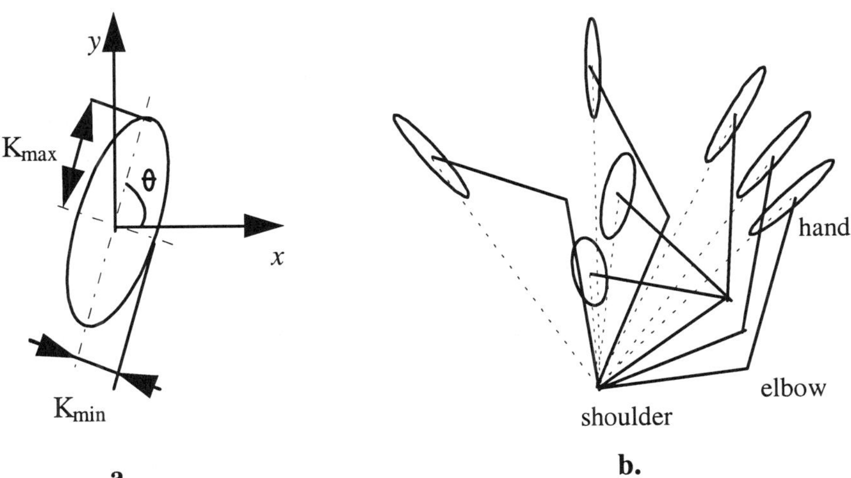

Figure 2. (a) The stiffness ellipse and (b) typical changes in its shape along with change in hand configuration under no-load conditions.

The results of experiments performed using the system described [11, 13] can be summarized as follows:

- When there is no preload acting on the hand (no-load conditions), the hand position along the radial direction, having the shoulder as reference (the proximal-distal axis), influences the stiffness field in a predominant way (Figure 2b).
- The stiffness field is almost isotropic near the shoulder. When increasing the distance between the hand and the shoulder, its shape changes, becoming more elongated.
- By increasing the radial distance between the shoulder and the hand, there is a slight tendency of the primary axis of the stiffness ellipse to rotate in the counter-clockwise direction.
- Under no-load conditions, the direction of the stiffness field (direction of the major axis of the stiffness ellipse) is almost the same as the radial direction, defined as the proximal-distal direction between the shoulder and the hand. This characteristic slightly changes even when different preloads are induced.
- When a preload is introduced, the stiffness changes. This includes mostly changes in the size, and less in the shape of the ellipse, but very little changes in the orientation.
- As the position of the hand changes, when moving from side to side at the same distance from the shoulder and at the same loading, the relative angle between the major ellipse axis and the radial axis remains almost unchanged. In addition, the area size and shape of the stiffness ellipse are only slightly changed.

The above mentioned findings were used to produce the input functions to the learning model to be described later.

1.2. Methods of learning

Learning may be defined as acquiring through experience the required capabilities needed to achieve adequate performance of some task. In the context of machine learning, a more precise definition is as follows: a machine is said to learn from experience with respect to some class of tasks and performance measure, if its performance at the defined tasks, as measured by the performance measure, improves with experience [38]. The need to learn varies inversely with the quantity of knowledge [30]. Thus there is no need to learn what is already known, so the experts in specific fields can use their vast knowledge as a means for saving a lot of unnecessary computational effort.

There are two major procedures of learning: supervised and unsupervised. Unsupervised learning [8, 18, 31] is done using only raw training samples. It directly couples the input with the output, having no output targets available. Usually an extensive training stage is required, leading to some kind of a clustering operation, which makes it possible to categorize the input patterns into a finite number of classes. Although this seems difficult and unreliable, many of our biological systems use this kind of learning when no supervision is available.

Conversely, the supervised learning (SL) [17, 18] is a goal-directed method of learning. The learning rule is provided with a set of examples of proper system behavior. The system can be described by using an artificial computing network. As inputs are applied to the network, the network outputs are compared with the known correct answers, attempting to minimize an unknown expected cost or error function. The SL rewards or punishes a neural network by increasing or decreasing the components of a vector of weights and biases to move the network outputs closer to the targets. This is the reason that it is sometimes called learning with a "teacher." Error is defined as the difference between the "desired" and "actual" performance. The desired behavior is determined by "supervision," which provides an error or "teaching" signal. Although it seems implausible to have such learning at the level of individual synapses, it is possible that parts of our brain, for example, the cerebellum, will use it for motor control and motor learning [1, 2, 27].

Another kind of learning, part of the SL family, is reinforcement learning (RL) [6, 26]. It is very similar to SL, except that instead of being provided with the correct output for every input, the algorithm is given only a grade. This type of learning performs estimated gradient descent by using an error scalar instead of an error vector [7, 18, 46]. It is also called learning with a "critic", because the critic reinforces actions done to a certain environment (in either a positive or a negative way) by using overall evaluative signals, making no direct connection between the pairs of input-output [37, 52]. The critic is meant to lead the system to an action policy that maximizes the total reward it will receive from any starting state [38]. Sometimes the system uses a feedforward model to pre-evaluate the environment [22, 36]. Although not as widely used as SL, RL is quite popular in many fields such as computer science, statistics, psychology, and neurophysiology. It is a valuable tool for producing autonomous systems, able to improve by means of achieving additional experience. Nevertheless, this kind of learning is more difficult to apply from a computational point of view and appears to be most suitable for control system applications [10] and for applications within a biological context.

Algorithmically, there is a close relation between the signed error vectors used in SL and the evaluative signals used by RL. It is always possible to convert one into the other. Thus, SL can always be used for RL problems and vice versa [22]. The situation is different when discussing learning paradigms, which depend on the natural frame of representation of certain problems, with no connection to the algorithm used for solving it. Using a RL algorithm to solve a SL problem may be inefficient, because it does not take into consideration the advantage of directional information. Conversely, using a SL algorithm to solve a RL problem is likely to be inefficient because of the need to translate the evaluative signals to a signed error vector, which makes the calculation method more cumbersome. Thus, SL algorithms may be translated to RL and vice versa, although this may cause some inefficiency in the learning process.

1.3. Using a neuro-fuzzy system to solve the learning problem

The basic principles of fuzzy logic and control are described thoroughly in the literature [29, 43, 45, 57], including applications in the field of expert systems [24] and robotics [19, 32, 42, 48, 52]. Here we intended to show only the relevance of fuzzy logic in the context of building our adaptive model. The use of a fuzzy inference system seems natural here for several reasons. First, the parallel action of the fuzzy rules is meant to achieve modularity and avoid interference between stored patterns [30]. Second, the overlapping between membership functions (MFs), which describe the input variables, decreases the sensitivity to the chosen shapes of the membership functions, and increases the ability to learn and control a system smoothly. Third, even when no direct connection exists between the rules and the exact state of the input variables, a fuzzy system tends to produce a meaningful description of an unknown system, including robustness regarding changes in the input [54]. Last, using fuzzy rules enables a flexible fitting of rules, allowing a choice among many possibilities [28].

Fuzzy systems include the capability of self-tuning by trial and error, as well as using the precious prior knowledge of human experts for partitioning the space of input and output, thus making the inference process more accurate and less complex [15, 16]. However, fuzzy systems lack the ability to learn. Neural networks, on the other hand, are able to learn from examples, but they lack the ability to use prior knowledge, and their "black-box" behavior makes results difficult to interpret [41]. Thus, it is only natural to combine a fuzzy system and a neural network to make an adaptive system able to retain the advantages of both. Moreover, learning may be accelerated by using hybrid neuro-fuzzy systems that are computationally efficient, like ANFIS [20], GARIC [15], NEFCON [41], and others [4, 30].

Here we chose to use ANFIS because of its fast-convergence properties, its good capability in matching nonlinear data, and its functional equivalence to Radial Basis Function (RBF) approximation methods [39, 44], which may also have biological significance.

2. Main issues

The present work was intended to examine several issues. First, is it possible to use SL or RL, together with a fuzzy adaptive system, to solve motor learning problems of humans in the context of limb movement? Another interesting issue is how to build such a system, and last, to determinate how appropriate is it to solve a given learning problem. The interaction between these issues is challenging and holds a strong potential for solving complicated problems involving learning. This potential comes from the capability of combining the attractive attributes of fuzzy logic in describing input variables and making a robust "inference engine," together with the powerful adaptation and learning abilities of a neural network. The purpose here was to build an application of a neuro-fuzzy learning system in the context of human motor learning. This may serve as the basis of future models intended to create a deeper understanding of motor learning and control with humans.

Because of the existing analogy between motor learning and control with humans and that of robot manipulators, the methodology and the mathematical tools developed here may be useful in other areas concerning robotic manipulators, with or without redundancy. There are numerous works cited in the literature, which deal with robotic control based on fuzzy [19, 31] or hybrid learning systems [41, 55]; however, in practice, such systems in the context of motor learning are seldom used.

3. The model

Based on experimental results presented by Flash and Gurevich (1997) and Gomi and Osu (1996), as reviewed earlier, we considered the stiffness surface (S) to be approximated by the following parametric representation:

$$S(A,\rho,\Theta \mid R,F,\Phi) = g(R) + h(F,\Phi) \tag{5}$$

where A, ρ, and θ are the area, shape, and orientation of the stiffness ellipse, respectively (Figure 2a). These have a functional dependence on the parameters R, F, and Φ, which are the radial distance, preload size, and preload direction, respectively (Figure 1). The meaning of this functional relation is that under no-load conditions the parameters of the stiffness ellipse depend mainly on the radial distance [12], decreasing in an approximately nonlinear but smooth way. The influence of the tangential shifting of the static positions from one side to another was assumed negligible. Under preloading conditions, an additional term expressing the effect of the preload and its direction, influences the overall stiffness characteristics. This term is supposed to change as described by Gomi and Osu [13].

Although the stiffness characteristics are known to change from person to person, their pattern remains the same. For this reason, we looked into a normalized data set that captured the main characteristics without being limited to the real values of the variables. Combining the above guidelines and the results of postural stiffness experiments [12, 13], we were able to build complex surfaces in four dimensions, each of them representing one of the stiffness ellipse characteristics:

$$A(r,f,\Phi) = g_1(r) + h_1(f,\Phi)$$
$$\rho(r,f,\Phi) = g_2(r) + h_2(f,\Phi) \qquad (6)$$
$$\Theta(r,f,\Phi) = g_3(r) + h_3(f,\Phi)$$

where r, f, and ϕ are, respectively, the normalized radial distance, preload size, and preload direction.

These surfaces were used to generate a training and test set of data. The data enabled us to determine the possibility of building a neuro-fuzzy system that would be able to capture the stiffness characteristics.

Our simulation model is based on a neuro-fuzzy network. The fuzzy system is of the Takagi-Sugeno-Kang type [20, 50, 52, 56] called, in short, the Sugeno type. It has five parts (Figure 3):

- A rule base containing a set of if-then rules, characterized by functional type consequents that are linear combinations of weighted input variables plus a constant term. Having three inputs (x,y,z) and one output (r), the rules have the following form: "If x is A and y is B and z is C, then $r = ax + by + cz + d$", where a,b,c and d are called consequent parameters.

- A knowledge base containing *a priori* knowledge about the variables behavior and specifications about the fuzzy MFs to be used by the fuzzy rules.

- An inference "engine" defining the inference process regarding the rules.

- A fuzzification interface partitioning the input space and translating the crisp input to MFs with well-defined linguistic values.

- A defuzzification interface transforming the output of the inference engine into crisp output, using knowledge based on the physical structure of the system. When the fuzzy rules used are the Sugeno type, the final output is the weighted average of each rule's output.

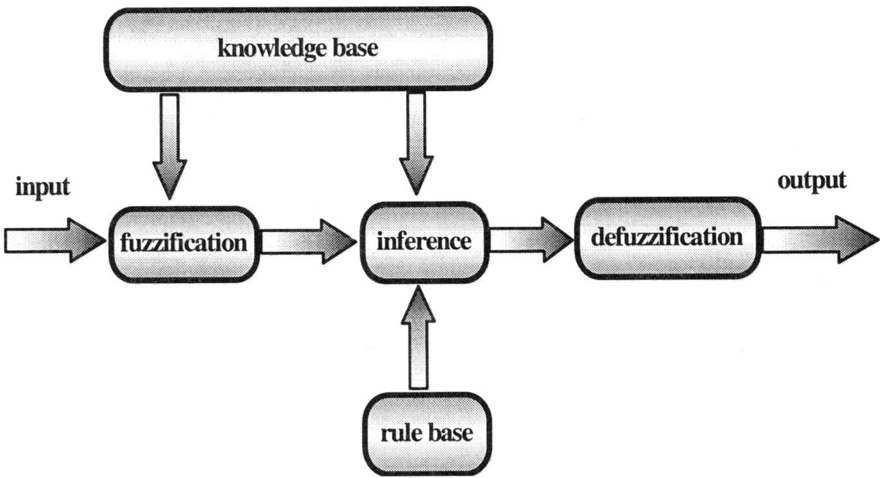

Figure 3. The structure of the inference fuzzy system.

The stages of the fuzzy inference process are the following:

- Fuzzification, by translating the crisp data from the input to MFs, in order to set membership values to the linguistic labels.
- Integration of the input membership values, setting for each rule a certain weight.
- Generating a result, either crisp or fuzzy, for every rule, taking into account its weight.
- Defuzzification, unifying all the results to make a crisp output.

The three input variables of the system were normalized to the range $[0,1]$. The first input is the radial distance between the shoulder and the hand ($r = R/(L_1+L_2)$), expressed in polar coordinates, where R designates the actual distance and L_1, L_2 are the lengths of the two parts of the arm. The second input is the size of the preload ($f = F/F_{max}$) acting on the hand (as explained earlier), where F is the actual preload and F_{max} is the maximum preload used in the experiment set. The third input is the direction of the preload ($\phi = \Phi/2\pi$), where Φ is the actual angle measured in radians. The input variables were fuzzified using Gaussian MFs of the form

$$f(x; \mu,\sigma) = \exp\left[-1/2(x-\mu)^2/\sigma^2\right] \tag{7}$$

having x as the variable and μ, σ as parameters. These parameters, directly influencing the shape and the location of the Gaussian function over the input grid, are also called nonlinear or premise parameters because their initial values are changed through the learning process. The final MFs will catch best local features of the training data set.

The output includes three normalized variables, namely,

- the characteristic area of the stiffness ellipse ($a = A / A_{max}$), where A_{max} is the maximal value of the ellipse area in the data set,
- the ratio between the main axes of the ellipse ($\rho = \lambda_1 / \lambda_2$), and
- the normalized relative orientation of the stiffness ellipse, $\theta = (\theta_e - \theta_r)/(\pi/4))$, expressing the ratio between the direction of the principal axis of the ellipse (θ_e) and the radial direction (θ_r), both measured in radians.

Here, we preferred to have the link between the inference rules and the output done by a Sugeno-type fuzzy inference system (FIS) rather than a Mamdani type system [35]. Although less intuitive and perhaps less suited to human expert input, the Sugeno FIS makes more compact and computationally efficient representations than a Mamdani system, therefore being more appropriate for optimization and adaptive techniques, especially when interaction with a neural network is required. Thus, our FIS is based on a method using functional-type consequents instead of the fuzzy consequents used by Mamdani type systems. The crisp output inferred by the fuzzy model is defined as the weighted average of the set of crisp outputs of individual linear subsystems. A system of this type was found more appropriate for our model, since it makes possible the weighted output of every rule as input to a neural network in which the learning process is established. The neural network used is based on a forward model with an algorithm having the following stages:

- setting initialization parameters,
- estimating the error by calculating the difference between the estimated and the actual values of the input to the neural network,
- backpropagation of the error causing changes to values of the input variables, and
- iteration until convergence to the minimum error requested.

In order to achieve this, we used a hybrid inference system named ANFIS (Adaptive Network-based Fuzzy Inference System) [20]. This hybrid system combines the robustness of the fuzzy inference system with the learning ability of a neural network. Additional methods of building hybrid learning systems are described in the literature [28, 33].

The characteristics of the hand stiffness matrix were represented by smooth but highly nonlinear functions in four dimensions (Figure 4), based on the results of previous experiments cited in the literature [11, 13], as described earlier. The raw data describing the above functions was split into two groups: one for the learning stage and the other for the testing stage. The simulation system had three stand-alone subsystems, one for each stiffness characteristic.

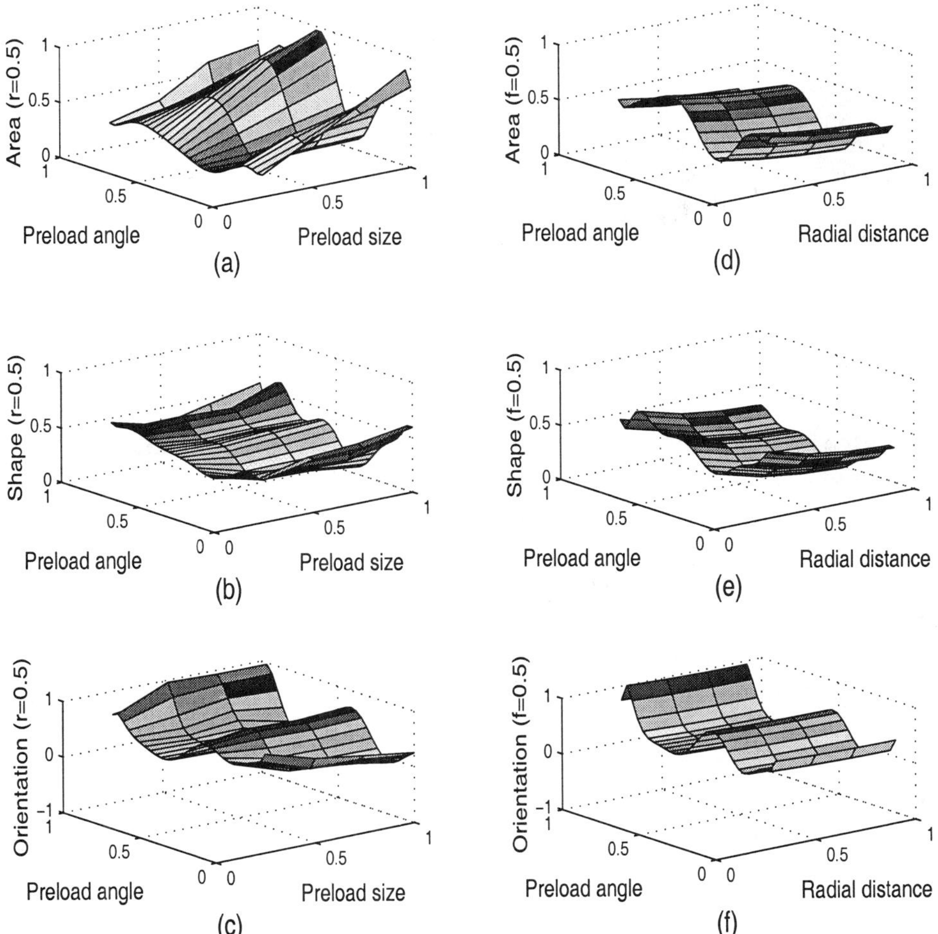

Figure 4. The highly nonlinear characteristics of stiffness (area, shape, and orientation) as a function of the normalized input values. Since the functions are four-dimensional, having three inputs and one output (Figures a-c), the radial distance is kept constant ($r = 0.5$), whereas in the subsequent Figures (d-f), the force is kept constant ($f = 0.5$).

The overall learning achieved was actually the result of combining these parts. The whole system is described in Figure 5. The three FIS have basically the same structure. Each had three inputs: radial distance, size of preload, and the direction of the preload, and one output, representing one of the stiffness ellipse characteristics: area, shape, or orientation.

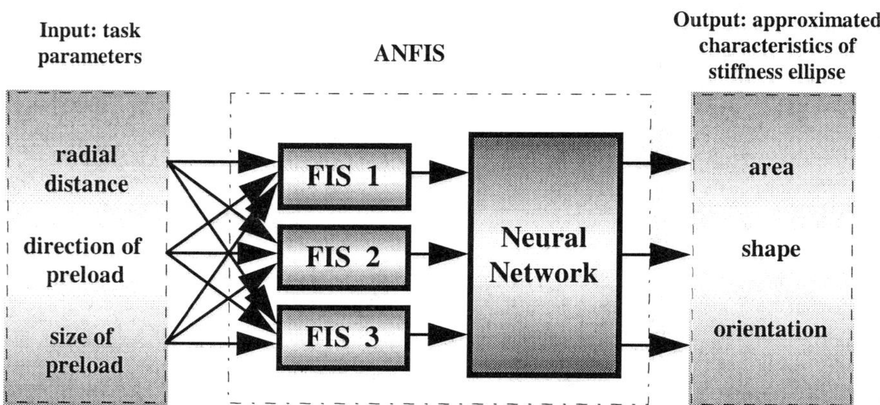

Figure 5. Block diagram of the whole inference system. FIS 1, FIS 2, and FIS 3 stand for Area FIS, Shape FIS, and Orientation FIS, respectively.

An SL method was used to train the ANFIS neural network. It was based on a two-pass algorithm [20], using a forward model with a least square estimation on the first pass and then a gradient error descent for backpropagation of the error. We used this method to establish a straightforward connection between the pairs of input-output data resulting from the experiments. However, it may be interesting to use a neuro-fuzzy system based on RL [4, 16, 34], in order to solve the same problem. Theoretically, the representation of the model in terms of RL is possible [22], but it remains to be proven whether or not it is computationally efficient.

4. Simulations and results

The input and the output range of the normalized data was [0,1] except for the orientation output, which was normalized in the range of [-1,1] because of the negative values it can take. From the grid of points of the range $[0,1] \times [0,1] \times [0,1]$ within the input space, 482 data vectors were obtained. An amount of 125 data vectors, picked at random among the complete data set, were reserved as a test set. This data set was used to provide an unbiased estimate of the generalization error. The other 357 data vectors were used to train ANFIS.

The initialization of the three FIS was done by using, for all the inputs, the same number of MFs, three, three, and four, respectively. This seemed to be reasonable from a heuristic point of view, keeping in mind the surface structure of the functions to be learned.

Actually, the optimal configuration was found to be as follows. The inputs of the Area FIS were fuzzified with four, three, and five MFs (Figure 6 a-c), respectively, and assigned to the input variables. It contained 60 rules, having 264 parameters, composed of 240 consequent parameters and 24 premise parameters. The inputs of the Shape FIS were fuzzified with only three MFs for the first two input variables and four MFs for the last one (Figure 7 a-c). It contained 36 rules, having 164 parameters, composed of 144 consequent parameters and 20 premise parameters. The inputs of the last FIS, the Orientation FIS, were fuzzified in the same way as the Shape FIS except for the third input variable, which was fuzzified using five MFs (Figure 8 a-c). It contained 45 rules, having 202 parameters, composed of 180 consequent parameters and 22 premise parameters.

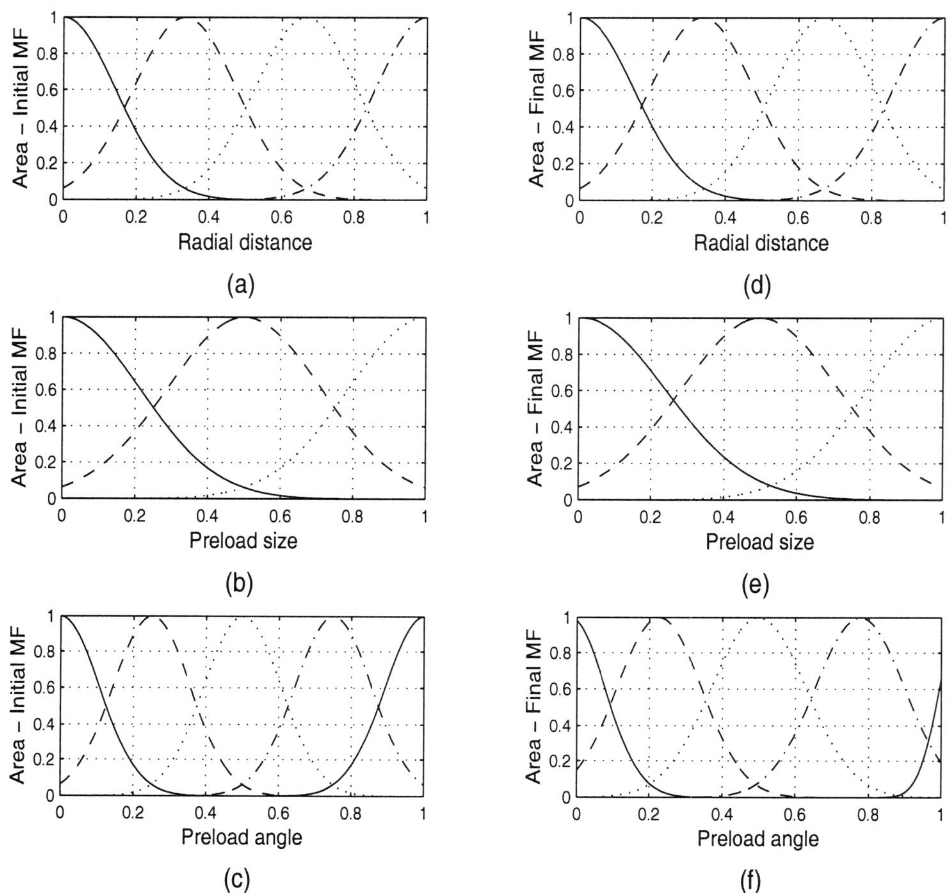

Figure 6. Membership functions describing the inputs to the Area ANFIS (a-c) before and (d-f) after learning.

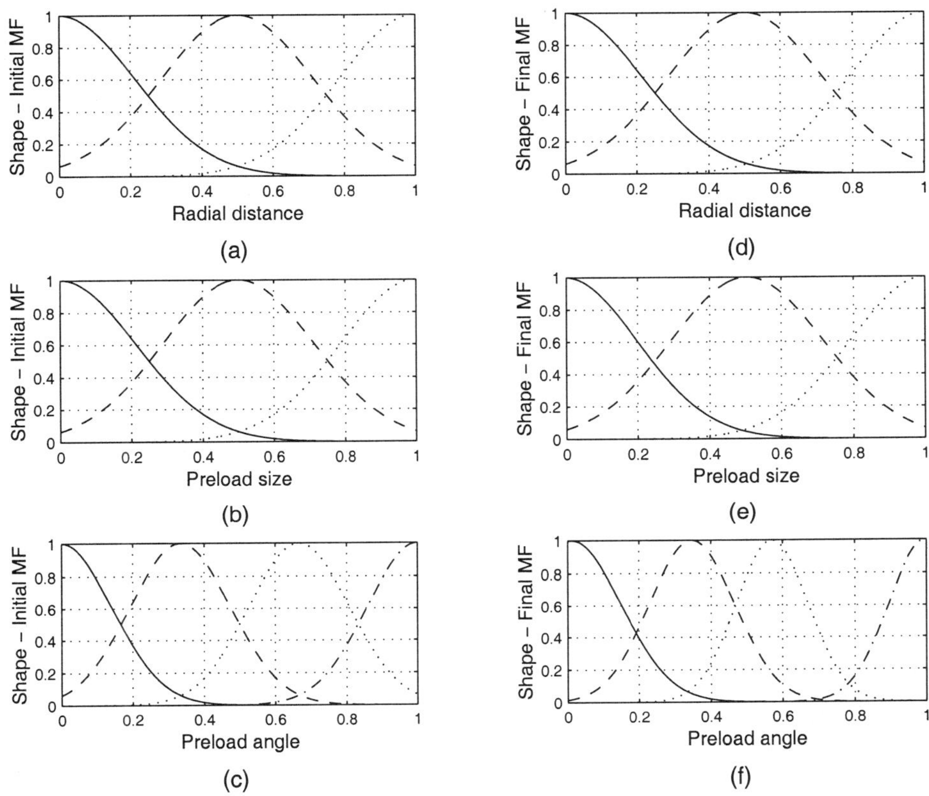

Figure 7. Membership functions describing the inputs to the Shape ANFIS (a-c) before and (d-f) after learning.

During the learning stage, the MFs are adapted. The final MFs of the radial distance inputs (Figures 6d, 7d, 8d) remain unchanged. This might be expected due to the small variations induced by this parameter on the output as may be seen in Figures 4 d-f. Different numbers of MFs were tried with the same result.

The final MFs of the preload size are just slightly changed in Area FIS (Figure 6d) and are unchanged in the two other FIS, because their influence on the output is also small, although slightly larger than that of the radial distance, as can be seen from Figures 4 a-c. Conversely, the final MFs of the preload angle have significant changes. The cause for this may be the relatively larger size variations in the output as a function of this parameter (Figures 4a-c), so that major changes are required to capture the best representation of this input variable.

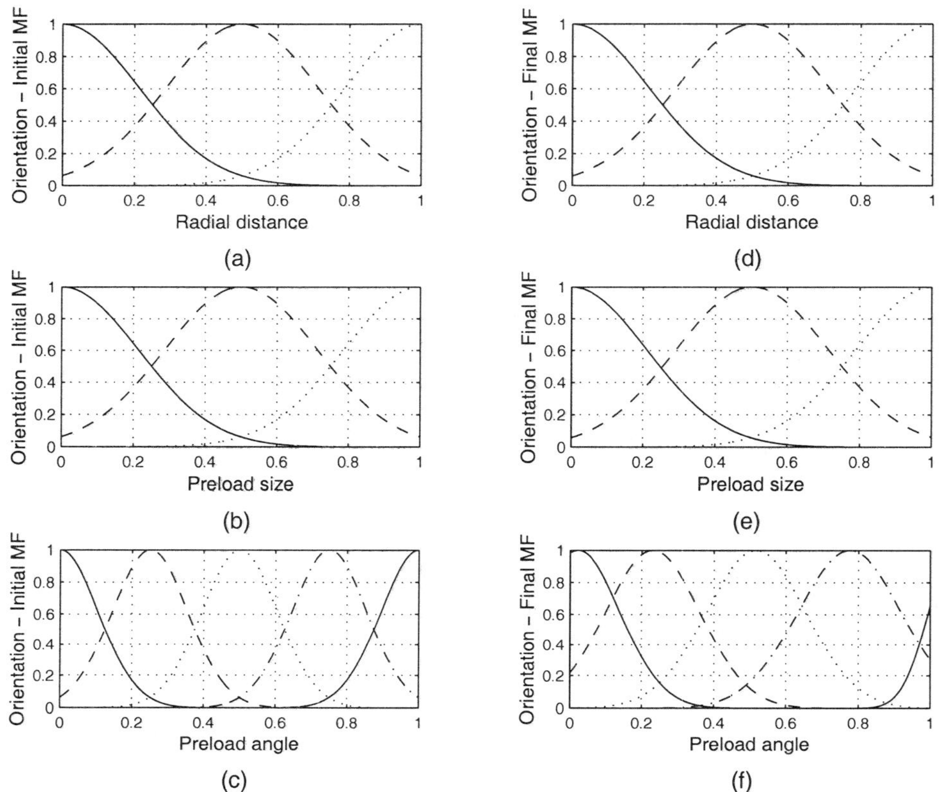

Figure 8. Membership functions describing the inputs to the Orientation ANFIS (a-c) before and (d-f) after learning.

The change of training and test root mean square error (RMSE) along the iteration process is shown in Figure 9 a-c for the three FIS in our system. After 30 epochs, the error of the training set and the test set become almost constant. The minimal training RMSE is in the range of 1.1 to 2.3%, whereas the minimal testing RMSE is in the range of 3.2 to 4.2%. The step size profiles, representing the length gradient transition in the parameter space, are shown in Figures 9 d-f. The initial step size is 0.01. The step size increases during the first 10 epochs and then decreases until the end of the learning process, showing the tendency to converge.

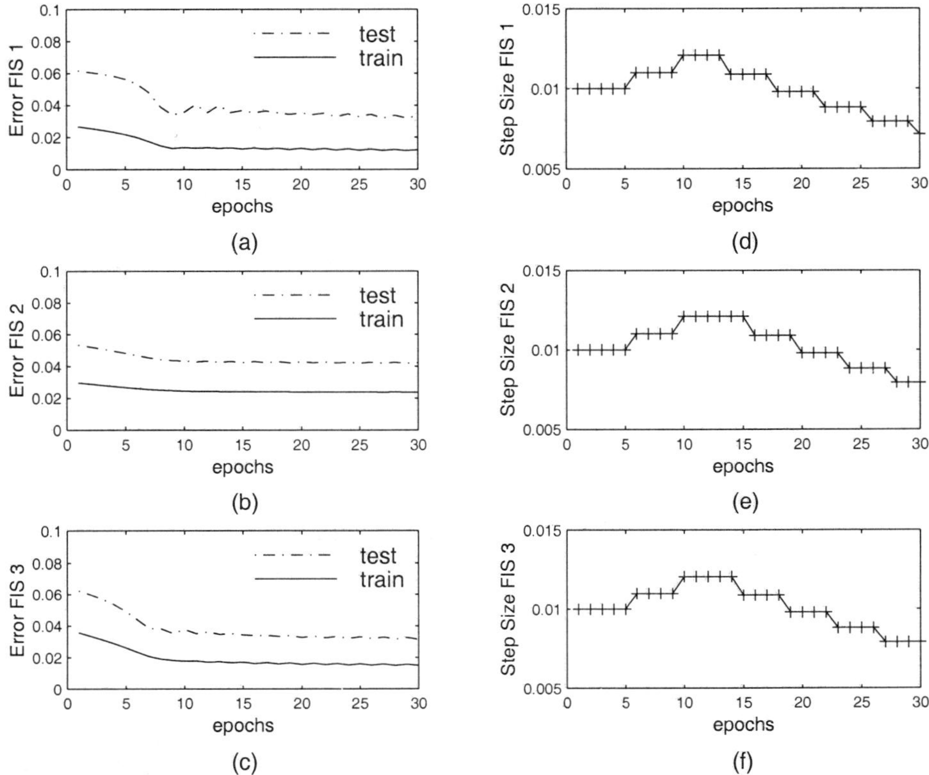

Figure 9. Rate of change of the error (a-c) in the training set of each ANFIS (solid line) and in the training set (broken line) along iterations. Figures (d-e) show the change in the size of the step, first increasing and then decreasing as the convergence is achieved.

5. Discussion

The results of the simulation clearly demonstrate a good capability for learning by maintaining consistency between the data used for learning and the data used for testing purposes. The learning features of the system led to a change in the initial MFs of the input, according to the degree of influence on the output variables. This made it possible to tune the MFs to most resemble the given data set. Although the MFs shown were of a Gaussian type, the simulation was also run with linear MFs (triangles) and nonlinear MFs (generalized bell-functions) with almost the same results, showing the high robustness of the approximation system.

The use of Gaussian MFs made it possible to compare ANFIS to radial basis functions (RBF) techniques [39, 44], the latter being considered as a special case of the former [52]. The RBF networks are of great importance in the neurophysiological context, as they are able to represent locally tuned, overlapping receptive fields, which have great relevancy in the areas of motor sensing and control. The functional equivalence between radial basis function networks and fuzzy inference systems [21] makes it possible to better understand each of them, in the physiological context, and to apply learning techniques developed for either of them to the other.

The number of MFs in the input may be set by trial and error or, in our case, by using the experience gathered as a result of carrying out large sets of experiments, such as measuring the stiffness of the human arm. There is a close connection between the number of inference rules, the modulation of their shapes, and the number of inference rules needed to build an accurate enough model. Thus, using the knowledge of an expert may significantly decrease the computational complexity of the system.

It is worth noting that for building specific models, there is an optimal number of inference rules to be used. Using many more or too few rules usually makes a poor semantic description of the problem. Moreover, this may distort the knowledge base so that the model tends to be a "black-box" analogy, as occurs when using neural-networks only. Here, the low number of MFs used to partition the input space also keeps the rule number low. Although optimization of the rule set was not investigated, the relatively small changes in the shape of the MFs, after the learning stage, showed that here the partition chosen for the input space was effective and the system used an appropriate number of rules. The compact partition of the input space may suggest a low extent representation of the afferent signals to the human motor cortex, possibly required to define the postural stiffness.

Satisfying learning features were achieved after 30 epochs, showing the high convergence capacity of ANFIS on mapping functions with high degree of nonlinearity, like the one that characterizes stiffness, in a very efficient way. The simulation results showed that learning was achieved through changing the initial representation of the input, described by the initial MFs, so that the local features of the input in the training set were caught best. The results, showing good resemblance between the output of the model and the testing data set, allow us to use such a system for approximating the postural stiffness of the human hand, based on experimental results.

The fuzzy inference rules can usually be written by human "experts" to represent their knowledge and experience in the specified field of interest, which in many cases makes it possible to predict, at "low-cost," the behavior of a system. However, this behavior can also be described by governing equations, if these are available. In our case, a combination between these two has been used. Human expertise was used to set the appropriate number of MFs in the input, whereas the governing equations making the link between the input and the output were found empirically, based on the results of a large set of experiments.

Further work should try to apply the above learning system to a radial basis function network for similar or more complex environments. In addition, it is worthwhile trying to make a model based on RL, implement it to the same problem, and check whether or not it is superior to the SL method. The comparison could be based on such criteria as the assurance of convergence to the optimum, the rate of convergence, and the performance index.

Although similar computational models to the problem discussed here are not available, it may be interesting to compare the results obtained using the proposed system with results obtained using other computational methods. Finally, it may be beneficial to use the basic architecture of ANFIS in order to design a computationally efficient hybrid learning system based on a hierarchy of experts [23, 46].

Acknowledgments

We are grateful to Tamar Flash and to Irena Gurevich for bringing the information concerning the stiffness field to our attention. The comments of Dario Liebermann were also very helpful.

References

[1] Albus, J.S., A theory of cerebellar function, *Mathematical Biosciences*, 10: 25-61, 1971.

[2] Albus, J.S., A new approach to manipulator control: The Cerebellar Model of Articulation Controller (CMAC), *Journal of Dynamic Systems, Measurement and Control*, Transactions of the ASME, 97: 220-227, 1975.

[3] Asada, H. and Slotine, J.-J. E., *Robot Analysis and Control*, John Wiley & Sons, New York, pp. 189-199, 1986.

[4] Berenji, H.R. and Khedkar, P., Learning and tuning fuzzy logic controllers through reinforcement, *IEEE Transactions on Neural Networks*, 3(5): 724-740, 1992.

[5] Barto, A.G., Reinforcement learning, in *The Handbook of Brain Theory and Neural Control*, Arbib, M.A., (Ed.), MIT Press, 1995.

[6] Barto, A.G., Reinforcement learning in motor control, in *The Handbook of Brain Theory and Neural Control*, Arbib, M.A., (Ed.), MIT Press, 1995.

[7] Barto, A.G. and Jordan, M.I., Gradient following without back-propagation in layered networks, in *Proceedings of the IEEE First Annual Conference on Neural Networks*, Candill, M. and Butler, C., (Eds.), San Diego: IEEE, pp. 11629-11636, 1987.

[8] Bishop, C.M., *Neural Networks for Pattern Recognition*, Clarendon Press, Oxford, 1995.

[9] Craig, J.J., *Introduction to Robotics*, Addison Wesley, Reading, Massachusetts, 1986.

[10] Crites, R.H. and Barto, A.H., Improving elevator performance using reinforcement learning, *Neural Information Processing Systems,* Vol. 8, Touretzky, D.S., Mozer, M.C., and Hasselmo, M.E. (Eds.), MIT Press, pp. 1017-1023, 1996.

[11] Flash, T. and Gurevich, I., Models of motor adaptation and impedance control in human arm movements, Morasso, P. and Sanguineti, V., (Eds.), in *Self Organization Computational Maps and Motor Control*, to appear 1998.

[12] Flash, T. and Mussa-Ivaldi, F.A., Human arm stiffness characteristics during the maintenance of posture, *Experimental Brain Research*, 82: 315-326, 1990.

[13] Gomi, H. and Osu R., Task dependent spatial characteristic of human arm stiffness in interaction with environments, *Technical Report ISRL-96-4*, 1996.

[14] Gurevich, I., Strategies of motor adaptation to external loads during planar two-joint arm movement, Ph.D. Thesis, Department of Applied Mathematics and Computer Science, The Weizmann Institute of Science, 1993.

[15] Hall, L.O. and Pokorny, M.A., Averaged reward reinforcement learning applied to fuzzy rule tuning, FUZZY'97.

[16] Hall, L.O. and Pokorny, M.A., Reinforcement tuning of fuzzy rules, NAFIPS'97, pp. 124-129, Syracuse, NY.

[17] Haykin, S., *Neural Networks - A Comprehensive Foundation*, Prentice-Hall, Englewood, New Jersey, 1994.

[18] Hertz, J., Krough, A., and Palmer, R., *Introduction to the Theory of Neural Computation*, Addison-Wesley, Reading, Massachusetts, 1991.

[19] Hirota, K., Fuzzy control robot playing two-dimensional ping-pong game, *Fuzzy Sets and Systems*, 32: 149-159, 1989.

[20] Jang, J.-S.R. and Sun, C.-T., ANFIS: Adaptive-Network-Based Fuzzy Inference Systems, *IEEE Transactions on Systems, Man and Cybernetics*, 23(3): 665-685, 1993.

[21] Jang, J.-S.R. and Sun, C.-T., Functional equivalence between radial basis function networks and fuzzy inference systems, *IEEE Trans. Neural Networks*, 4: 156-159, 1993.

[22] Jordan, M. and Rumelhart, D.E., Forward Models: Supervised learning with a distal teacher, *Cognitive Science*, 16: 307-354, 1992.

[23] Jordan, M.I. and Jacobs, R.A., Hierarchical mixtures of experts and the EM algorithm, *Neural Computation*, 6: 181-214, 1994.

[24] Kandel, A., Editor, *Fuzzy Expert Systems*, CRC Press, Boca Raton, Florida, 1995.

[25] Kandel, E.R., Schwartz, J.H., and Jessel, T.M., (Eds.), *Principles of Neural Science*, Elsevier Science Publishing, Amsterdam, 1991.

[26] Kaebling, L.P., Littman, N.L., and Moore, A.W., Reinforcement learning: a survey, *Journal of Artificial Intelligence Research*, 4: 237-285, 1996.

[27] Kawato, M. and Gomi, H., A computational model of four regions of the cerebellum based on feedback-error learning, *Biological Cybernetics*, 68: 95-103, 1992.

[28] Kim, S-H., Kim, Y-H., Sim, K-B., and Jeon, H-T., On developing an adaptive neural fuzzy control system, *Proceedings on the 1993 IEEE/RSJ International Conference on Intelligent Robots and Systems*, Yokohama, Japan, pp. 950-957, 1993.

[29] Klir, G.J. and Yuan, B., *Fuzzy Sets and Fuzzy Logic*, Prentice-Hall, Englewood Cliffs, New Jersey, 1995.

[30] Kosko, B., *Neural Networks and Fuzzy Systems*, Prentice-Hall, Englewood Cliffs, New Jersey, 1992.

[31] Kung, S.Y., *Digital Neural Networks*, Prentice-Hall, New Jersey, 1993.

[32] Lim, C.M. and Hiyama, T., Application of fuzzy logic control to a manipulator, *IEEE Transactions on Robotics and Automation*, 7(5): 688-691, 1991.

[33] Lin, C-T., A neural-fuzzy control system with structure and parameter learning, *Fuzzy Sets and Systems*, 70: 183-212, 1995.

[34] Lin, C-T. and Lee, C.S.G., Reinforcement structure/parameter learning for neural-network-based fuzzy logic control systems, *IEEE Transactions on Fuzzy Systems*, 2(1): 46-63, 1994.

[35] Mamdani, E.H. and Gaines, B.R., (Eds.), *Fuzzy Reasoning and Its Applications*, Academic Press, London, pp. 311-334, 1981.

[36] Marchalleck, N.J., *Improving Simulation Technology Through Reinforcement Learning*, Ph.D. Thesis, University of South Florida, Tampa, FL, 1997.

[37] Miller, W.T., Sutton, R.S., and Werbos, P.J., (Eds.), *Neural Networks for Control*, MIT Press, Cambridge, Massachusetts, 1990.

[38] Mitchell, T.M., *Machine Learning*, McGraw-Hill, New York, 1997.

[39] Moody, J. and Darken, C. J., Fast learning in networks of locally tuned processing units, *Neural Computation*, 1: 281-294, 1989.

[40] Mussa-Ivaldi, F.A., Hogan, N., and Bizzi, E., Neural, mechanical, and geometrical factors subserving arm posture in humans, *The Journal of Neuroscience*, 5: 2732-2743, 1985.

[41] Nauck, D. and Kruse, R., Designing neuro-fuzzy systems through backpropagation, in *Fuzzy Modelling Paradigms and Practice*, Pedrycz, W., (Ed.), Kluwer Academic Publishers, Boston, 1996.

[42] Palm, R., Control of a redundant manipulator using fuzzy-rules, *Fuzzy Sets and Systems*, 45: 279-298, 1992.

[43] Pedrycz, W., *Fuzzy Sets Engineering*, CRC Press, Boca Raton, Florida, 1995.

[44] Poggio, T. and Girossi, F., Regularization algorithms for learning that are equivalent to multilayer networks, *Science*, 247: 978-982, 1990.

[45] Ross, T.J., *Fuzzy Logic with Engineering Applications*, McGraw-Hill, New York, 1995.

[46] Sabes, P.N. and Jordan, M.I., Reinforcement learning by probability matching, *Neural Information Processing Systems,* Vol. 8, Touretzky, D.S., Mozer, M.C., and Hasselmo, M.E., (Eds.), MIT Press, pp. 1081-1086, 1996.

[47] Shadmehr, R., Mussa-Ivaldi, F.A., and Bizzi, E., Postural force fields of the human arm and their role in generating multijoint movements, *Journal of Neuroscience*, 13(1): 45-62, 1993.

[48] Stoica, A., Learning eye-arm coordination using neural and fuzzy neural techniques, (in this volume).

[49] Takagi, T. and Sugeno, M., Fuzzy identification of systems and its application to modeling and control, *IEEE Transactions on Systems, Man, and Cybernetics*, SMC-15(1): 116-132, 1985.

[50] Terano, T., Asai, K., and Sugeno, M., *Fuzzy Systems Theory and Its Applications*, Academic Press, New York, 1992.

[51] Tsuji, T., Morasso, P.G., Goto, K., and Ito, K., Human hand impedance characteristics during maintained posture, *Biological Cybernetics*, 72: 475-485, 1995.

[52] Wang, L-X., *Adaptive Fuzzy Systems and Control*, Prentice-Hall, Englewood Cliffs, New Jersey, 1994.

[53] Wang, L-X., Stable adaptive fuzzy controllers with applications to inverted pendulum tracking, *IEEE Transactions on Systems, Man and Cybernetics - Part B: Cybernetics*, 26(5): 677-691, 1996.

[54] Watanbe, K., Tang, J., Nakamura, M., Koga, S., and Fukuda, T., Mobile robot control using fuzzy-gaussian neural networks, *Proceedings of the 1993 IEEE/RSJ International Conference on Intelligent Robots and Systems*, Yokohoma, Japan, pp. 919-925, 1993.

[55] Whitehead, S.D. and Lin, L.-J., Reinforcement learning of non-Markov Decision Process, *Artificial Intelligence*, 73: 271-306, 1995.

[56] Yager, R.R. and Filev, D.P., *Essentials of Fuzzy Modeling and Control*, Wiley, New York, 1994.
[57] Zimmermann, H-J., *Fuzzy Set Theory*, Kluwer Academic Publishers, Boston, 1991.

Appendix 1. Symbols and Abbreviations

F_x, F_y - elastic restoring forces
d_x, d_y - displacements imposed by the manipulandum
K - the stiffness matrix
K_{min}, K_{max} - minimum and maximum stiffness, as lengths of the primary and secondary axes of the stiffness ellipse
S - stiffness surface
ρ - shape of the stiffness ellipse
θ - orientation of the stiffness ellipse
R - radial distance measured from the shoulder to the hand
r - normalized radial distance of the stiffness ellipse
L_1, L_2 - the lengths of the upper and lower parts of the arm, respectively
F - preload size
F_{max} - maximum preload size
f - normalized preload size
Φ - direction of the preload
ϕ - normalized direction of the preload
x - variable of the Gaussian membership function
μ, σ - parameters of the Gaussian membership function
A - area of the stiffness ellipse
A_{max} - maximal value of the stiffness ellipse area
a - normalized value of the stiffness ellipse area
λ_1, λ_2 - main axes of the stiffness ellipse
θ_e - direction of the principal axis of the stiffness ellipse
θ_r - radial direction with the shoulder as origin

ANFIS - adaptive network-based fuzzy inference system
FIS - fuzzy inference system
MF - membership function
RBF - radial basis function
RMSE - root mean square error
RL - reinforcement learning
SL - supervised learning

Chapter 4

Fuzzy reduction control of acceleration and vibration of a stretcher-cart on an ambulance

Mikio Maeda and Shuta Murakami

When an emergency car carries a dangerous object or a patient in critical condition, it should provide safe and smooth conveyance, free of swaying and swinging. However, while the car (i.e., an ambulance or an emergency vehicle) is running, these movements actually cannot be reduced by passive control only, using springs and dampers. Therefore, an active method of acceleration and vibrations reduction is needed. We describe a fuzzy control to reduce the acceleration and vibration that a patient (or the object) receives on the ambulance. The fuzzy controller is designed based on human driver-type knowledge. The fuzzy control uses three sets of rules to reduce vibrations in three orthogonal directions, namely, in the forward-backward direction, in the lateral direction, and in the longitudinal direction. In addition, we describe two different approaches based on fuzzy control algorithms, namely, the indirect fuzzy control method and the direct fuzzy control method. Experimental measurements and control simulation results are discussed; several conclusions end the chapter.

1. Introduction

Recently, automobile engineering and medical technology have both experienced a remarkable development, as a result of the application of electronic products in these fields. In vehicle technology, applied integrated circuits products are commonly used in electronic fuel injection units, electrical braking systems, four-wheel steering, and four-wheel drive by almost all automobile companies. On the other hand, medical technology is applied to patient monitoring systems in intensive care units, digital processing of medical images, and diagnosis and treatment systems, among others.

In a highway network, an ambulance can rapidly reach the accident site. For first-aid medical care, seriously wounded patients need immediate treatment in the ambulance and must be gently carried to a hospital or emergency room. Nevertheless, a patient in a car receives loads including sway, swing, shock from the road surface, the stop motion, and the steering action of the car. E. Picard reported that complications in a circulatory organ system have appeared in six percent of transported patients because they receive the vehicle vibration [1]. Also, Okada reported that when a patient receives acceleration within a frequency from 1 [Hz] to 14 [Hz], organism response and sympathy of internal organs have appeared [2]. Hearing impairment, increased intra-abdominal pressure, abdominal pain, restriction of respiratory movement, and left chest pain occurred in the presence of vibrations in the range of 4~8 [Hz].

Therefore, different stretcher systems which can reduce these loads (acceleration and vibration in the region of 1~14 Hz) have been developed [3, 4]. They consist of a set of springs and dampers fixed under the stretcher to absorb the impacts. The medical aspects related to the effects of the accelerations and vibrations to which a patient is submitted on the stretcher in an ambulance were analyzed in detail in [5]. In addition, various types of passive vibration control were addressed in several papers [3, 4, 5]. This research has been rigorously conducted and is helpful in assessing the damage inflicted to the patient. However, such analyses are of limited use if systems more effectively damping the vibrations are not built based on them. The passive control of vibrations has limited capabilities. It is difficult to reduce the shocks or loads that a patient receives from the stretcher movement only by using a mechanical structure.

Active control is needed for the effective attenuation of the stretcher's swinging and swaying corresponding to the usual environmental conditions. In this chapter, we discuss the use of fuzzy control in order to reduce the patient's load on ambulances and other critical vehicles. This method has been adopted because heuristic - "natural" - rules obtained from human knowledge can easily be adapted, redesigned, and applied to a nonlinear controller for the purpose of vibration reduction.

L. A. Zadeh first proposed fuzzy logic as an engineering tool [6], and Mamdani applied this approach to the temperature control of a steam engine [7]. The fuzzy control is implemented in a computer, and the control rules are described using fuzzy linguistic variables and labels. The structure of the fuzzy control rules consists of an antecedent part ("if" part) and a consequent part ("then" part), that is, *"if ...then ..."*. These rules are called the control knowledge rule set. The fuzzy labels, such as *positive big*, *zero*, and *negative small,* are characterized by membership functions. These rules are produced based on the driver's human knowledge.

By using fuzzy control, it is possible to keep the cart position on a reference point and to reduce the swing and sway that a patient receives from the road surface and the behavior of the vehicle (the ambulance or the emergency car). Those vibrations include the acceleration, the deceleration, and the lateral acceleration [8] and have appeared around three axes: roll, yaw, and pitch. In this chapter, we take into account the acceleration and the vibration of the sick person on the stretcher; moreover, we consider lateral, front, and back loads. Second, we discuss methods to reduce the pitching of cart. Springs and dampers can reduce high frequency pitch of the stretcher. The use of fuzzy active control rules for reducing the sway and swing of the stretcher is presented for two different approaches. One approach is an indirect fuzzy control method using the fuzzy truth-value, and the other is a direct fuzzy control method using the numerical truth-value.

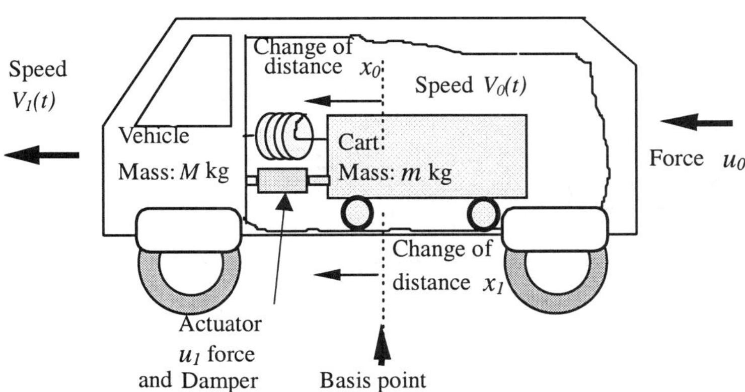

Figure 1. Cart model on ambulance.

The fuzzy control rules consist of three kinds of rule sets: the protection rules on the forward and backward direction, the rules for lateral direction, and the rules for longitudinal direction. The pitching control employs only the direct fuzzy control method. In this chapter, that control is simulated on a computer. For the results of various simulations, the usefulness of this control is discussed from the viewpoint of the comfort on the vehicle (stretcher), the degree of acceleration, and the position of the stretcher-cart. However, three dimensions control is not simulated in this chapter. At first, the front and rear direction control and the lateral direction control are simulated, and after that, only the longitudinal direction control is simulated.

2. Fuzzy control system for reduction of acceleration and vibration

2.1. Fuzzy control system

The position of the stretcher cart in the ambulance is shown in Figure 1. When the ambulance is running at a speed v_1 [Km/h], the cart is moving at speed v_0 [Km/h] in relation to the ground. The masses of the vehicle and the cart are M [Kg] and m [Kg]. The force applied to the vehicle, u_0, is changed by the driver. It is possible for the cart to move freely forward and backward and in the transversal direction within a limited area around the desired position of the cart.

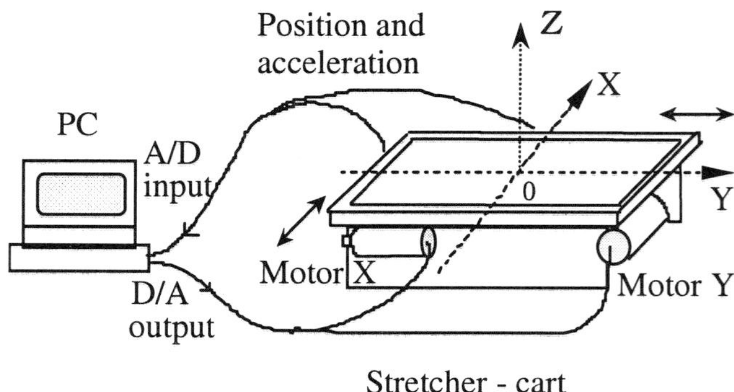

Figure 2. Stretcher control system.

The aim of this control is to keep the cart position on the target point without the acceleration and the vibration which a patient receives on the stretcher. Figure 2 schematically shows the control system designed by us for the real cart control. The swaying and swinging in the lateral direction, in the front and rear direction, and in the longitudinal direction are measured by acceleration servo sensors and position sensors and are converted into voltages. These signals are acquired by the control computer through an A/D converter. The control errors are derived with respect to the reference values (set point for the X coordinate, Y coordinate, and Z coordinate of the cart's position) by using integration and difference operators. The fuzzy controller (control algorithm) computes the forces to the (X, Y, Z) axis motors using the control values, the fuzzy control rules, and fuzzy reasoning (i.e., an indirect method and a simplified method). The signals corresponding to the forces are sent to the cart via a D/A converter.

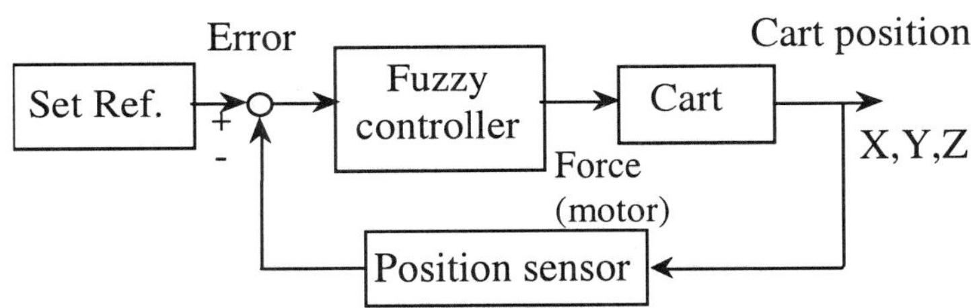

Figure 3. Fuzzy control system.

The configuration of the fuzzy control system used to reduce the sway and swing of the stretcher-cart is shown in Figure 3. This is a standard design of a fuzzy control system. However, two signals are input to the cart as the forces for the X-axis and Y-axis controls. The set reference value is the basis point (X, Y) of the cart and is assigned the null value $(0, 0)$. For longitudinal vibration control, the fuzzy control is applied to the three points that support the cart to keep it horizontal. We simulate the fuzzy control for vibration reduction on longitudinal direction (Z-axis) and independently on the X-axis and Y-axis.

2.2. Fuzzy logic controller design

In this section, we present two designs of the fuzzy controller for sway and swing reduction. Both controllers are implemented by software on the control computer. These controllers are described by linguistic control rules. The differences between the two controllers are the structure of the control rules and the fuzzy reasoning method for the calculation of the force. Regarding the fuzzy inference method used, one of the controllers is called the indirect method fuzzy controller [9, 10], while the other is called the direct method fuzzy controller (simplified method) [11-14]. The indirect method uses a fuzzy truth-value, while the direct method uses a numerical truth-value. These are shown in detail in the following subsections.

2.2.1. Indirect fuzzy controller [15]

The fuzzy controller using the *indirect* method for reduction of the sway and the swing includes two sets of fuzzy control rules, namely,

(1) The front-rear position control rule set (Y-axis)

$$
\begin{aligned}
&\text{If } e^p_k \text{ is } P_1 \text{ then } u^p_k \text{ is } Pu_1 \\
&\text{If } e^p_k \text{ is } N_1 \text{ then } u^p_k \text{ is } Nu_1 \\
&\text{If } \Delta e^p_k \text{ is } P_2 \text{ then } u^p_k \text{ is } Pu_2 \\
&\text{If } \Delta e^p_k \text{ is } N_2 \text{ then } u^p_k \text{ is } Nu_2 \\
&\text{If } \Delta^2 e^p_k \text{ is } P_3 \text{ then } u^p_k \text{ is } Pu_3 \\
&\text{If } \Delta^2 e^p_k \text{ is } N_3 \text{ then } u^p_k \text{ is } Nu_3
\end{aligned}
\tag{1}
$$

(2) The lateral position control rule set (X-axis)

$$
\begin{aligned}
&\text{If } e^l_k \text{ is } P_4 \text{ then } u^l_k \text{ is } Pu_4 \\
&\text{If } e^l_k \text{ is } N_4 \text{ then } u^l_k \text{ is } Nu_4 \\
&\text{If } \Delta e^l_k \text{ is } P_5 \text{ then } u^l_k \text{ is } Pu_5 \\
&\text{If } \Delta e^l_k \text{ is } N_5 \text{ then } u^l_k \text{ is } Nu_5 \\
&\text{If } \Delta^2 e^l_k \text{ is } P_6 \text{ then } u^l_k \text{ is } Pu_6 \\
&\text{If } \Delta^2 e^l_k \text{ is } N_6 \text{ then } u^l_k \text{ is } Nu_6
\end{aligned}
\tag{2}
$$

Here, k is the sampling instant, and

$$
\begin{aligned}
\Delta e^p_k &= e^p_k - e^p_{k-1}, \\
\Delta^2 e^p_k &= \Delta e^p_k - \Delta e^p_{k-1}, \\
\Delta e^l_k &= e^l_k - e^l_{k-1}, \\
\Delta^2 e^l_k &= \Delta e^l_k - \Delta e^l_{k-1},
\end{aligned}
\tag{3}
$$

e^p_k the position error between the center of cart and the target position on the Y-axis (front and rear direction),

Δe^p_k the first difference of the position error,

$\Delta^2 e^p_k$ the second difference of the position error,

e^l_k the lateral position error between the center of cart and the target position on the X-axis,

Δe^l_k the first difference of the lateral position error,

$\Delta^2 e^l_k$ the second difference of the lateral position error.

The P_i, N_i, Pu_i, and Nu_i (i = 1, 2, 3) in control rules are the fuzzy labels. The membership function type in the antecedent parts is the arctangent as shown in Figure 4 (a). The membership functions of the consequent parts is linear (triangular), as shown in Figure 4 (b).

The position error is positive if the center of the cart is located in back of the target position (X-axis), and it is negative if it is located in front of the target position. The lateral position error is positive if the center of the cart is located on the right side of the target position (point at intersection with the Y-axis), while it is negative if it is on its left side. The axes related to the system are shown in Figure 5. The stretcher is set on one side of the floor in the vehicle and can be controlled inside the movable area.

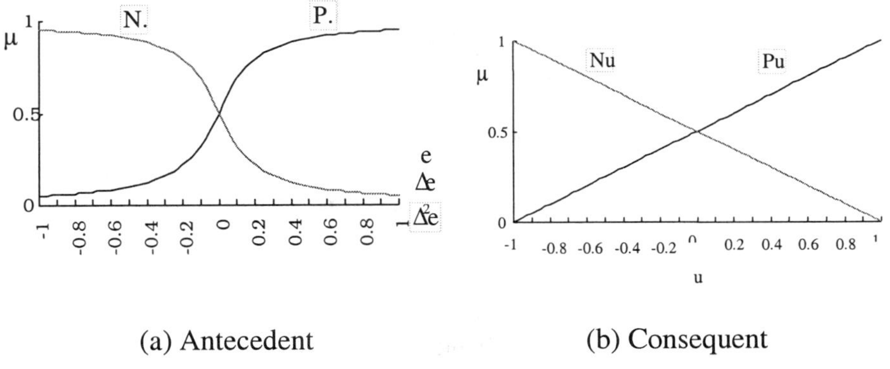

(a) Antecedent   (b) Consequent

Figure 4. Membership functions (fuzzy labels).

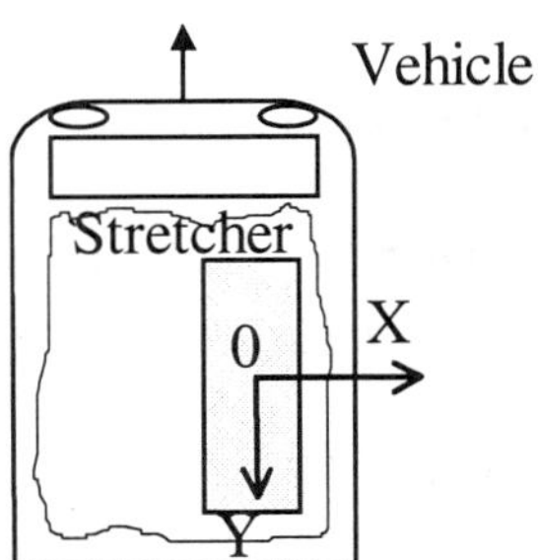

Figure 5. Stretcher-cart on ambulance.

By using the previous control rules (1) and (2), we assume that the characteristics of the fuzzy controller are as shown in Figure 6 when the inputs to the fuzzy control rules are the control errors. As shown in Figure 6, this controller has some saturation areas for the variable (the force); the control surface is smooth.

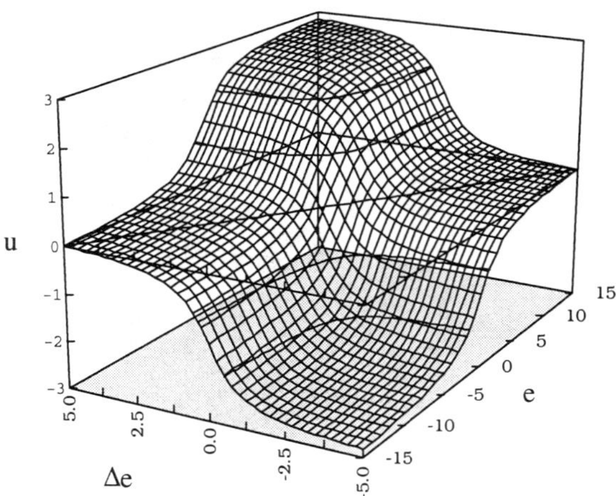

Figure 6. The characteristic (input-to-output function)
of the fuzzy controller.

The control characteristic surface is changed by adjusting the fuzzy labels. Generally, by changing the controlled object (type of car), the characteristics of the fuzzy controller must be changed. The fuzzy control rule set of the indirect fuzzy controller is tuned by the adjustment of the fuzzy labels, that is, the tuning of parameters of the membership functions which characterize the fuzzy labels. These fuzzy labels are tuned by evaluating simulation results and experimental results with a certain frequency of vibration.

2.2.2. Direct fuzzy controller

The fuzzy controller using the *direct* method for the reduction of the sway and the swing includes the fuzzy control rule sets as follows.

The front and rear position control rule set (Y axis):

$$\text{If } e^p_k \text{ is } PB \text{ and } \Delta e^p_k \text{ is } PB \text{ then } u^p_k \text{ is } PB \tag{4}$$

These rules are shown in Table 1.
The lateral position control rule set (X-axis) consists of rules in the form:

$$\text{If } e^l_k \text{ is } PB \text{ and } \Delta e^l_k \text{ is } PB \text{ then } u^l_k \text{ is } PM \tag{5}$$

These rules are shown in Table 2, and e^p_k, Δe^p_k, u^p_k, e^l_k, Δe^l_k, and u^l_k have already been explained in Equation (3).

Table 1. Front-rear position control rules.

u^p	e^p						
	NB	NM	NS	ZO	PS	PM	PB
PB	ZO	PS	PM	PM	PM	PB	PB
PM	NS	ZO	PS	PM	PM	PM	PB
PS	NS	NS	ZO	PS	PS	PM	PM
Δe^p ZO	NM	NS	NS	ZO	PS	PS	PM
NS	NM	NS	NS	NS	ZO	PS	PS
NM	NB	NM	NM	NM	NS	ZO	PS
NB	NB	NB	NM	NM	NM	NS	ZO

Table 2. Lateral position control rule set.

u^l	e^l						
	NB	NM	NS	ZO	PS	PM	PB
PB	ZO	NS	PM	PB	PB	PB	PM
PM	PM	ZO	PS	PM	PM	PB	PS
PS	PB	NS	ZO	PS	PS	PM	PS
Δe^l ZO	NS	NM	NS	ZO	PS	PM	PS
NS	NS	NM	NS	NS	ZO	PS	NB
NM	NS	NB	NM	NM	ZO	ZO	NM
NB	NB	NB	NB	NB	NS	PS	ZO

Table 3. Longitudinal position control rules.

u^v	e^v				
	NB	NS	ZO	PS	PB
PB	PS	PS	PM	PB	PB
PS	PS	ZO	PS	PS	PM
Δe^v ZO	ZO	ZO	ZO	ZO	ZO
NS	NM	NS	NS	ZO	NS
NB	NB	NB	NM	NS	NS

v: Vertical

In these rule sets, each part of the antecedent has two fuzzy linguistic variables: the control error and its first difference, which is different from that of the indirect controller. In addition, the antecedent parts in Table 1 and Table 2 describe the pairs of fuzzy labels that belong to the fuzzy variables and show all possible patterns of the state of the control object. Therefore, the possible patterns of the control state must be entirely expressed. The membership function type of each fuzzy label of the antecedent part is triangular, while that of consequent part is a singleton. The simplified method proposed by Maeda et al. [13] is used for the fuzzy reasoning. It has been shown that the computing time decreases and the control results improve with respect to other methods. Furthermore, the rule sets of Table 1 and Table 2 are mutually independent, and they are also easily tuned by an adjustment algorithm or the expert's knowledge. Table 3 shows the fuzzy control rules used to reduce the longitudinal vibration and acceleration of cart. Here, superscript v implies a vertical (longitudinal) direction.

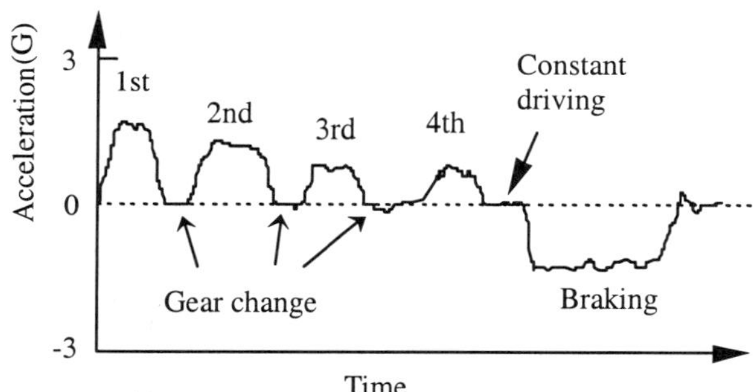

Figure 7. Vehicle response of cart by shift changing and braking. (Measuring unit for acceleration is the gravitational acceleration, G.)

3. Measurement of vehicle acceleration and vibration

The vehicle used in this study is supposed to have automatic and manual transmission. Figure 7 shows the response of a stretcher-cart on the vehicle with a manual-shift (an ambulance; Nissan E-KMGNC2, 1.99 t.). The variable in Figure 7 indicates the acceleration degree the patient receives on the stretcher. In this experiment, the vehicle speeds up from 0 [Km/h] to about 40 [Km/h], braking and coming to a stop. The patient has varying loads of acceleration with the gear changes (shift changes) and the braking stop. When the vehicle brakes to a stop, the cart catches a negative acceleration; then the acceleration decreases to zero.

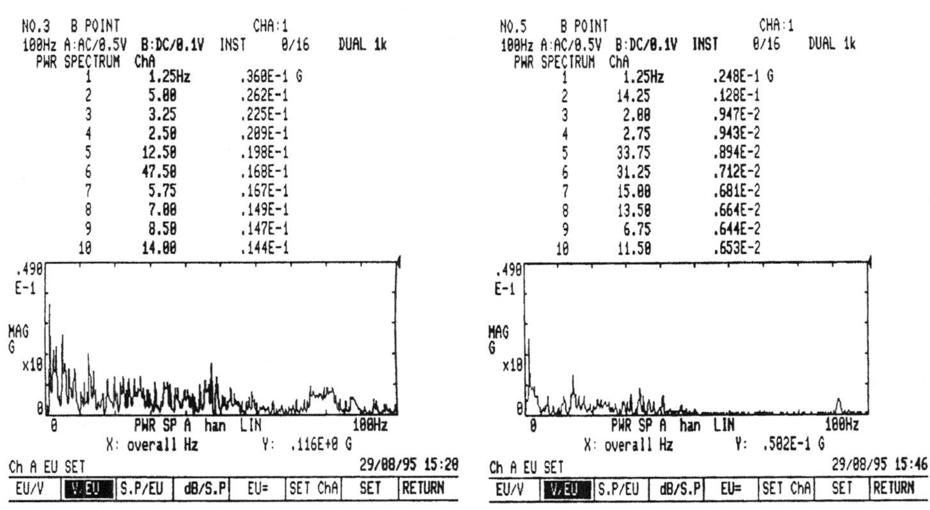

(a) Longitudinal   (b) Forward and backward

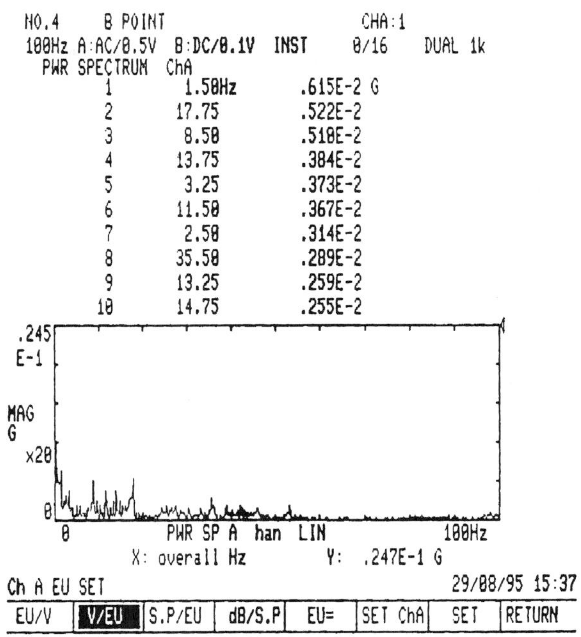

(c) Lateral vibration

Figure 8. Power spectra for the vibrations.

After that, the cart receives a slightly positive acceleration and vibrates for a short time. Due to this phenomenon, the cart moves backward quickly. Note that the change of acceleration of an automatic car is smaller than that of a manual-shift car.

The power spectra of vibrations for pitching, yawing, and rolling are shown in Figure 8. The spectra exhibit vibrations in the low frequency region. These vibrations have to be reduced by the fuzzy control.

4. Control simulations

The design of the models that include all the loads is difficult. Therefore, we restrict ourselves to simplified models. We formulate the vehicle model and the stretcher-cart model in only a bidimensional space (*X-Y* plane), as follows.

4.1. Models

Vehicle model [10, 14]
The equations deriving the speed (speed model) of the vehicle are

$$
\ddot{x}(t) = -0.634 \cdot \dot{x}(t) - 0.034 \cdot x(t) + 1.228 \cdot u_1(t),
$$
$$
y(t) = \int_0^t x(t)dt, \tag{6}
$$
$$
V_1(t) = x(t)
$$

The notations in Equations (6) are

$x(t)$: the vehicle speed
$u(t)$: the vehicle throttle power
$y(t)$: the vehicle displacement from a basis point.

A steering model is developed in [14].

Stretcher-cart model
The model is

$$
m\ddot{z}(t) - b[\dot{y}(t) - \dot{z}(t)] - k[y(t) - z(t)] = T_0 u_0
$$
$$
e(t) = y(t) - z(t) \tag{7}
$$

In Equations (7) the notations are:

$z(t)$:   the cart displacements from a basis point
$e(t)$:   the position error of the cart from a target point
u_0:   the cart force (motor driver current)
T_0:   the coefficient of cart force (this coefficient is equal to 1)
$m =$ 200 [Kg] (typical value used in simulations)
k: the spring coefficient
b: the damping coefficient.

The derivation of the vehicle model is presented in [8, 15]. In Equations (7) the state variable expresses the X or Y coordinates of the position of the cart. The mass m is affected by the patient's weight, which is fixed in simulations. Note that the longitudinal model of the cart has the same structure as in Equations (7).

4.2. Control of vibrations in the X-Y plane

A result of the fuzzy control's reduction of the acceleration of the cart in the front and rear direction is presented in Figure 9. Here, the vehicle's speed reached a set point: 60 [Km/h] from the stop: 0 [Km/h] (the dynamical state); afterward, the car stops by braking from the steady state (in which the vehicle keeps a constant speed). In this case, the indirect method was used, and the coefficients of spring and damper were, respectively, 100 [N/m] and 10 [Ns/m]. A speed controller, whose performance is shown in Figure 9 (b), controls the vehicle speed. Note that the position errors are kept within ± 15 [cm], the cart has been approaching a target point, and the acceleration of the vehicle is smooth. Consequently, the cart-stretcher control accomplishes the necessary comfort for the patient. Figure 10 shows the control simulation without a spring in the same conditions as simulation 1 (see Figure 9). The results obtained are similar to the previous ones. However, in this case, the force is smaller than in the case without a spring.

In real vehicle control, the vibrational effect of the manual shift-change is strong. Therefore, in order to be close to the real driving situation, the control was simulated with braking acceleration and disturbance instead of shift-change. This result is also shown in Figure 10. Due to the disturbance, which is assumed as the shift change, the vehicle's speed and the force to the cart fluctuate. However, the position errors are settled in the allowance area (± 15 cm). Based on these results, a robust control system was designed.

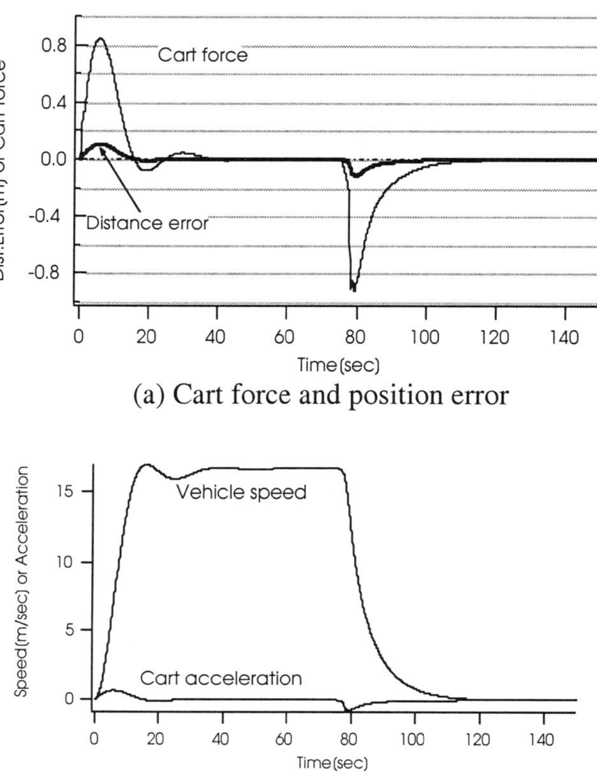

(a) Cart force and position error

(b) Vehicle speed and acceleration of cart

Figure 9. Simulation result 1 using an indirect method.

Figures 11 and 12 show the simulation results using the direct method. Figure 11 shows a result in the front and rear direction, while the vehicle reached a target speed of 60 [Km/h] from the stopping position at 0 [Km/h] (the dynamical state). Then it decelerates from the steady state to about 40 [Km/h]. The position errors in this figure are larger than those of the simulation result using the indirect method.

The simulation results of the lateral position and acceleration control are shown in Figure 12. In this case, the vehicle is running on a turning road (i.e., a curve which has a radius of 40 [m]) while the vehicle is decelerating from 40 [Km/h] to 30 [Km/h]. Using the direct method, the acceleration was reduced (compared to a method without acceleration control), but the position errors exceed the allowance area and become large.

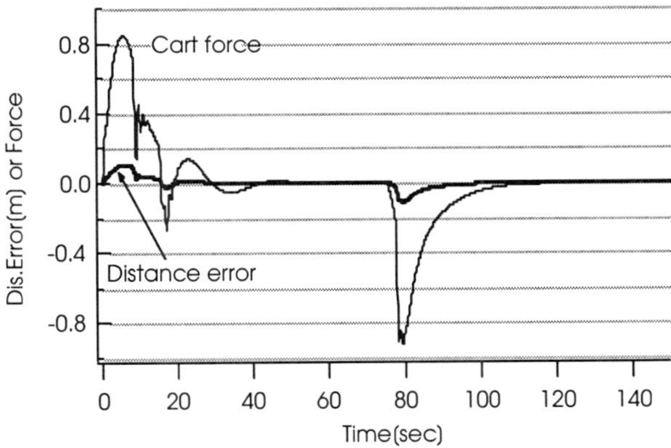

(a) Cart force and position error

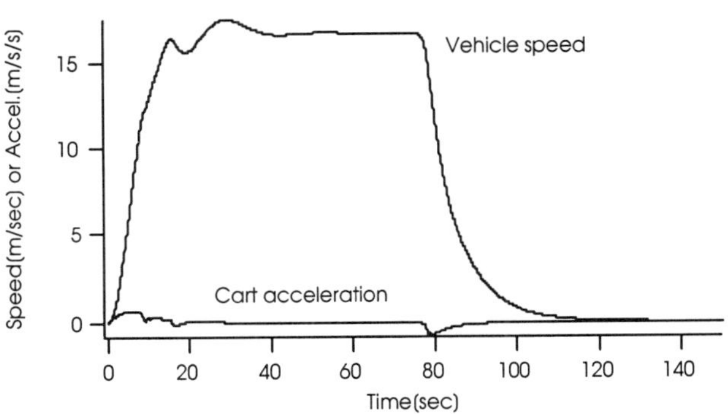

(b) Vehicle speed and cart acceleration

Figure 10. Simulation result #2 with disturbance.

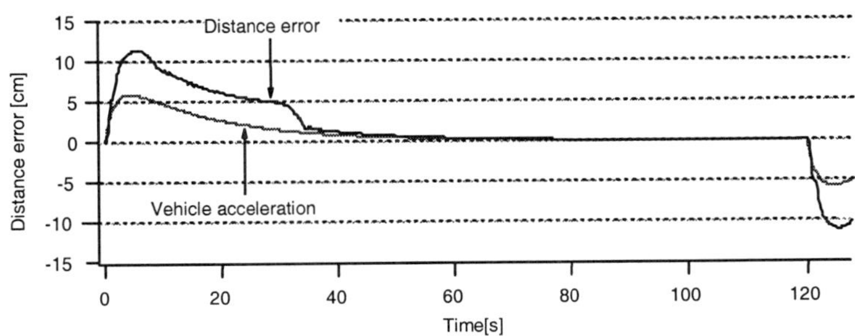

Figure 11. The control result of cart in front-rear direction.

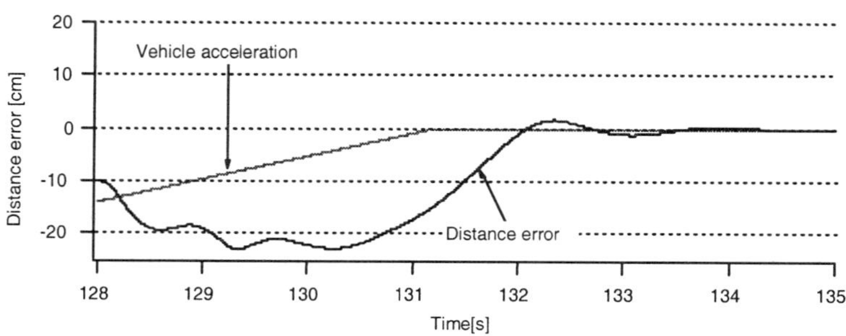

(a) The position error and acceleration in front and rear

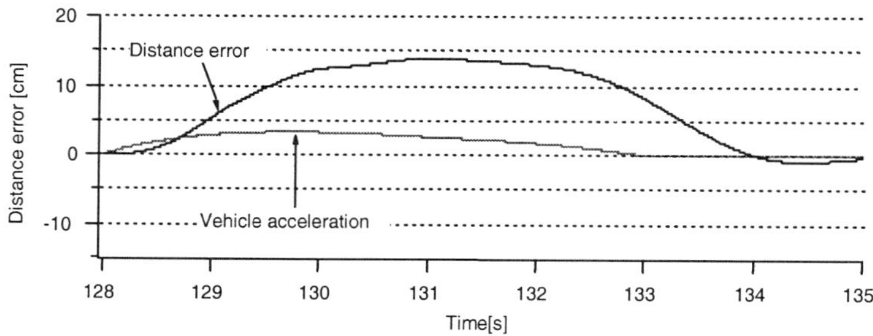

(b) The lateral position and acceleration

Figure 12. The acceleration and position errors of the cart, when using a direct control method.

The results of acceleration and vibration control using the direct method are worse than the results of the control using the indirect method. The reason is that the control rules are imperfect and the selection of the object variables is unsatisfactory. Therefore, we must consider adjusting the control rules and including the second difference of position error to the object variables of the antecedent parts.

In the next paragraphs we show simulation results of acceleration reduction by fuzzy control for the case of the longitudinal vibration or acceleration. In this simulation, the fuzzy controller applies to the three points that support the stretcher cart. Each point is connected to the vehicle floor by a damper and spring system with a linear motor. The three points A, B, and C correspond to a triangle under the cart surface. Figure 13 shows a control result at point A. At each point a random disturbance is impressed. Its range of disturbance is between 0 [N] and +4 [N]. The vibration amplitude at point A decreased when the vibration control was applied. Similar results were obtained at all points.

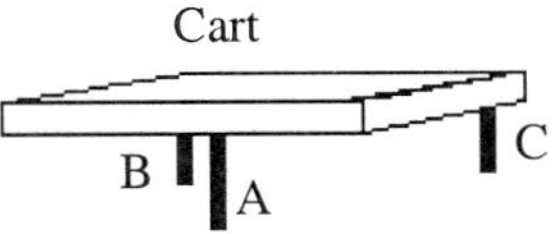

(a) Control points (support points) of the cart

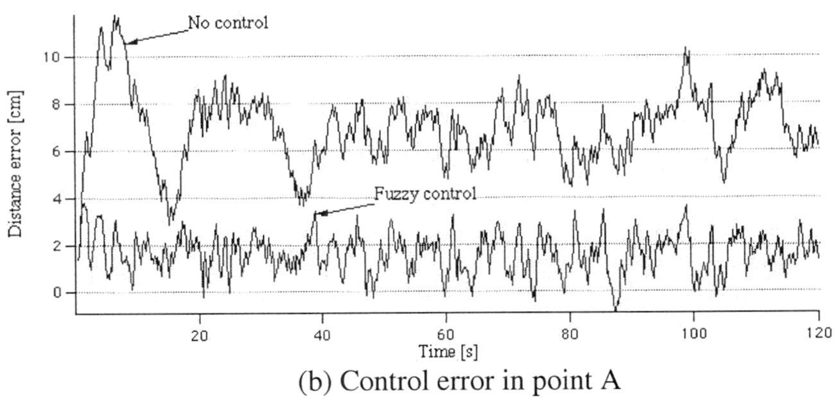

(b) Control error in point A

Figure 13. Longitudinal vibration control.

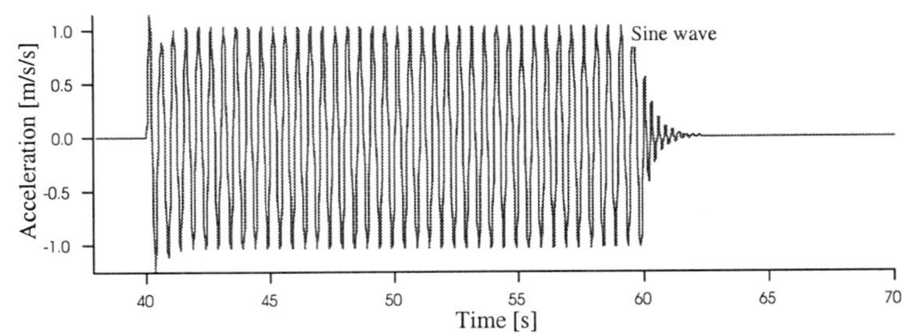

(a) Vibration with no control

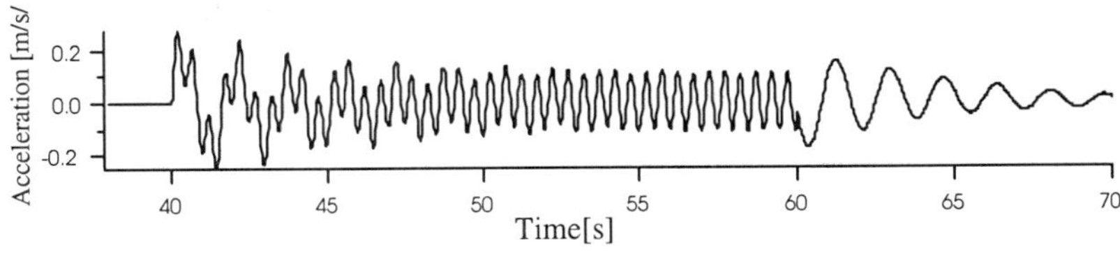

(b) Control result

Figure 14. Cart vibration under a disturbance.

Finally, in order to ascertain that the fuzzy controller effectively reduces the vibration, we added a sine curve at 5 [Hz] to the control object (a stretcher-cart model in front and rear direction). Figure 14 shows a simulation result for that object. The response in Figure 14 (a) implies a motion and an acceleration of the cart without controlling. Figure 14 (b) shows the control result: the vibration is significantly reduced by using fuzzy control.

Note that the results in Figures 11, 12, 13, and 14 were obtained under different conditions. Forward and backward direction (Figure 11); forward and backward direction, and lateral direction, at the same time (Figure 12); longitudinal direction, with no control for forward and lateral directions (Figure 13); disturbance control for only the forward and backward direction (Figure 14).

5. Conclusions

In this chapter we presented the design of a fuzzy control system used to reduce the acceleration and vibration of the movable stretcher-cart in an ambulance. It was found that the cart position could be kept in an allowance area reducing the acceleration that a sick person receives. By analyzing the measurement results of the acceleration and vibration of the stretcher-cart system, the control rules were improved and resulted in almost complete suppression of the effect that the cart receives from shift-change and braking.

First we presented the simulation of the fuzzy control for reduction of the vibration along the forward and backward directions and for the lateral directions. Then the vibration reduction control was performed on three control points by using the longitudinal control rules. The purposes of controls are to keep a cart in the allowance areas around reference points and to reduce the vibrations of the cart.

Finally, to determine the quality (robustness) of the fuzzy controller, we presented the simulated results for the control against the vibration impressed by a sine curve with a frequency of 5 [Hz]. In the simulations for the reduction of sway and swing of the cart, the fuzzy active control of the cart position was shown useful, and the control system demonstrated applicability to the real system.

Three-dimensional control simulations for forward and backward, lateral, and longitudinal directions must be performed in the future. In addition, a trial product machine (stretcher-cart system) must be designed to test the real-life use of the fuzzy active control of vibrations on emergency cars with movable carts.

References

[1] Picard, E., The effect of acceleration and vibration on sick person during transport, *Rev Corps Santé*, (11), 611, 1970.

[2] Okada, A., Physiological effects of acceleration on human body, *Journal of the Society of Automotive Engineers of Japan, Inc.*, 25 (10), 1082, 1971.

[3] Leyshow, D.R. and Stammers, C.W., The development and performance of an ambulance stretcher suspension, *Proceedings of Institutional Mechanical Enginering, Part D*, 200 (4), 249, 1986.

[4] Ishida, S. et al., Vibration measurements of a newly developed vibration-absorbing stretcher, *JJAM*, (1), 103, 1990.

[5] Hakamada, T., Study of vibration and absorption mechanism, *Annual Report of Fire Research*, (21), 1, 1992.

[6] Zadeh, L.A., Outline of a new approach to the analysis of complex system and decision processes, *IEEE Trans. on Systems, Man and Cybernetics*, 3 (193), 28, 1965.

[7] Mamdani, E.H., Application of fuzzy algorithms for control of simple dynamic plant, *Proceedings of the Institute of Electrical Engineers*, 121, 1588, 1974.

[8] Maeda, M. et al., Fuzzy control for reduction of vibration and acceleration of a stretcher-cart on an ambulance, *Journal of Biomedical, Fuzzy, and Human Sciences*, 3 (1), 21, 1997.

[9] Maeda, M. et al., A design of fuzzy logic controller, *Research Report of KIT (Engineering)*, (49), 43, 1984.

[10] Maeda, M. and Murakami, S., A speed control of an automobile by using fuzzy logic controller, *Journal of Transactions of SICE*, 21 (9), 984, 1985.

[11] Takagi, T. and Sugeno, M., Fuzzy identification of systems and its application to modeling and control, *IEEE Transactions on Systems, Man, and Cybernetics*, 15 (1), 116, 1985.

[12] Maeda, M. and Murakami, S., Steering control and speed control for an automobile with a fuzzy logic, *Proceedings of the 3rd IFSA Congress*, Seattle, WA, August 23, 1989.

[13] Maeda, M. et al., A self-tuning fuzzy controller, *Fuzzy Sets and Systems*, 51 (1), 29, 1992.

[14] Maeda, M., Fuzzy drive expert system for an automobile, *Information Sciences, Applications*, 4 (1), 29, 1995.

[15] Maeda, M. et al., Fuzzy control for reduction of sway and swing of seat or object carried on vehicle, *Proceedings of 15th SICE Kyushu Branch Annual Conference*, Saga, Kyushu, November 23, 1996.

Part 2.

Medical Diagnosis and Health Care

Chapter 5

Computational intelligence for medical information analysis and refinement

Patrik Eklund, Lena Kallin, and Gustaf Selén

In this chapter we describe an architecture for a workstation that combines data mining tools with analysis tools in building new decision support systems and automatically integrates the new system into a diagnosis classification skeleton. The workstation is intended to support fast and efficient navigation toward a correct diagnosis and consists of modules each capable of supporting the diagnosis of specific diseases.

The production line within which domain experts can generate decision support systems for a specific disease will be described together with one of the analysis tools used in the production line, the generalised pre-processing perceptron (GPP). The GPP has a structure that allows results comparable to a multilayer perceptron, yet perceiving parameter interpretations relevant within the medical domain.

1. Introduction

1.1. Models of motor control and skill learning and their use in studies of human motor behavior, bioengineering, and robotics

From a systems engineering point of view, this chapter describes the production line within which domain experts can generate clinical decision support. The systems architecture includes facilities for database navigation, data analysis in a wide range of tools, and a systems integration module to enable end-user system development without involving programming efforts.

From a data analysis point of view, we add to the *religious* discussion on appropriate analysis methods by suggesting considering the combination of numerical and logical methods. This will provide a connection between numerical values as found, respectively, in the computational model and the medical domain. In particular, we have demonstrated the use of the *generalized preprocessing perceptron*, which shows a remarkable discriminating power as compared to the multilayer perceptron, yet preserving parameter interpretations relevant within the medical domain.

The chapter is structured as follows. In Section 2, we discuss the overall information scope for our work, together with a presentation of typical case studies, and how information is organized within a health care system. In Section 3, we present the Clinician's Workstation from a general systems perspective. Section 4 presents some detail for techniques used when constructing a particular expert system. The focus is on the relationship between numerical and logical feedforward approach. In Section 5, the Clinician's Workstation together with the expert systems production line is presented in detail.

2. Information scope and management

The overall objective of information handling, within the medical domain, is to use interconnected information systems to support patient care management in order to enable communication and information flow between home care units, primary care units, and hospitals.

In a workflow scenario describing patient care management (see Figure 1), patient information is always instantly available for the general practitioner as well as the specialist.

Information systems within patient care management should promote large-scale access to information sources, both related to patient specific information as well as supporting information required during the health care situation. Patient specific information resides mainly in patient record systems, and supporting documentation and decision support are integrated into multimedia systems.

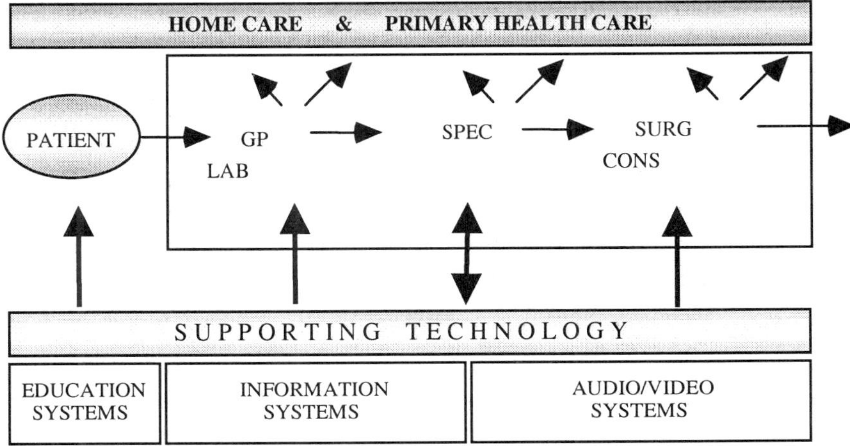

Figure 1. Patient care management.

In general, information retrieval involves a long-term broad coordination of different health care registers and databases to support region-wide information exchange and utility, thereby supporting a more flexible database management and providing a platform for developing distributed information systems. Database management systems (DBMSs) range from patient record systems in primary care units, through hospital information systems, to other public organization information systems and demographic backbones.

Patient records require ease-of-use and instant information access while still enabling the practitioner to maintain focus on the patient. For refinement purposes, data pools need to be available to a broad user community.

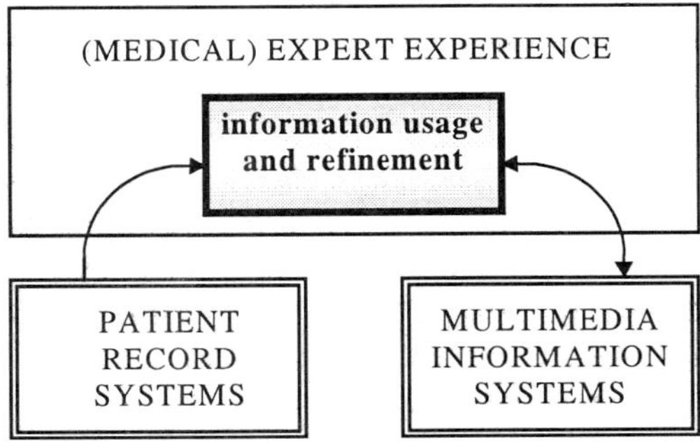

Figure 2. Information systems usage, maintenance, and refinement.

Multimedia information systems need an architectural organization to be available for immediate integration of generated information packages and decision support systems. In the data refinement scenario, data mining is supported through a data analysis workbench, including tools both within statistics and computational intelligence, together with supporting tools to enable system integration (Figure 2).

2.1. The patient's view of health care

The contacts between a patient and the health care management can be very different from time to time. This section presents a few examples of different interactions; see also Figure 3.

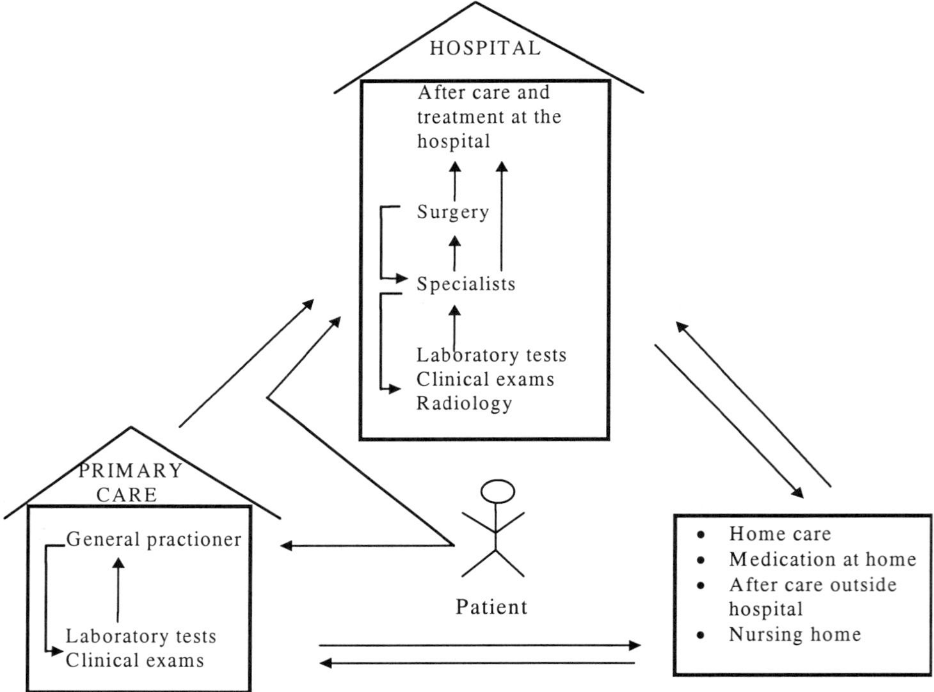

Figure 3. Different paths a patient can take through the health care system.

A patient can visit a health care center for two different reasons, either the patient has been summoned to preventative care or he/she is feeling sick. In both cases, a doctor will examine him/her and laboratory samples might be taken. If the doctor suspects a fracture somewhere, most health care centers are able to take X-rays. After the examination, the doctor makes a diagnosis and the patient is either sent home or referred to a hospital. The patient is sent home if he/she is healthy or if the treatment can be provided at home, (e.g., medication at home or home-care given by district nurses). If the patient is treated at home, he/she is often summoned to another visit to the doctor to make sure that treatment has given the expected results.

If the doctor at the health care center wants to consult specialists or if the patient needs treatment that cannot take place in the patient's home, the patient is referred to a hospital. A patient can also be directly admitted to a hospital e.g., if there has been an emergency. At the hospital specialists examine the patient, and laboratory tests and/or X-rays are taken. The hospital has the ability to perform surgery if needed, and the patients are often admitted to the hospital during a period of time for after care. In cases that are more difficult, the patient might need rehabilitation and to see a physiotherapist after the stay at the hospital. If a patient has a difficult chronic disease or is unable to take care of himself/herself, the patient might be admitted to a nursing home.

2.2. The clinician's view of health care

From the clinician's point of view, the travel through the health care system is to take the steps necessary for making the correct diagnosis as quickly as possible. On the way through the system, a patient can meet three different kinds of clinicians: the general practitioner, the specialist, and the surgeon.

In primary health care a general practitioner uses a computerized patient record system in order to store the information about a patient in a way that makes it easy to change, append, or retrieve. The general practitioner might also have access to education and/or information systems that act as assistants during the decision process. The systems in the primary health care are often local, and they can be different in different places. This makes it hard to compare and/or combine the data stored about a patient at a health care center and at a hospital.

The specialists at the hospitals have the same kind of supporting technology as the general practitioners. They can also have access to more sophisticated equipment such as CAT-scans (Computerized Axial Tomography) and decision support systems. When a specialist needs to consult other specialists, the contacts can be made using telecommunication systems.

Telecommunication can also be used by surgeons during operations. A specialist can be able to see and hear the actions in the operating theatre and be able to provide help and support without being there in person.

2.3. Case studies and scenarios

In this section we will present some case studies to illuminate the ways in which data and information are available and analyzed. Expert systems for some of the case studies have been developed and can be found on the World Wide Web; an example is shown in Figure 4. We refer to medical journals and books for more complete descriptions of diseases.

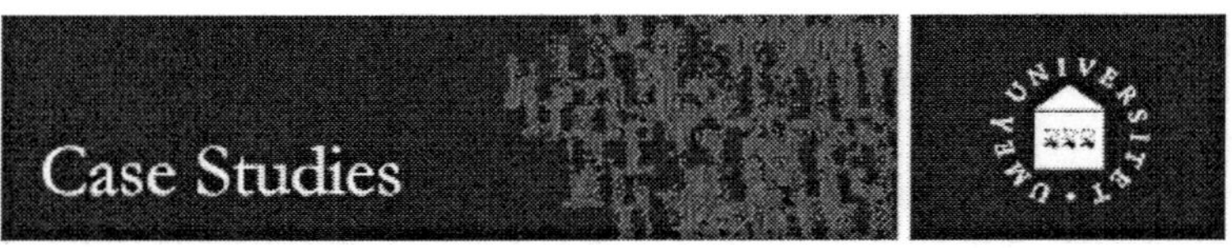

The GeDeMeDeS research group has contributed to the following cases (including ICD-9-CM codes):

Appendicitis
Down's syndrome (758.0)
Myocardial infarction
Nephropathia Epidemica (078.6)
Polycystic ovary syndrome (256.4)
Thyroedea
Urinary tract infection

Information on other case studies using DiagaiD and systems alike as performed by other groups will be made available also through this www-server as appropriate.

Respective case studies can also be reached through the ICD-9-CM classification system.

Back to:
[GeDeMeDeS main page] [Department of Computing Science] [Umeå university]

30-07-1996
Lena Kallin
(kallin@cs.umu.se)

Figure 4. Case studies on the World Wide Web[1].

2.3.1. Myocardial infarction

Myocardial infarction (MI) is the death of heart-muscle cells from reduced or obstructed blood flow through the coronary arteries. Traditionally, the diagnosis of MI is made using signs such as sweating, nausea, pain in the chest, changes in the ECG, and raised levels of biochemical markers. The symptoms can vary a great deal among different patients and thus various treatments are used in different stages of MI. The time factor is critical in the diagnosis process; 50% of the patients die within two hours after the first symptoms, so it is important to find a quick and reliable way to make the diagnosis.

The diagnosis of MI requires at least two of the following criteria: a history of characteristic chest pain, evolutionary changes on the ECG, or elevation of serial cardiac enzymes [2]. The values of the enzymes are

---

[1] This page can be found on the World Wide Web at the address:
  http://www.cs.umu.se/~medinfo/GeDeMeDeS/CaseStudies.html

measured from samples taken at regular intervals within the first 24 hours after the infarction. Markers used are, for instance, CK-MB, myoglobin, and tropinin.

In the case of MI, the level of CK-MB increases 2-3 hours after the MI has started, reaches a peak 10-24 hours after the MI, and returns to normal within 3-4 days afterward. The myoglobin level is increased 2-3 hours after the start, peaks at 6-9 hours, and returns to normal within 18-24 days. The value of troponin is increased at 4-6 hours, peaks at 10-24 hours, and is back to normal within 10-15 days.

Observations related to data as indicated above should be used as a basis for specifying combinations and transformations of data. Apart from data modeling, it is also interesting to investigate whether or not biological modeling, e.g., of CK-MB behavior, is possible. We know that the value of the markers increases, peaks, and decreases, but the values differ from patient to patient. Reasons for the different values are that the patients are seeking treatment at different stages of their MI. The treatment given, e.g., intravenous drip and/or drugs, affects the values, and physical activity can raise the level of CK-MB without being a sign of MI. Clearly, intravenous drip when started also needs to be considered in data modeling.

2.3.2. Down's syndrome

The most common form of the chromosomal abnormality, Down's syndrome, is also known as Trisomy 21, because it involves an extra copy of the 21st chromosome. Individuals with Down's syndrome possess varying degrees of mental retardation, from very mild to severe. Women over age 35 have a significantly increased risk of having a child with Down's syndrome. A 35-year-old woman has a one in 400 chance of conceiving a child with Down's syndrome, and this chance increases gradually to one in 110 by age 40. At age 45 the incidence becomes approximately one in 35 [9].

The most commonly used biochemical markers are AFP (alpha-foetoprotein) and hCG (human chorion gonadotropin), especially its free subunit, beta-hCG. There are several factors that have an influence on AFP and beta-hCG levels, e.g., insulin diabetes, race, smoking, and overweight of the mother. Therefore, it can be expected that when adding more anamnestic information to be taken into consideration, especially those known to have an influence on marker levels, it is possible to get more specific and sensitive information to find the group that is at risk of having a DS baby. A more detailed description of the syndrome, as far as data analysis is concerned, can be found in [7].

Based on computational methods as indicated in this chapter, we have implemented a decision support system [7] which evaluates a risk for the syndrome given the three inputs: the mother's age, AFP, and beta-hCG. The system shows improved performance over the multiple Gaussian formula, one of the most common statistical formulas used in software today.

2.4. Information organization

Large hospitals in the industrial countries store information about patients' health status, like laboratory test results, medications, and diagnoses, in vast databases. Many important medical observations have been done by studying patient history, and much more could be done if scientists would have faster and broader access to the knowledge that can be found in these huge databases.

Hospital information systems (HIS) are in practice focused on insertion and retrieval of data concerning one particular patient. The identifying key is usually the Social Security Number (especially in the Nordic countries) or a patient number. This makes it easy to find information about one single patient at the time. However, when conducting scientific research, there is a need for grouping patients together, combining symptoms, diagnoses and treatments. However, as HIS are not designed for this, the computer departments at the hospitals are forced to take an active part in the database searches. This makes data mining a complicated and time-consuming process. Our aim is to make it possible for the scientist to easily perform the data mining, with inexpensive tools.

We have, in other words, a "conflict" between the scientific and the administrative viewpoint in some cases. The administrative interest is to find information about one patient at a time, inserting or retrieving data concerning one particular patient. The scientific interest is, however, to combine information concerning patients' health status rather than focus on individual patients. Larger groups that have certain things, e.g., the same diagnosis, in common are the focus. Summarized information is also of interest for administrative purposes, but such information concerns e.g., how much an average patient costs or which hospital wards consume the most resources. The scientific viewpoint has generally not been considered when building the hospital databases, but this trend is changing.

Information/knowledge can be presented in many ways other than being found in hospital databases, viewed on on-line terminals, or printed on paper. There exists a wide variety of expert systems and information bases, but they are seldom connected to each other. Multimedia systems are also popular, but in many cases they can be described as merely presenting a book in a more fashionable way. However, there is huge potential in this approach, and one can only imagine the possibilities of, e.g., a virtual clinic. The textual information, pictures, laboratory test results, medications, diagnoses, and graphical interfaces together as a whole eventually form the data.

3. A medical information systems perspective

When characterizing medical information systems, we need to distinguish between user groups represented by patients typically using education systems and health care professionals. The latter group is subdivided into practitioners and administrators. In this work we focus on practitioners using systems that combine medical patient records with clinical information systems.

In particular we can consider a multimedia approach, e.g., to implement a web-like system for information found in any textbook of medicine. Note, however, that such a system is static and does not provide added value other than broader availability and (perhaps, but not obviously) faster navigation toward reaching some diagnosis.

Our focus in this chapter is to demonstrate the possibility of adding value to textual information by including disease specific expert systems arising from data analysis performed on data relevant to a particular disease. The extraction of data must, of course, be supported by extraction software connected to patient records or to some information pool collecting unidentifiable data from patient records, as described in Section 2.4.

In this section we will address the particular problem of decision making when arriving at a (differentiating) diagnosis for a patient. From a disease classification point of view, a disease can be seen as being within the ICD-9-CM International Classification of Diseases [10, 11]. (In Sweden the standard has been updated to ICD-10, but the underlying ideas described can still be applied.) A short printout from the Classification of Diseases is shown below.

Diseases of the Skin and Subcutaneous tissue (680-709)
Diseases of the Musculoskeletal System and Connective Tissue
(710-739)
Congenital Abnormalities (740-759)
Certain Conditions Originating in the Perinatal Period
(760-779)

The Down's Syndrome is a Congenital Abnormality and part
of the subgroup for Chromosomal Anomalies (with ICD-9-
CM code 758)

758 Chromosomal anomalies
    758.0 Down's syndrome
    758.1 Patau's syndrome
    758.2 Edwards' syndrome
    758.3 Autosomal deletion syndromes
    758.4 Balanced autosomal translocation in normal
        individual
    758.5 Other conditions due to autosomal anomalies
    758.6 Gonadal dysgenesis
    758.7 Klinefelter's syndrome
    758.8 Other conditions due to sex chromosome
        anomalies
    758.9 Conditions due to anomaly of unspecified
        chromosome

Under the Down's Syndrome subtitle, information about this particular
disease can be made available (Figure 5). In the extended view of a multimedia
information handbook, we need to present information not just related to
description of disease, but also to data material used and analyzed, data
analyses and knowledge acquisition algorithms used, and test results. Further,
the resulting expert system can also be included (Figure 6). The web view,
traversing from the ICD-9 list all the way down to specific information on a
particular disease, is presented in the following figures.

This demonstrates the availability of disease-specific information that can
be used for patients being "processed" with respect to questions concerning
Down's Syndrome. The data analysis and engineering task of developing
expert systems for particular diseases are initially discussed in Section 4 with a
focus on the computational view and further in Section 5 related to the
engineering task. It will be seen that a particular expert system can, in fact, be
generated in a fully automatic way, including data analysis as well as
generation code, both for the user interface as well as for the inference
mechanism of the expert system.

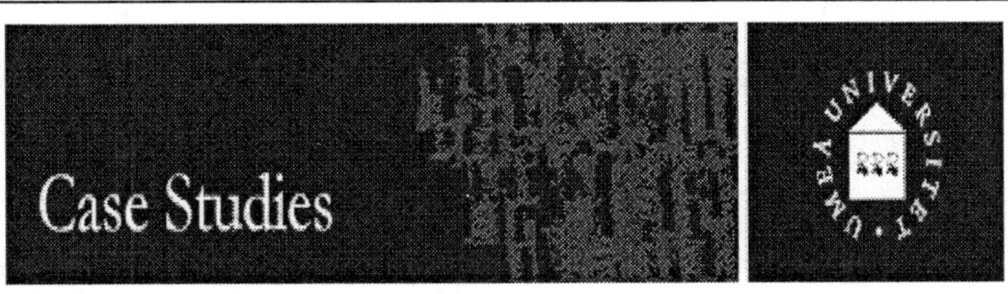

Many countries offer pregnant women the possibility of testing for Down's syndrome. Previously it was based on an early (in the second trimester) amniocentesis, which was preformed only on mothers over the age of 35. Biochemical screening methods have been developed elsewhere, which enables cost-effective screening for all mothers.

There are different numerical techniques used to interpret the results of the biochemical screening method. The goal is to calculate the risk for a chromosomal abnormality as exact as possible. Three techniques have been tested on data collected in Europe and USA. The techniques include the multiple Gaußian formula (MGF), the multi-layer perceptron (MLP), and the preprocessing perceptron (PPP), all using inputs related to the mother's age and the hormones AFP and free β-hCG.

Even if Wald's formula is one of the most common statistical formulas used in software today, the neural techniques MLP and PPP demonstrate improved performance, both in discriminance and detection rate.

- Description of the disease
- Material and Methods
- Results
- Discussion
- Contacts
- Expert system

Figure 5. Example of how information about a particular disease might look.

Note that in this particular "diagnosis" view, we have no support for the navigation process toward specifying an appropriate diagnosis. In differentiating diagnostics, a typical case occurs in infectious diseases, where patients' general symptoms of infections together with particular symptoms arising from the particular effects the virus applies to the body.

This immediately calls for an "ICD front-end" where a practitioner is supported in his/her navigation toward an appropriate diagnosis. The emphasis is on 'support' in the sense that the navigation process is highly interactive and strongly dependent on the expert. However, a well-structured intelligent front-end can provide a significant speed-up of the navigation process and act as a kind of watchdog for the consideration of all possible patient situations.

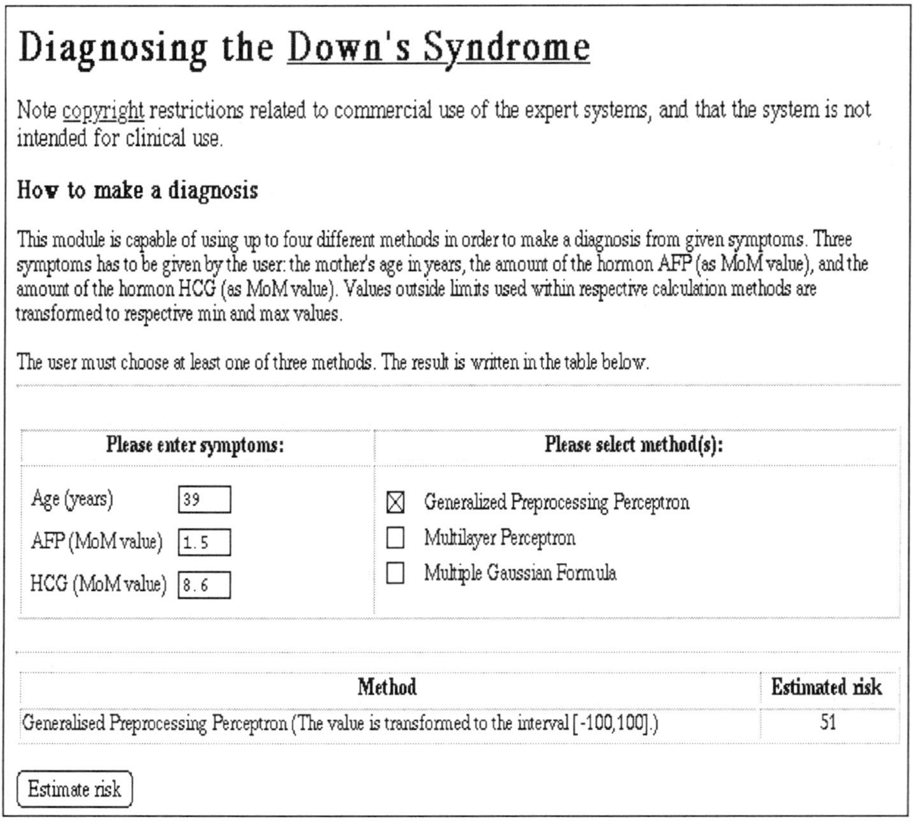

Diagnosing the Down's Syndrome

Note copyright restrictions related to commercial use of the expert systems, and that the system is not intended for clinical use.

How to make a diagnosis

This module is capable of using up to four different methods in order to make a diagnosis from given symptoms. Three symptoms has to be given by the user: the mother's age in years, the amount of the hormon AFP (as MoM value), and the amount of the hormon HCG (as MoM value). Values outside limits used within respective calculation methods are transformed to respective min and max values.

The user must choose at least one of three methods. The result is written in the table below.

Please enter symptoms:		Please select method(s):
Age (years) `39`	☒	Generalized Preprocessing Perceptron
AFP (MoM value) `1.5`	☐	Multilayer Perceptron
HCG (MoM value) `8.6`	☐	Multiple Gaussian Formula

Method	Estimated risk
Generalised Preprocessing Perceptron (The value is transformed to the interval [-100,100].)	51

[Estimate risk]

Figure 6. Example of how an expert system might look.

The front-end can also be seen as a pattern matching system, where input of clinical and laboratory information provides a list of possible diagnosis or diagnosis classes. When bounded to only a few possibilities for diagnosis, the system provides advice as to which diseases are more properly matched and which further measurements and examinations are recommended in order to arrive at higher certainty degrees with respect to a disease.

Overall, the system view as presented above aims at showing how particular expert systems, arranged within a disease classification schema, together with an appropriate front-end, can provide an innovative decision support as a Clinician's Workstation to aid experts in reaching a diagnosis more effectively and efficiently. An important observation is also that added value to the system in the form of developed expert systems is done by the experts themselves in the production line that is integrated into the system.

From the software organization point of view, the production line consists of three different modules. First, we have a data and information retrieval module to provide fast and comfortable extraction of patient data to prepare for and enable a variety of data analysis experiments. Second, we require a data analysis workbench, integrating and interconnecting our favorite data analysis tools. Most of these tools usually include structure identification facilities of different degrees of sophistication. Third, we envision the existence of system generation support.

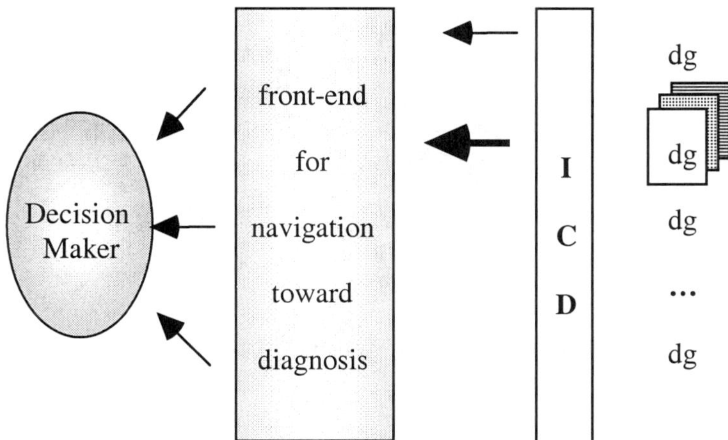

Figure 7. A model of the Clinician's Workstation.

Once the structures of the system are identified in the analysis phase, the domain expert needs to be relieved from technicalities in end-user system developments and integration.

4. Implementing an expert system

In this section we consider an isolated situation where we need to implement a particular expert system for a single diagnosis. The main question in any expert system is the following: Given symptoms and signs of a patient, how do we infer a diagnosis either in the form of a binary value (yes/no) or as a certainty degree?

The inputs need to be preprocessed/transformed before being entered into the feedforward structure. A pure linearization (or even binarization) that transforms data into the unit interval (or into symptom-ON/symptom-OFF binary values) is not sufficient for obtaining optimal success rates together with explainable parameters in feedforward systems. It is also important to note that laboratory and other methods are usually not uniform world-wide and differ from region to region. Thus, it is vitally important to be aware of, for example, which markers have been used for some particular laboratory tests and how the values have been transformed prior to insertion into the patient record systems.

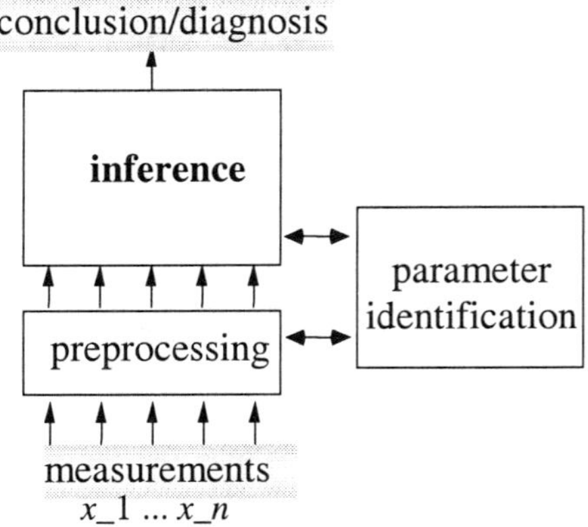

Figure 8. Preprocessing, feedforward, and learning.

Learning, or parameter identification, affects parameters not only in the feedforward mechanism but can (or should) be extended to also cover preprocessing. The selection of preprocessing functions relates to some extent to assumptions on probability distributions. As an example, the sigmoidal transformation functions,

$$g[\alpha,\beta](x) = \frac{1}{1+e^{-\beta(x-\alpha)}}$$

are obtained for exponential likelihood ratios

$$LR(x) = e^{\beta x}$$

as the transformation to probabilities gives

$$p = \frac{LR}{1+LR} = \frac{1}{1+\dfrac{1}{LR}}$$

Since the parameters for the transformation curves are trainable, what remains is the type of function to be used. Preprocessing is obviously separated from feedforward systems which can be understood from logical, numerical, or probabilistic perspectives. In addition, whatever feedforward style is selected, different learning algorithms can be applied as a pure parameter identification procedure. This is of course a very general statement and raises doubts, especially as far as the probabilistic networks are concerned. Logical and numerical style feedforward, however, can be seen to be strongly related [5], and indeed optimization techniques of various orders apply very similarly for neural-like structures as well as for rule bases [8]. In case of probabilistic networks, recent work [6] also use the feedforward independent parameter identification techniques.

The relation between numerical and logical feedforward is rather obvious. Suppose a transformed measurement, i.e., the logical value of the symptom, is given by S. From feedforward point of view, we need to determine a diagnosis value D, given some certainty value w with respect to a conclusion, i.e., we need to specify the $D = D(w, S)$. From the logical point of view, we reason it in the presence of w being specified as the implication in

$$S \overset{w}{\Rightarrow} D$$

In the approach using neural networks, we would have the implication semantics according to $D(w, S) = wS$.

$$y = \bigcup_i \varphi_i \left(w_i, g_i[\alpha_i, \beta_i] \cdot (x_i) \right)$$

As we realize the relation between numerical and logical feedforward, we arrive at the Generalized Preprocessing Perceptron. [1, 3, 4] have the structure shown in Figure 9, with respective dysjunction and implication operators.

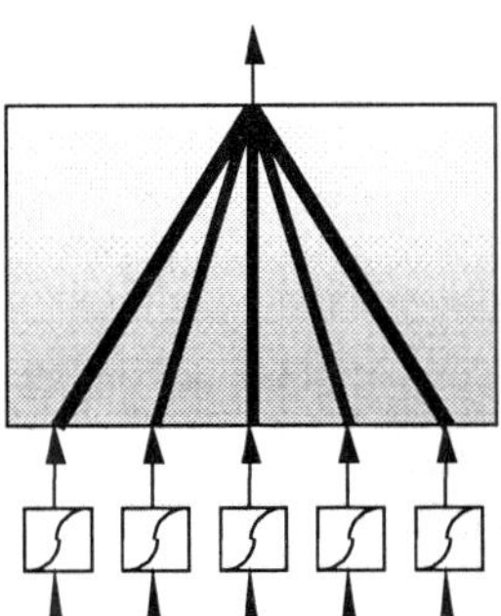

Figure 9. The Generalized Preprocessing Perceptron.

This should be compared with a preprocessing perceptron

$$y = act\left(\sum_i w_i \cdot g_i [\alpha_i, \beta_i] \cdot (x_i) \right)$$

wherein a logical interpretation of the weighted sum suddenly seems rather restricted. Of course, it is doubtful whether these simple networks can compete at all with multilayer perceptron. However, as has been demonstrated, e.g., in [3], preprocessing is clearly a key factor for obtaining high success rates. Even more so, several case studies show clearly that MLPs with only linear data preprocessing cannot outscore simpler networks provided with appropriate preprocessing. Reasons for this are certainly manifold, but one reason is obviously the monotonicity with respect to inputs of the feedforwarding function.

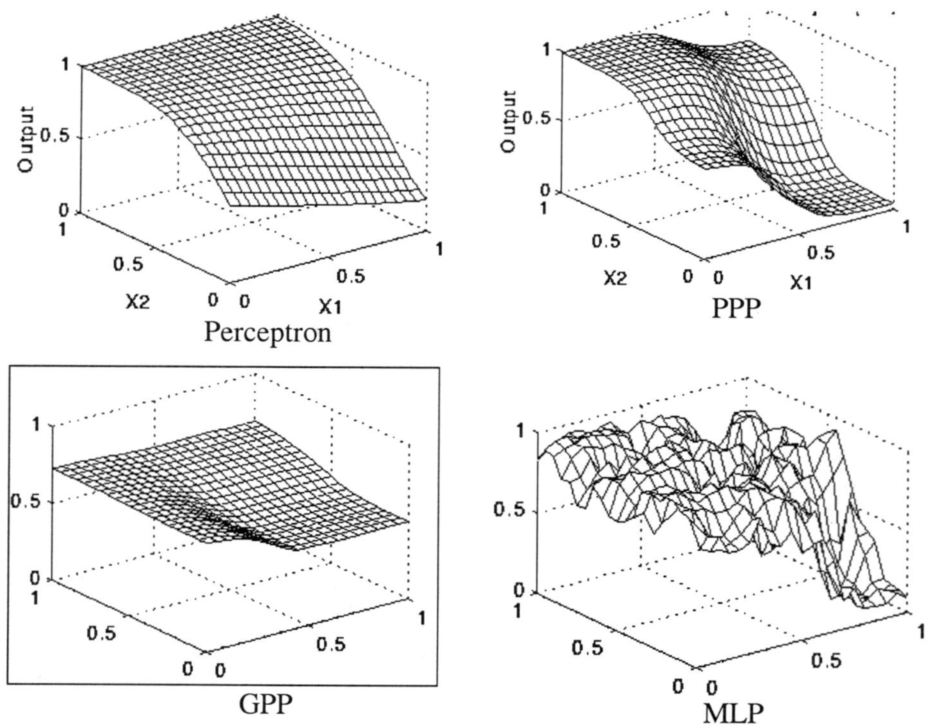

Figure 10. Comparison of surfaces for example networks.

We should also note that a single GPP is not the suggestion for a logical counterpart of multilayer perceptrons, but rather configurations thereof. It can be expected that such configurations significantly reduce the network size as compared to MLPs. In comparison Figure 10 shows surfaces for the classic networks represented by a perceptron, preprocessing perceptron (PPP), generalized preprocessing perceptron (GPP), and a multilayer perceptron (MLPs). The "point-chasing" capacity of MLPs is obvious and at the same time clearly undesirable. Certainly far from all MLPs are of this nature, but in network design we need to pay attention to, e.g., size of layers in order to find a reasonable trade-off between robustness and discriminating capacity.

Note that the basic motivation for using GPPs is clearly the ambition to obtain knowledge from each parameter in the network. Our experience shows that cut-off values in preprocessing functions are very evident and relate directly to reference values. Slope values are more difficult to interpret but still give reasonable information. As for the inference mechanism, the subject is important for knowledge modeling, but for diagnostics, the role of logical concepts is not obvious.

To conclude this section we point out that whatever feedforward style adopted, corresponding software tools should support parameter identification and code generation to contribute to the automation of the production line.

5. The architecture of the Clinician's Workstation

As described in Section 3, the Clinician's Workstation consists of a lot of small decision-support systems connected together in an "ICD front-end" and the purpose of the system is to speed up the navigation process toward an appropriate diagnosis. This section will describe the architecture of the Clinician's Workstation in general and then give a more thorough description of the architecture of the production line.

5.1. The Clinician's Workstation

The system is built out of a large number of small modules. Each one of these small modules is capable of estimating the risk factor for a given disease. The modules are connected together in a system with a graphical interface showing the possible diseases and the risk factor for each one. For a description of how the modules are built and connected to the system, see Section 5.2. The graphics changes as the user presents new facts to the system and the clinician can interact and decide how the results should be presented. The system is able to give support and advice concerning what test or examination to do next.

As a prototype Clinician's Workstation, we experimented with a World Wide Web structure (see also Section 3) where the user can find the ICD-9-CM classification system. From there, the user can navigate toward more information about the disease and find an expert system giving a risk value for the specific disease.

5.2. The production line

The general outline of the production line is shown in Figure 11. In the extraction phase the data are extracted from the information bank and pre-processed into forms that are easy for a computer to work with. In the analysis step, the data are analyzed and a decision support system is trained. The resulting decision support system is integrated in the Clinician's Workstation at the synthesis step of the production line.

In this section, we describe the architecture of the production line, using Down's syndrome as an illustrative example. The following subsections show the progress from raw data to a decision-support system, which is integrated in the Clinician's Workstation.

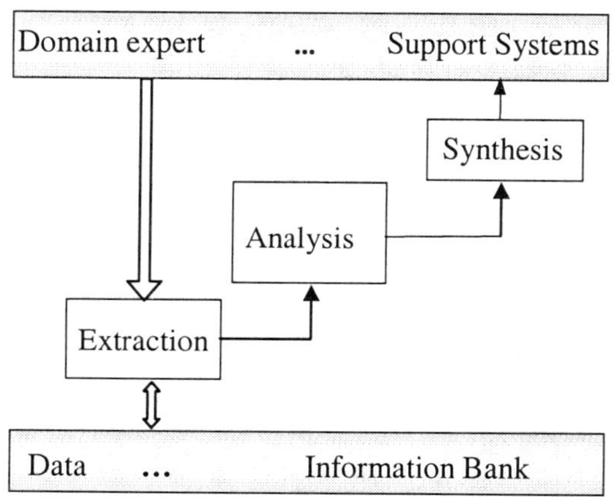

Figure 11. Decision-support systems production line.

5.2.1. The extraction phase

In this phase the goal is to obtain data for later use. The clinician gives a physical disease description of the expected symptoms, signs to the system, and specifies the amount of data needed. This is done by selecting diagnosis from a lookup table (in our case, we want information about only one diagnosis: Down's Syndrome), selecting the measurements needed (the age and the values of the hormones AFP and beta-hCG), and perhaps also giving some restricting criteria (e.g., only female patients with age in the range 15 to

50). It is also possible to tell the system to get data only if the measurement lies in a specified interval.

A specification file is generated from the given disease description and this file is used to create an extraction program for the given database (the database program can be written in SQL, MUMPS, etc.). The data returned from the database is in raw format and might contain empty fields and sometimes unnecessary information depending on the structure of the database. The clinician is able to give the system instructions as how to organize and combine the data in order to produce the expected data files. This phase of the production line is implemented as prototype software that has been in use at, e.g., Turku University Central Hospital.

5.2.2. The analysis phase

When the data has been extracted, the analysis phase begins. In this phase, the data is used to construct a decision support system for the given disease. The analysis tools used can be statistical, logical, neural, or hybrids of two or more approaches (see Section 4 for more details). In this part, the clinician has a toolbox with different approaches at hand and can easily test and evaluate different decision support systems. The generalized preprocessing perceptron has also been implemented and used in data analysis. Regardless of what system the clinician chooses, the result is a set of parameters that has to be conformed into a module and integrated in the Clinician's Workstation.

5.2.3. The synthesis phase

Finally, the information from the analysis part must be integrated into the existing system during the synthesis phase. Assume that the clinician has decided to use the generalized preprocessing perceptron (GPP) as a decision support system for the Down's syndrome. The analysis phase has produced parameters telling what kind of functions to use in the GPP and the values of the parameters in the network.

When automatically creating a decision support system module, the following happens: the parameters, given by the program, are written as constants into an include-file. The include-file is linked together with a template program in order to produce a new instance of the GPP-program in C-code, specialized for the Down's syndrome.

The integration into the existing system (the World Wide Web pages) is made by a program using template HTML-pages and the program given to construct a graphical user interface for the decision support system module. The program also makes information pages providing a short description of the disease and an explanation of the materials and methods used. A page presenting the results is also made by the converting program. Finally, an index-file for the disease is constructed (i.e., the index-file for Down's Syndrome as shown in Figure 5). All this can be performed automatically and the resulting files written in a special library, then moved to the web-servers file system. All that is left to do is to make a link between the name of the disease in the ICD-file and the index-file in the library.

6. Conclusions

In this chapter we presented the information flow through a health care system and examples of how clinicians use supporting technology in their work. We proposed a production line for generating decision support systems and showed a case study of how such a system would look.

We discussed how a decision support system would be built and described the generalized preprocessing perceptron. In order to compare different kinds of networks, we looked at the surfaces of example networks and pointed out the smoothness of the preprocessing perceptron as compared to the "point-chasing" capacity of multilayer networks.

The architecture of a workstation was depicted that combines data mining tools with analysis tools in building new decision support systems and automatically integrates the new system into a diagnosis classification skeleton. The workstation is intended to support fast and efficient navigation toward a correct diagnosis; it consists of modules, each able to support the diagnosis of a specific disease. The use of various soft-computing techniques at various levels of such health care systems is discussed in several of the subsequent chapters.

References

[1]   Anttila, L., Eklund, P., Kallin, L., Koskinen, P., and Penttilä, T-A., The generalized preprocessing perceptron for medical data analysis: a case study for the polycystic ovary syndrome, *Proceedings of EMCSR '96* (Ed. R. Trappl), Vienna, Austria, April 9-14, 1996, 597-602.

[2]   Apple, F.S., Acute myocardial infarction and coronary reperfusion - serum cardiac markers for the 1990s, *A. J. C. P.*, Vol. 97, No. 2, 1992.

[3]   Eklund, P., Network size versus preprocessing, *Fuzzy Sets, Neural Networks and Soft Computing* (Eds. R. Yager, L. Zadeh), Van Nostrand, NY; 1994: 250-264.

[4]   Eklund, P. and Forsström, J., Computational intelligence for laboratory information systems, *Scandinavian Journal of Clinical Laboratory Investigations,* Vol. 55 (222), 1995, 21-31.

[5]   Eklund, P. and Klawonn, F., Neural fuzzy logic programming, *IEEE Transactions of Neural Networks*, 1992; 3: 815-818.

[6]   Jensen, F., *An Introduction to Bayesian Networks*, UCL Press Limited, 1996.

[7]   Kallin, L., Räty, R., Selén, G., and Spencer, K., A comparison of numerical risk computational techniques in screening for Down's Syndrome, *International Conference on Artificial Neural Networks, Industrial Conference (Medicine),* Paris, France, 9-13 October 1995.

[8]   Zhou, J. and Eriksson, J., Suitability of fuzzy controller fine-tuning: a case study for a chemical plant, *Proceedings of EMCSR '96* (Ed. R. Trappl), Vienna, Austria, April 9-14, 1996, 324-328.

[9]   http://www.ndss.org/gen.html. (The homepage of the National Down Syndrome Society).

[10]   ICD-9, Klassifikation av sjukdomar 1987 - Systematisk förteckning, Socialstyrelsen   1986. ICD-10, Klassifikation av sjukdomar och hälsoproblem 1997, Socialstyrelsen, 1997.

[11]   Homepage for the Central Office on ICD-9-CM has the address http://www.icd-9-cm.org/index.html.

Chapter 6

Intelligent diagnostic systems in maternal and fetal medicine

Sinan Beksac, Aydan J. Erkmen , Sezer Aksel, Ugur Halici,
Kemal Leblebicioglu, Meral Beksac, Volkan Atalay, and
Lakhmi C. Jain

The aim of maternal and fetal medicine is to reduce perinatal morbidity and mortality as much as possible. This can be achieved by diagnosing genetical disorders and fetal health problems at an early stage. The easy availability of low-cost, high-capacity microcomputers has facilitated the development of artificial intelligent diagnostic systems. These systems are intended to overcome problems arising from the application of low-level decision-making systems depending on classical medical practice and conventional bio-statistics to manage such ill-defined, complicated biological phenomena. Application of better data acquisition, feature extraction (signal/image processing), classification, and automation techniques will enable the development of more efficient intelligent diagnostic systems. We believe that these intelligent systems will bring objectivity to clinical decision making and will take their place in the field of maternal and fetal medicine.

1. Introduction

The structure of medical data used in decision making in routine clinical practice is complicated. In most cases the exact biological rationale behind the medical parameters are multifactorial, and subjective approaches are, therefore, used in order to make a medical decision. This lack of objectivity necessitates the application of intelligent systems. Progress in technology enabled scientists to use computerized systems in medicine [13, 15, 17, 19, 25, 26, 56, 64, 68]. The accepted roles of computers have expanded from the traditional data retrieval, storage, and processing to the area of what is often called intelligent systems [4-7, 9, 11, 14, 16]. Recently, simple decision-making programs have been replaced by intelligent learning systems which utilize various medical data in different forms according to the medical discipline [6, 7, 11, 16].

One of the most important issues is obtaining reliable medical parameters (features) with which to set up the systems [3], [8], [10], [12], [29]. In earlier systems, features defined by medical experts were widely used and reasonable results obtained [3, 8, 10, 12, 13, 18, 19, 26, 29, 64]. However, limitations inherent in the previous approaches forced the development of automatic data processing to obtain better features [4-6, 9, 11, 14]. Various signal and image processing methods were then introduced for improved reliability [3, 4, 6, 8, 12, 14, 29]. Neural networks and adaptive fuzzy systems brought new dimensions to this field and intelligent systems that improve their decision-making capability through learning were developed [5-11, 14, 16]. In this chapter, various applications of such intelligent systems to routine clinical practice in maternal and fetal medicine are presented.

2. Data structure and decision making in maternal and fetal medicine

Decision making in "Maternal and Fetal Medicine" is composed of various subsystems and their components [10]. The first subsystem is data acquisition and feature extraction. Table 1 shows the usual sources used for gathering the necessary information. The structure of this data is very complex and heterogeneous. Hereditary and obstetrical information as well as signs, symptoms, and physical examination findings make up part of the main data used in decision making. However, the main tool in decision making is fetal observation, and fetus-originated data is essential for a correct diagnosis. Mother-originated information plays a secondary role in predicting fetal well-being [10].

The purpose of "Prenatal Diagnosis" is to eradicate genetic disorders [11]. Measurements of some biochemical markers in maternal blood, fetal ultrasonography, fetal karyotyping, and application of molecular genetics methodologies together constitute the data collection procedures for prenatal diagnosis [7, 11]. On the other hand, the situation is slightly different with "Perinatal Surveillance" data [28]. The fetus is our patient, but there are serious limitations in approaching the fetus. The clinical goal is to detect fetal hypoxia in order to prevent perinatal morbidity or mortality [10]. Perinatal surveillance starts with detailed fetal imaging using ultrasonography [14]. Following this are the other fetal-monitoring technologies [4, 5, 16]. The ideal data are acid-base measurements via fetal blood sampling [10]. However, fetal blood sampling is an invasive procedure and must be performed as a final resort. Fetal blood sampling enables biochemical measurements as well as acid-base measurements resulting in numerical data.

The technology used in perinatal surveillance necessitates image processing and the processing of various fetus-originated signals. Various transducers and sensors are used to collect fetal data in order to estimate or predict fetal well-being [5, 9, 16].

Table 1. Types of medical data in maternal and fetal medicine

Information Obtained by Questioning
- Family History
- Personal Information

Data Obtained by Inspection and Observation

Data Obtained by Physical Examination

Laboratory Findings
- Biochemical Measurements
- Data Obtained by Imaging Techniques (Obstetrics and Fetal Ultrasonography)
- Data Obtained by Cytogenetics and Molecular Genetics Techniques

Fetus-Originated Signals and Related Data
- Fetal Monitoring (Antepartum Fetal Heart Rate Testing $\cong$ Non-Stress Testing)
- Doppler Velocimetry
- Others (Fetal ECG, Pulse Oximetry, Laser and Infrared Spectroscopy)

There are two main problems associated with the data used in decision making. The first is the type of data. The medical expert uses his/her clinical experience to sift through patient history, signs, symptoms, clinical findings, images, and laboratory results during the course of decision making. Medical expert decision making uses subjective, objective, and heuristical tools, and needs some bio-statistical support (Tables 1 and 2). The second problem is the predictive values of these data. Some data are clear-cut in decision making, as in fetal karyotyping. However, in most cases, representative values and the predictive roles of the data are limited or unclear.

Table 2. Type of data used in decision making

Specific Data 　　　　e.g., Results of Karyotyping Studies. **Fuzzy Data** 　　　　e.g., Blood Flow Velocity Waveforms **Probabilistic Data** 　　　　e.g., Triple Test Results

The data used in prenatal diagnosis and perinatal surveillance are different, and each should be handled in a different way [5, 7, 11, 16]. In prenatal diagnosis the medical expert is looking for chromosomal abnormalities, gene disorders, and congenital abnormalities; hence, the results of diagnostic tools are more reliable and clear-cut [11]. The result of fetal karyotyping clearly describes any chromosomal abnormality, and the same is true with molecular genetics methodologies in describing gene disorders. Ultrasonography gives well-defined results in describing congenital abnormalities [14]. Less clear-cut are biochemical markers of maternal serum, which are used in prenatal screening [7]. Here, the predictive values of these markers are unclear, and more sophisticated approaches are needed in order to achieve successful results. High levels of education and training are necessary in the field of prenatal diagnosis, which is limited to certain high-risk pregnancies. Trained medical staff does not have much difficulty in decision making. Intelligent diagnostic systems are necessary when the medical staff is not sufficiently trained in this area. Fetal ultrasonography and evaluation of metaphase chromosomes are the province of well-trained medical experts [11, 14]. Image processing and analysis technologies may compensate for the absence of such medical experts [4, 30]. However, there is a serious problem with prenatal screening programs which are widely used in routine practice by less experienced medical units [7]. Mother-originated data are sometimes used in predicting fetal genetic disorders or maternal ovulation day for HCG administration for the artificial insemination in the conception phase of a fetus. The reliability of this data is insufficient, and so there is a need for more advanced decision-making methodologies.

The situation in perinatal surveillance is completely different. The goal is to detect fetal hypoxia or a decrease in essential nutrients due to maternal health problems, such as hypertensive states of pregnancy and carbohydrate metabolism disorders in pregnancy [10]. Normally the fetus is healthy but at risk due to maternal and utero-placental factors. As described above, fetal blood sampling and acid-base measurements are effective in diagnosing fetal hypoxia at a later stage, but are not preferable because of their invasive nature. Furthermore, these measurements require a high level of experience and training. Noninvasive methodologies must be employed in perinatal surveillance by inexperienced medical staff. This medical practice is employed for all pregnancies and is usually used to select fetuses at risk. However, high-risk pregnancies should be under perinatal surveillance programs right from the beginning.

The fetus is our patient, but direct communication with such a patient is not possible; nor is it possible to examine it at close proximity. The medical staff reaches a fetus by imaging techniques, usually with fetal ultrasonography [14]. This means that fetal medicine requires advanced technology in order to reach its patient. High-resolution ultrasound transducers enable better fetal evaluations [4-5, 9, 14]. Recent fetometric studies enable obstetricians to detect intrauterine growth retardation. The aim is to detect growth-retarded fetuses and hypoxia in order to prevent unwanted fetal losses. This necessitates the use of various fetus-originated signals and images in order to decide upon the timing of the delivery. One should deliver the fetus before irreversible tissue damage occurs due to long-term hypoxia resulting in acidemia. There are various perinatal surveillance methodologies for this purpose, such as Doppler Velocimetry, Antepartum (AP) Fetal Heart Rate (FHR) testing (nonstress testing), fetal electrocardiography, pulse oximetry, and laser/infrared spectroscopy [5, 16]. All these methodologies need advanced techniques for data acquisition. Due to technical limitations, only Doppler velocimetry and AP-FHR testing are widely used in clinical practice [4-5, 9, 13-14, 16]. The problem with these methodologies is the nature of the acquired data. Although these data are the results of advanced fetal monitors and ultrasound technology, the biological rationale behind them is unclear [5, 9-10, 16].

The FHR signals obtained by AP-FHR testing and blood flow velocity waveforms obtained by Doppler velocimetry necessitate various signal/image processing and analysis techniques for better feature extraction [3-4, 8, 29]. Medical experts have serious difficulties in the interpretation of such data. Classical bio-statistics is also limited in the evaluation of Doppler velocimetry and AP-FHR testing data. At this point pattern recognition and intelligent diagnostic systems become necessary [5, 9-10].

3. Intelligent techniques

The so-called "knowledge-based" and "intelligent" techniques are those that are inspired by understanding information processing in biological systems. The popular intelligent techniques are expert systems, neural networks, fuzzy logic, genetic algorithms, chaos engineering, and the fusion of various techniques. The basic idea is to design systems that can mimic the performance of a human expert by transferring his/her expertise to the computer in a limited way [41].

3.1. Signal processing and feature extraction

3.1.1. Signal processing

Decision-making systems base their decisions on the available "information" already stored in databases that reflect *a priori* experiences and experiments and the information extracted from incoming data. In order to reach better decisions, one has to obtain the features of patterns to be identified which are implicit in the given data. It is possible to work directly on the original data as well as its transformed representations. Input data or signals are transformed to construct new signals from which it may be possible to obtain more or better features to characterize the signal pattern.

Many signals are nonstationary (or "evolutionary"). The power spectrum of a signal can be time varying. For example, radar signals with frequency modulation have a time-dependent spectrum. In speech, the formant frequencies vary for different segments of a spoken word. A complete characterization of nonstationary signals in the frequency domain must, therefore, include the time aspect, resulting in the time-frequency (TF) analysis of a signal. Among the most prominent TF transforms are the short-time Fourier transform [23], the Wigner distribution [23], and the wavelet transform [22, 24].

In the last ten years, time-frequency analysis [23], and in particular the wavelet transform [22, 24], has become indispensable in all kinds of signal processing jobs. To account for the special importance of wavelet analysis in signal processing and feature extraction, a short section is included here to give basic definitions about wavelets, together with an historical development of the subject.

The wavelet transform

Starting with the announcement by J. Fourier in 1807 that any periodic function can be represented as a series of sines and cosines, the spectral analysis of functions using Fourier series and integrals has been the source of numerous mathematical problems [33]. In general these problems could be simplified so that it was impossible to describe the local properties of functions in terms of their spectral properties, which could be viewed as an expression of the Heisenberg uncertainty principle. Other problems arise because Fourier series may diverge in many of the usual function spaces.

Similar difficulties appear in the areas of analog and digital signal processing, particularly when signals represent evolutionary phenomena. Engineers as well as mathematicians have investigated and tested analytic methods that were better adapted to their problems and that attempted to avoid the difficulties inherent in the classical Fourier analysis. Some of these methods were very close to spectral analysis. For example, D. Gabor introduced a "sliding-window" technique [34]. He first multiplied the signal by a "window," for which he used a Gaussian function g and then calculated its Fourier transform. Thus the analyzing function becomes

$$g_{a,b}(x) = e^{jax}g(x\text{-}b), \quad a,b \in \Re \tag{1}$$

which is a "time-frequency" expression. While these methods are useful for certain applications, this analyzing function has the disadvantage that its spatial resolution is limited by the fixed size of the Gaussian envelope.

In the early 1980s, J. Morlet, who was a geophysicist, had the idea to base the analysis on one function, h, that would be well localized in both time and frequency [54]. This function, which Morlet called a "wavelet," was then dilated and translated to form a family of analyzing functions. These are normalized as follows:

$$h_{a,b}(x) = a^{-\frac{1}{2}} h(\frac{x-b}{a}), a \in \Re^{+}, b \in \Re \tag{2}$$

With this technique, small values of the parameter *a* provide a local analysis of f and the function of two variables,

$$WT_{f}(a,b) = \int a^{-\frac{1}{2}} f(x) h^{*}(\frac{x-b}{a}) \, dx = <f, h_{a,b}> \tag{3}$$

where h^* is the complex conjugate of h and a time-scale representation of $f(x)$ called a "continuous time wavelet transform." If the wavelet h satisfies the admissibility condition

$$C_h = 2\pi \int \frac{|H(w)|}{|w|} dw < \infty \tag{4}$$

where H is the Fourier transform of h, that is

$$H(w) = \int h(x)e^{-jwt} dt \tag{5}$$

then the transform can be inverted with the reconstruction formula

$$f(x) = \frac{1}{C_h} \iint WT_f(a,b) \, h_{a,b}(x) \frac{1}{a^2} dadb \tag{6}$$

An interesting property of this formula is that it converges in many function spaces where the Fourier transform fails to do so.

In 1985 Y. Meyer discovered [52] (by carefully choosing the analyzing function and by taking $a = 2^j$ and $b = 2^j k$, $(j,k \in Z)$ as discrete values for the parameters a and b) that one could obtain orthonormal bases for $L^2(R)$ (i.e., square integrable functions), of the type

$$\Psi_{j,k}(x) = 2^{j/2} \Psi(2^j x - k), \; j,k \in Z \tag{7}$$

and the expression

$$f = \sum_{j,k \in Z} < f, \Psi_{j,k} > \Psi_{j,k} \tag{8}$$

for decomposing a function in these orthonormal wavelets converged in many function spaces. In Equation (8) the expression

$$< f, \;_{j,k} > = DWT_f(j,k) = 2^{j/2} \int (2^j x - n) f(x) dx \tag{9}$$

is called a "discrete wavelet transform" of f.

A particular example of orthonormal wavelets has been known for a long time and was first introduced by A. Haar in 1910 [36]. Unfortunately the Haar wavelets are discontinuous and consequently poorly localized in frequency.

S. Mallat made a decisive step in the theory of wavelets in 1987 when he proposed a fast algorithm for the computation of wavelet coefficients [48]. He identified his algorithm with pyramidal schemes that decompose signals into subbands. These techniques were developed by several engineers in the 1970s to reduce quantization noise. The framework that unifies these algorithms and the theory of wavelets is the concept of a multiresolution analysis. Briefly a multiresolution analysis is an increasing sequence of closed, nested subspaces $\{V_j\}_{j\in Z}$ that tends to $L^2(\Re)$ as j increases. In addition, one assumes that V_j is obtained from V_{j+1} by a dilation of factor 2, and there exists a function φ whose $\{\varphi(x\text{-}k)\}_{k\in Z}$ form is an orthonormal basis for V_0. It follows that φ satisfies a relation of the form

$$\varphi(x) = 2 \sum_{n\in Z} h_n \varphi(2x - n) \tag{10}$$

where h_n is a coefficient that may take complex values. This "two-scale" equation plays an essential role in the theory of wavelet bases. By writing

$$\Psi(x) = 2 \sum_{n\in Z} (-1)^n h^*_{1-n} \varphi(2x - n) \tag{11}$$

one generates a function whose translated form $\{\Psi(x\text{-}k)\}_{k\in Z}$ is an orthonormal basis for the orthogonal complement W_0 of V_0, in V_1. It follows that the complete family $\{\Psi_{j,k}\}_{j,k\in Z}$, as defined by Equation (7) forms a Hilbert basis for $L^2(\Re)$. All known wavelet bases are obtained this way. Thus the scaling function φ, which is sometimes called the father wavelet, plays a key role in this theory. Linear combinations of its translated form provide the "V_0-approximation" for functions f in $L^2(\Re)$, while the scaled form of the function ψ carries the details that allow the approximations to be refined to the next scale, that is, to the "V_1-approximation."

On the other hand, the algorithms identified by S. Mallat use discrete, sampled data that are analyzed as if they were "approximation coefficients" $h_n = <f(.), \varphi(.\text{-}k) >$ at a scale of $j = 0$. As a consequence of relations (10) and (11), Mallat's algorithms depend on the coefficients h_n rather than on the functions φ and Ψ. In turn these coefficients are identified with the impulse response of a conjugate quadrature filter (CQF) whose transfer function $m_0(w)$ satisfies the relation

$$\left|m_0(w)\right|^2 + \left|m_0(w + x^*)\right|^2 = 1 \tag{12}$$

These filters were introduced by Smith. Their complete classification, when the coefficients h_n are real and finite numbers, was given by I. Daubechies in the context of constructing wavelet bases with compact support [24].

3.1.2. Feature extraction

Feature extraction and data projection are two important issues in pattern recognition and exploratory data analysis [65]. Feature extraction can eliminate the *curse of dimensionality*, improve the generalization ability of classifiers, and reduce the computational requirements of pattern classification. Data projection enables us to visualize high dimensional data in order to better understand the underlying structure, explore the intrinsic dimensionality, and analyze the clustering tendency of multivariate data. Consequently feature extraction and data projection have received considerable attention for the past 25 years, and hundreds of methods have been developed in various branches of pattern recognition. In the early approaches, statistical techniques were quite popular. In recent years the tendency is toward a) the use of neural networks for feature extraction [44, 51], b) the fusion of classical and modern approaches such as performing linear/nonlinear discriminant analysis using multilayer perceptrons [69], and c) the use of new techniques in signal processing to form new structural methods for feature extraction [10, 16, 40, 60].

Mathematically, feature extraction and/or data projection can be formulated as a mapping ψ from an n-dimensional input space to an m-dimensional output space,

$$\psi: \Re^n \rightarrow \Re^m, \ m<n \tag{13}$$

such that some criterion C is optimized. This formulation is similar to a function approximation problem where the mapping function is estimated from training patterns, which are input-output pairs whose desired outputs are known. In feature extraction and data projection, however, the desired outputs are often not available even for supervised approaches (e.g., linear discriminant analysis). Feature selection, which is used for choosing an optimal subset of features, can be viewed as a special case of feature extraction where ψ is a linear $m\times n$ permutation matrix. For data visualization purposes, the value of m is usually set to two or three.

A large number of approaches for feature extraction and data projection are available in the pattern recognition literature [51, 65]. These approaches differ from each other in the characteristics of the mapping ψ, how ψ is learned, and what optimization criterion C is used. The mapping function can be either linear or nonlinear and can be learned through either supervised or unsupervised methods. The combination of these two factors results in the following four categories of feature extraction and data projection: i) supervised linear, ii) supervised nonlinear, iii) unsupervised linear, and iv) unsupervised nonlinear. Within each category the methods differ in the criteria function C being used. In general, linear methods are attractive because they require less computation than nonlinear methods and analytical solutions are often available for linear methods. On the other hand, nonlinear methods are more powerful. But since their analytical solutions are often not available, a numerical optimization method must be used in order to obtain the solution. This is usually computationally demanding. Furthermore the optimization procedure often gets trapped into a local minimum. It is also generally true that supervised methods perform better than unsupervised methods.

Various neural networks, including self-organizing feature maps (SOM) [44] and multilayer perceptrons (MLP) [30, 69], are used for feature extraction and data projection. The principal component analysis (PCA) is one of the most important classical techniques, and it is still among the most powerful and frequently used techniques in feature extraction [32].

Principal component analysis (PCA)

PCA, also called the Karhunen-Loeve (K-L) transform, is a well-known statistical method for feature extraction, data compression, and multivariate data projection. PCA has been widely used in communication, signal and image processing, pattern recognition, and data analysis. It is a linear orthogonal transform from an n-dimensional input space to an m-dimensional space, $m \leq n$ such that the coordinates of the data in the new m-dimensional spaces are uncorrelated and a maximal amount of the variance of the original data is preserved by only a small number of coordinates [39, 45].

PCA finds the representation of the input vectors in terms of the eigenvectors of their covariance matrix. Given an ensemble of M real-valued vectors, $\mathbf{x}^k \in \Re^n$, $1 \leq k \leq M$, their covariance matrix $\mathbf{R}_x$ is calculated as

$$\mathbf{R}_x = \frac{1}{M} \sum_{k=1}^{M} (\mathbf{x}^k - \hat{\mathbf{x}})(\mathbf{x}^k - \hat{\mathbf{x}})^T \tag{14}$$

where

$$\hat{\mathbf{x}} = \frac{1}{M} \sum_{k=1}^{M} \mathbf{x}^{k} \tag{15}$$

The unit length eigenvectors of $\mathbf{R}_x$ are the orthogonal basis for the K-L transform and are obtained by solving the following equation:

$$\mathbf{R}_x \Psi = \Psi \Lambda \tag{16}$$

where Λ is a diagonal matrix having the eigenvalues of $\mathbf{R}_x$ for its diagonal elements and Ψ is the modal matrix having eigenvectors of $\mathbf{R}_x$ for its columns ordered in decreasing eigenvalues, $\lambda_1, \lambda_2, .., \lambda_n$. After determining Ψ, the K-L transform of any vector can be found as follows:

$$\nu = \Psi^{T} \mathbf{x} \tag{17}$$

Reducing Ψ to Ψ^{m} by eliminating the last $(n\text{-}m)$ eigenvectors results in an m-dimensional subspace spanned by the remaining m eigenvectors in Ψ^{m}. The subspace spanned by these eigenvectors is called the "principal subspace." The components of the projection of a vector into the principal subspace are called the "principal components." This results in dimensionality reduction if Ψ^{m} is used instead of Ψ in Equation (17). If the mth eigenvalue is small when compared to the first eigenvalue, the principal components carry approximately the same information as the original vector, although the dimensionality is reduced. It is easy to show that the covariance matrix of the transformed data is a diagonal matrix, $\text{diag}(\lambda_1, \lambda_2, .., \lambda_m)$, which means that the components of the transferred data are uncorrelated [65]. The variance of the original data retained in the new m-dimensional space is

$$\text{var} = \sum_{i=1}^{m} \ddot{e}_i \tag{18}$$

which is the largest retained value among all linear orthogonal transforms of the same output dimensionality. PCA is optimal in the mean square sense among all orthogonal linear transforms.

3.2. Decision making

3.2.1. Expert systems (ES)

The growing popularity of applied artificial intelligence (AI) has resulted in the implementation of extremely complex "rule-based" systems [20, 21, 38, 70]. Often such expert systems are being used either in critical environments where hazards can occur, the safety of a crew is an issue, or in transporting expert information to inexperienced people. Most often, expert systems are constructed and implemented without any formal analysis of the dynamics of how they interface with their environment or how the inference mechanism works over the information in the rule base. Currently many expert systems are evaluated a) in an empirical manner by comparing the expert system against human experts, b) by studying reliability and user friendliness, or c) by examining the results of extensive simulations. The basic structure of a rule-based expert decision making is illustrated in Figure 1.

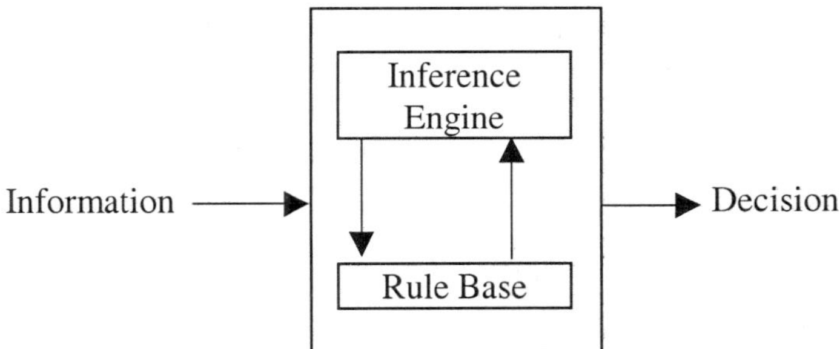

Figure 1. Basic structure of a rule-based system.

The rules R in the rule base are usually of the following form:

R: IF A, THEN B,

where the action B can be taken only if A is evaluated as being true. The inference mechanism usually consists of three general functional components [20].

1. **Match Phase:** The premises of the rules are matched to the current facts and to data stored in the rule base. The set of the enabled rules is called the "conflict set."

2. **Select Phase:** One rule is selected from the conflict set, and it is fired.
3. **Act Phase:** The actions indicated as a consequence of the fired rule are taken, and the inference engine state is updated.

The select phase is composed of "conflict resolution strategies," a few of which are listed below:

- **Refraction:** All rules in the conflict set that were fired in the past are removed from the conflict set. If firing a rule affects the matching data of the other rules' antecedents, then those rules are considered in the conflict resolution.
- **Recency:** Use an assignment of priority to fire rules based on the "age" of the information in the rule base that matches the premise of each rule. The "age" of the data that matches the premise of a rule is defined as the number of rule firings since the last firing of the rule that allows it to be considered in the conflict set.
- **Distinctiveness:** Fire the rule that matches the most (or most important) data in the rule base. (Many different types of distinctiveness measures are used in expert systems.)
- **Priority schemes:** Assign a priority ranking of the rules and then choose the highest priority rule to fire from the conflict set.
- **Arbitrary:** Pick a rule from the conflict set to fire at random.

It should be noted that if all the conflict resolution strategies are applied and more than one rule remains in the conflict set, then one of the remaining rules is chosen randomly and is fired. In an expert system it is not important whether or not the human cognitive structure and processes are actually emulated, but whether the expert decision-making system functions properly, achieving a high rate of correct decisions. Generally speaking, enhanced decision-making capabilities of the expert decision-making system will imply enhanced functionality and ability to meet conditions that are more demanding.

It is interesting to note that the knowledge representation and decision-making capabilities of the expert systems are more sophisticated than those of the standard fuzzy decision-making (FDM) systems. One can also use an expert system to provide intelligent sequencing of a number of FDM systems. In this way the expert system acts in a supervisory role to perform "meta-level reasoning" about how to choose the best FDM system to supply decisions. In addition, expert systems can be designed to exhibit some learning capabilities [2]. For example, automatic rule synthesis or deletion may be provided, and a learning rule selection mechanism can be added. Finally, an expert system automatically manages the data and decision fusion problems that are increasingly important as technology evolves. In medicine, for instance, a new sensor or a new kind of measurement system is introduced virtually every day, and a medical expert is confronted with a huge amount of apparently irrelevant data. In contrast, an expert system easily accomplishes this task by the use of its rule base. It is for these reasons that the development and use of expert systems in medicine is quite old, beginning in 1975 (i.e., PIP, CASNET, MYCIN, and INTERNIST) [11]. In recent years, expert systems based on the latest techniques of AI and signal/image processing have begun to appear in the literature. One of the first examples is given in [11], where neural networks and image processing techniques are used together with expert systems in the development of an automated cytogenetics system. Additional pioneering work by the same group in the development of expert diagnostic systems in various areas of medicine is reported in [5, 7, 9, 16, 30]. Most of these are intelligent decision-making units employing either neural networks or fuzzy logic to provide decisions.

3.2.2. Fuzzy logic and belief functions

In the past decade, fuzzy systems have supplanted conventional technologies in many scientific and engineering systems, especially in control systems and pattern recognition applications. In addition, a rapid growth has been witnessed in the use of fuzzy logic in a variety of consumer products and industrial systems. Well-known examples include washing machines, auto-focus cameras, ship navigators, and cement kilns. The same fuzzy technology, in the form of approximate reasoning, can also be used in information technology, where it provides decision-support and expert systems with powerful reasoning capabilities bound by a minimum of rules.

Fuzzy sets, introduced by Zadeh in 1965 as a mathematical means of representing vagueness in linguistics, can be considered as a generalization of classical set theory [73]. The basic idea of fuzzy sets is easy to grasp. In a classical crisp (non-fuzzy) set, an element of the universe either belongs to or does not belong to the set. That is, the membership of an element is crisp; it is either yes (in the set) or no (not in the set). A fuzzy set allows the degree of membership for each element to range over the unit interval [42, 55]. Thus the membership function of a fuzzy set maps each element of the universe of discourse to a unit interval.

One major feature of fuzzy logic is its ability to express the amount of ambiguity in human thinking and subjectivity (including natural language) in a comparatively undistorted manner. Fuzzy logic is appropriate when

- the mathematical model of the process does not exist, or it exists but is too difficult to encode, or it is too complex to be evaluated rapidly enough for real time evaluations,
- the system requires too much memory for the designated chip architecture, or
- the process involves human interaction, and an expert is available who can specify the rules underlying the system.

With these properties, fuzzy logic techniques find their applications in such areas as control, pattern recognition, quantitative analysis, inference (e.g., expert systems for diagnosis, planning, and prediction), and information retrieval (e.g., databases) [55].

Basic definitions

A classical (crisp) set is a collection of distinct objects. It is defined in such a way as to divide the given universe into two groups: members and non-members. A crisp set can be defined by the "characteristic function." The characteristic function $\mu_A(x)$ of a crisp set $A \subset U$ takes its values in $\{0,1\}$ and

$$\mu_A(x) = \begin{cases} 1, & x \in A \\ 0, & x \notin A \end{cases} \tag{19}$$

where U is the universe of discourse. A fuzzy set, on the other hand, introduces vagueness by eliminating the sharp boundary between members and nonmembers. Thus the transition from full membership to nonmembership is usually gradual rather than abrupt. A fuzzy set A in the universe of discourse U can be defined as a set of ordered pairs,

$$A = \left\{ \left(x, \mu_A(x) \right); \, x \in U \right\} \tag{20}$$

where $\mu_A(x)$ is the membership function of A mapping U into $[0,1]$. For a discrete universe of discourse $U = \{x_1, x_2,..,x_n\}$, a fuzzy set A can be explicitly represented using the ordered pairs below:

$$A = \left\{ \left(x_1, \mu_A(x_1) \right), \left(x_2, \mu_A(x_2) \right)..., \left(x_n, \mu_A(x_n) \right) \right\} \tag{21}$$

Using the support of a fuzzy set A, we can simplify the representation.

$$A = \frac{x_1}{\mu_A(x_1)} + \frac{x_2}{\mu_A(x_2)} + .. + \frac{x_n}{\mu_A(x_n)} \tag{22}$$

where + and / signs in Equation (22) have only a symbolic meaning of disjunction and assignment. If the universe of discourse is continuous, then (22) is replaced by

$$A = \int_U \mu_A(x_1)/x \tag{23}$$

Again the integral and division signs have symbolic meanings.

Operations of fuzzy sets

Let A and B be fuzzy sets in the universe of discourse U. The basic operations on fuzzy sets are given in the following:

1. **Complement:** The complement of A, denoted by $\bar{A}$, is defined by its membership function as

$$\mu_{\bar{A}}(x) = 1 - \mu_A(x), \quad \forall x \in U \tag{24}$$

2. **Intersection:** The intersection of two fuzzy sets A and B, denoted as $A \cap B$, is defined by

$$\mu_{A \cap B}(x) = \min\{\mu_A(x)\mu_B(x)\} \equiv \mu_A(x) \wedge \mu_B(x), \forall \ x \in U \tag{25}$$

where $\wedge$ indicates the minimum operation.

3. **Union:** The union of fuzzy sets A and B, denoted as $A \cup B$, is defined by

$$\mu_{A \cup B}(x) = \max\{\mu_A(x)\mu_B(x)\} \equiv \mu_A(x) \vee \mu_B(x), \quad \forall x \in U \tag{26}$$

where $\vee$ denotes the maximum operation.

4. **Equality:** *A* and *B* are equal if and only if

$$\mu_A(x) = \mu_B(x), \quad \forall x \in U \tag{27}$$

To check the degree of equality of two fuzzy sets, we can use a similarity measure:

$$E(A,B) = \text{degree}(A = B) = \frac{|A \cap B|}{|A \cup B|} = \frac{\sum_{x \in U} \mu_{A \cap B}(x)}{\sum_{x \in U} \mu_{A \cup B}(x)} \tag{28}$$

5. **Subset:** *A* is a subset of *B* if and only if

$$\mu_A(x) \leq \mu_B(x), \; \forall x \in U \tag{29}$$

It is clear that $A \subseteq A \cup B$, $A \cap B \subseteq A$, $A \cap B \subseteq B$, $A \subseteq A \cup B$, and $B \subseteq A \cup B$. To check the degree that A is a subset of B, we can use the subsethood measure

$$S(A,B) = \text{degree}(A \subset B) = \frac{|A \cap B|}{|A|} \tag{30}$$

More generally, triangular norms (t-norms and t-conorms or s-norms) are used to represent intersection, union, and complements [62-63, 71].

Fuzzy relations

A (binary) fuzzy relation between two sets X and Y is denoted by R(X,Y) and is a fuzzy set on $X \times Y$;

$$R(X, Y) = \{(\,(x,y), \mu_R(x,y)\,); (x, y) \in X \times Y\} \tag{31}$$

There are many operations between fuzzy relations, but the most important one is the composition operation. Basically there are two types of composition operators, max-min and min-max compositions. They can both be applied to relation-relation and set-relation compositions.

Let $P(X,Y)$ and $Q(Y,Z)$ be two fuzzy relations on $X{\times}Y$ and $Y{\times}Z$ respectively. The max-min composition of P and Q, denoted as $P(X,Y)$ and $Q(Y,Z)$, is defined by

$$\mu_{PoQ}(x,z) = \max_{y\in Y}\ \min\ \{\mu_P(x,y),\mu_Q(y,z)\},\ \forall x \in X,\ z \in Z \qquad (32)$$

Dual to the max-min is the min-max composition. The min-max composition of P and Q, denoted as $P(X,Y)\Diamond Q(Y,Z)$, is defined by

$$\mu_{P\Diamond Q}(x,z) = \min_{y\in Y}\ \max\ \{\mu_P(x,y),\mu_R(y,z)\},\ \forall x \in X,\ z \in Z \qquad (33)$$

As in the case of relation-relation compositions, we have max-min and min-max compositions for set-relation compositions. Let A be a fuzzy set on X and $R(X,Y)$ be a fuzzy relation on $X{\times}Y$. The max-min composition of A and R, denoted as AoR, is defined by

$$\mu_{P\Diamond Q}(x,z) = \min_{y\in Y}\ \max\ \{\mu_P(x,y),\mu_R(y,z)\},\ \forall x \in X,\ z \in Z \qquad (34)$$

The min-max composition of A and R can be defined similarly.

Fuzzy measures

To represent the kind of uncertainty known as ambiguity, a value in the unit interval [55, 61] is assigned to each possible crisp set to which the element under discussion might belong. This value represents the degree of evidence or belief or certainty of the element's membership in the set. Such a representation of uncertainty is known as a fuzzy measure. There are several different fuzzy measures such as belief measures, plausibility measures, and necessity measures.

The basic difference between fuzzy sets and fuzzy measures can be described as follows. Fuzzy sets are used to solve the vagueness associated with the difficulty of making sharp distinctions between objects. On the other hand, fuzzy measures are used to solve the ambiguity associated with making a choice between two or more alternatives. Here we provide the definition of fuzzy measures and then briefly present belief and plausibility measures.

A fuzzy measure is a set function g: $\beta \rightarrow [0,1]$ such that $\beta \subset P(X)$, where X is the universe of discourse, $P(X)$ is the power set of X, and g is a sigma field which satisfies three axioms.

A1: $g(\emptyset) = 0$, $g(X) = 1$
A2: (monotonicity): for every crisp set $A, B \in P(X)$,
    if $A \subset B$, then $g(A) \leq g(B)$.
A3: (continuity): for every sequence $\{A_i \in P(X), i \in N\}$ of subsets of X,
    if the sequence is monotonic,
    i.e., either $A_1 \subset A_2 \subset ...$, or $A_1 \supset A_2 \supset ...$,
    then $\lim_{i \rightarrow \infty} g(A_i) = g(\lim_{i \rightarrow \infty} A_i)$

A belief measure is a fuzzy measure Bel: $\beta \rightarrow [0,1]$ that satisfies the sub-additivity axiom:

$$\text{Bel}(A_1 \cup A_2 \cup .. \cup A_n) \geq \sum_i \left[\text{Bel}(A_i) - \sum_{i<j} \text{Bel}(A_i \cap A_j) + .. \right.$$

$$\left. + (-1)^{n-1} \text{Bel}(A_1 \cap A_2 \cap .. \cap A_n) \right], \quad n = 1,2,.. \quad (35)$$

for any collection of subsets of X. For each crisp set $A \in P(X)$, the belief measure Bel(A) is interpreted as the degree of belief that a given element of X belongs to the set A. The construction of belief functions for a special case is explained in detail in Section 4.1.1. Associated with each belief measure, one can define a plausibility measure Pl as

$$Pl(A) = (1 - \text{Bel}(\overline{A})), \quad \forall A \in B \quad (36)$$

where $Pl(A)$ represents the total evidence or belief that the element $x \in X$ belongs to the set A or to any of the various subsets of A, plus the additional evidence or belief associated with sets that overlap with A.

Fuzzy decision-making (FDM) systems

The basic idea behind FDM is to incorporate the "expert experience" of a human in decision making for a system whose input-output relationship is described by a collection of fuzzy (IF-THEN) rules involving linguistic variables rather than complicated expressions. FDM systems include fuzzy logic control systems and fuzzy pattern recognition/classification systems. The basic architecture of a FDM system is shown in Figure 2.

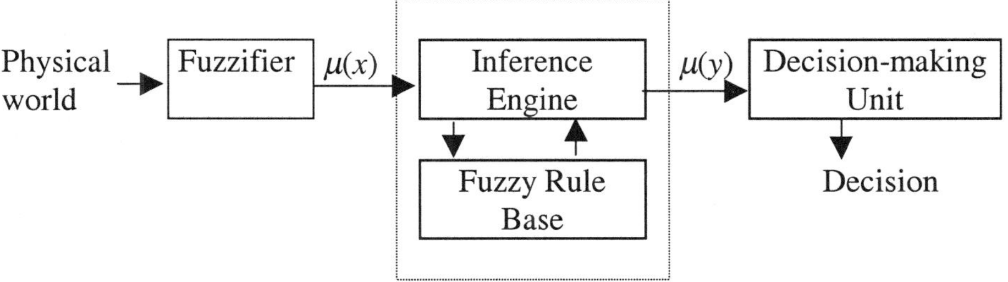

Figure 2. The basic architecture of a FDM system.

Of course, depending on the kind of application one has in mind, the basic structure can be modified accordingly. For example, in fuzzy logic control applications, the decision-making unit is simply a "de-fuzzifier" that produces a crisp action. The task of each block will now be described in some detail.

- **Fuzzifier:** A fuzzifier performs the function of fuzzification, which is a subjective valuation that transforms measured data into a subjective value. Hence, it can be defined as a mapping from an observed input space into labels of fuzzy sets in a specified universe of discourse.

- **Fuzzy rule base:** A collection of fuzzy IF-THEN rules in which the preconditions and consequents are linguistic variables. The general form of a fuzzy rule, R^i, is

$$\text{IF } x \text{ is } A_i \text{ AND .. AND } y \text{ is } B_i, \text{ THEN } z \text{ is } C_i, i = 1, 2, .., n \qquad (37)$$

where $x, .., y$ and z are linguistic variables representing the system inputs and decision, respectively. $A_i, .., B_i$ and C_i are the linguistic values of $x, .., y$ and z in the universes of discourse $U, .., V$ and W, respectively.

- **Inference engine:** This is the kernel in modeling human decision making within the conceptual framework of fuzzy logic and approximate reasoning. The generalized modus ponens plays an especially important role here.

$$\frac{\begin{array}{l} \text{Rule : IF } x \text{ is } A, \text{ THEN } z \text{ is } C \\ \text{Input : } x \text{ is } A' \end{array}}{\text{Output : } z \text{ is } C'} \tag{38}$$

In general, a rule R is a fuzzy relation which is expressed as a fuzzy implication R: $A \rightarrow C$. Then the conclusion C' can be obtained by taking the composition of fuzzy set A' and the fuzzy relation R.

$$C' = A' \text{o R} \tag{39}$$

There are various types of compositional operators that can be used in (39), in addition to various implications [47]. The most conventional for fuzzy implication is Mamdani's min operation [49]. If it is combined with (34) for compositions, then the membership function for B' is obtained as

$$\mu_{C'}(y) = \max_{x \in X}\left\{\mu_{A'}(x) \wedge \mu_A(x) \wedge \mu_C(y)\right\}, \ \forall z \in W \tag{40}$$

When the rule base contains more than one rule, the conclusion can be expressed as the union of individual conclusions of the form (40) (Mamdani's approach) [49]. For simplicity, let us assume that we have two rules as

$$\begin{array}{l} R^1: \text{ IF } x \text{ is } A_1 \text{ AND } y \text{ is } B_1 \text{ THEN } z \text{ is } C_1 \\ R^2: \text{ IF } x \text{ is } A_2 \text{ AND } y \text{ is } B_2 \text{ THEN } z \text{ is } C_2 \end{array} \tag{41}$$

Then the firing strengths α_1 and α_2 of these rules may be expressed as

$$\alpha_1 = \mu_{A_1}(x_o) \wedge \mu_{B_1}(y_o), \qquad \alpha_2 = \mu_{A_2}(x_o) \wedge \mu_{B_2}(y_o) \tag{42}$$

where x_o and y_o are the particular events. In Mamdani's approach, the ith rule leads to the conclusion

$$\mu_{C'_i}(\omega) = \alpha_i \wedge \mu_{C_i}(\omega) \tag{43}$$

The final inferred decision C is given by

$$\mu_C(\omega) = \mu_{C'_1} \vee \mu_{C'_2} = \max \{\mu_{C'_1}(\omega), \mu_{C'_2}(\omega)\} \tag{44}$$

This fuzzy reasoning and decision-making process is illustrated in the Figure 3.

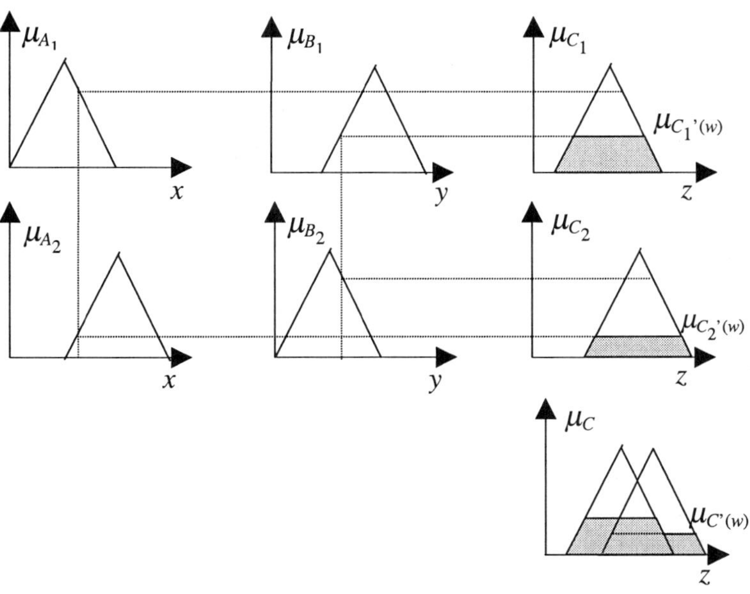

Figure 3. Fuzzy reasoning and decision-making process

Usually, after μ_C is detained, there is an additional stage in a FDM process. For example, a fuzzy controller needs a crisp value for the control input, and so a defuzzification operation [47] is added to finalize the decision. In classification methods based on fuzzy logic, the distance of $\mu_c(\omega)$ to fuzzy sets Ω_i in the feature space can be calculated for all known fuzzy features, and the minimum distance one is the decision. Further information about FDM systems can be obtained from [35, 47, 66].

3.2.3. Artificial neural networks (ANNs)

Artificial neural networks are computing structures containing elements that behave somewhat like the nerve cells in the brain. The transmission of signals in biological neurons through synapses is a complex chemical process in which specific transmitter substances are released from the sending side of the synapse. The effect is to raise or lower the electrical potential inside the body of the receiving cell. If this potential reaches a threshold, the neuron fires. It is this characteristic that the artificial neuron model proposed by McCulloch and Pitts [53] attempts to reproduce. This neuron model is the one that is widely used in artificial neural networks with some variations (Figure 4).

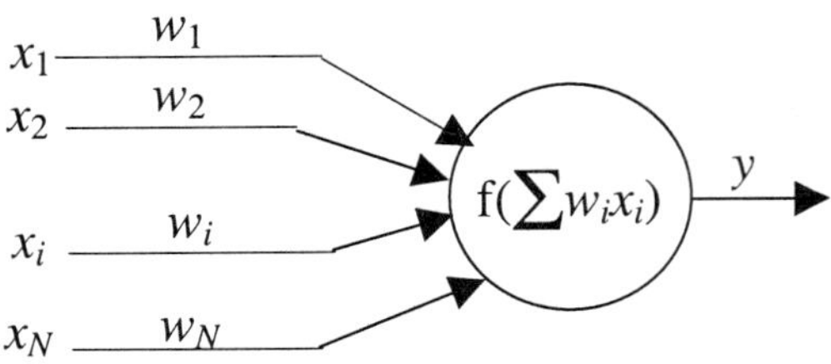

Figure 4. Artificial neuron

The artificial neuron shown in Figure 4 has N inputs, denoted as x_1, x_2, ...x_N, and each line connecting these inputs to the neuron is assigned a weight, denoted as w_1, w_2, ...w_N, respectively. The output value of the neuron is a function of the applied inputs and the connection weights.

A neuro-computing system is made up of a number of artificial neurons and a huge number of interconnections between them. According to the structure of the connections, we identify different classes of network architectures. In layered neural networks, the neurons are organized in the form of layers. The neurons in a layer get input from the previous layer and feed their output to the next layer. These types of networks are called feedforward networks, and output connections from a neuron to the same or previous layer neurons are not permitted. The input layer is made of special input neurons, transmitting only the applied external input to their outputs. The last layer of neurons is called the output layer, and the layers that are neither input nor output are called the hidden layers [37, 39, 45].

If there is only a layer of input nodes and an output layer, then the network is called a single layer network. Networks with one or more hidden layers are called multilayer networks. The multilayer perceptron is the well-known feedforward multilayer network upon which the backpropagation learning algorithm is widely implemented. Self-organizing maps and vector quantization networks are other examples of feedforward neural networks. Structures where connections to neurons in the same layer or to the previous layers are permitted are called recurrent networks. Hopfield network and Boltzmann machine are examples of widely used recurrent networks [37, 39, 45].

Among the many interesting properties of an ANN, the property that is of primary significance is the ability of the network to learn from its environment and to improve its performance through learning. A neural network learns about its environment through iterative processes of adjustments to its synaptic weights. The three basic classes of learning paradigms are supervised learning, reinforcement learning, and self-organized (unsupervised) learning. Supervised learning is performed when the related output patterns are known for training input patterns. Reinforcement learning is convenient for cases where the exact output pattern is not known, but we know if an output generated by the network is good or not. Unsupervised learning is used when no information is available on the output, and the purpose is to cluster the input patterns.

Self-organizing maps (SOM)

The SOM model was developed by Kohonen between 1979 and 1982 [44]. Kohonen's work is related to the earlier work of Willshaw and von der Malsburg. The essential difference between the SOM and many other networks is that the SOM learns without supervision. The major application of SOM is in clustering input data. SOM accepts n-dimensional input vectors and maps them to a lower (usually two) dimensional output plane. The topology for a typical SOM network is shown in Figure 5. It has n input nodes and m-by-m output nodes. Each output node j in the SOM network has a connection from each input node i, with w_{ij} being the connection weight between them.

There are two phases of operation in SOM: the training phase and the classification phase. In the training phase, the network finds an output node such that the Euclidean distance between the current input vector and the weight set connecting the input units to this output unit is minimum. This node is called the winner, and its weights and the weights of the neighboring output units of the winner are updated so that the new weight set is closer to the current input vector. The effect of the update for each unit is proportional to a neighborhood function, which depends on the unit's distance to the winner unit. This procedure is applied repeatedly for all input vectors until the weights are stabilized. The choice of the neighborhood function, the learning rate, and the termination criteria are all problem dependent. The classification phase is simple once the training phase is completed successfully. In this phase, after applying the input vector, only the winner unit is determined.

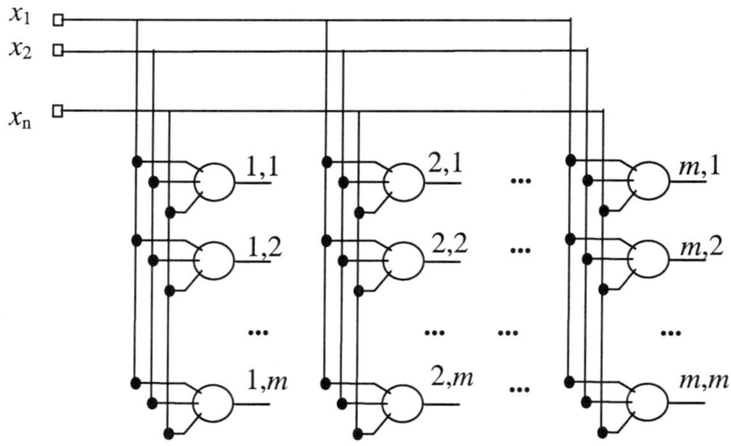

Figure 5: Network topology of the SOM

The training steps of SOM are as follows:

1. Assign small random values to the weights $\mathbf{w}_j = [\ w_{1j}\ ,w_{2j},\ ....w_{nj}]$, $j = 1, 2..m^2$;
2. Choose a vector $\mathbf{x}$ from the training set and apply it as input;
3. Find the winning output node d_{win} by the following criterion:

$$d_{win} = \arg\min_{j} \lVert \mathbf{x} - \mathbf{w}_j \rVert \tag{45}$$

where $\lVert . \rVert$ denotes the Euclidean norm and $\mathbf{w}_j$ is the weight vector connecting input nodes to the output node j;

4. Adjust the weight vectors according to the following update formula:

$$\mathbf{w}_j(t+1) = \mathbf{w}_j(t) + \eta(t)(\mathbf{x} - \mathbf{w}_j)N_{win}(j,t) \tag{46}$$

where $\eta(t)$ is the learning rate and $N_{win}(j,t)$ is the neighborhood function of the winner;

5.   Repeat Steps 2 to 4 until no significant changes occur in the weights.

The learning rate $\eta(t)$ is a decaying function of time; it is kept large at the beginning of the training and is decreased gradually as learning proceeds. The neighborhood function $N_{win}(j,t)$ is a window centered on the winning unit d_{win} found in Step 3, whose radius decreases with time. The neighborhood function determines the degree to which an output neuron j participates in training. This function is chosen such that the magnitude of weight change decays with increasing distance to the winner. This distance is calculated using the topology defined on the output layer of the network. The neighborhood function is usually chosen as a rectangular, 2-dimensional Gaussian or Mexican hat window.

Learning vector quantization (LVQ)

The LVQ network is a classification network proposed in [43]. An LVQ network contains an input layer, a Kohonen layer, which learns and performs the classification, and an output layer (Figure 6).

The input layer contains N neurons, each corresponding to an input parameter. The output layer contains M neurons, each corresponding to a class. K neurons are assigned to each class in the Kohonen layer. The Kohonen layer and the input layer are fully connected. In the output layer, each node is connected only to the Kohonen nodes assigned to the related class. At any time, only a single neuron, called the winner, is active in the Kohonen layer. An output neuron is active, if the winner of the Kohonen layer is within the related class.

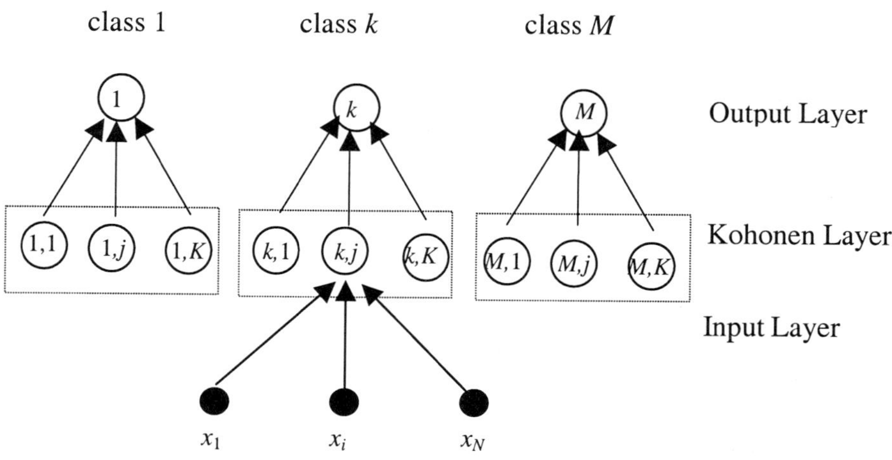

Figure 6. Learning Vector Quantization Network

There are two phases of operation in LVQ: the training phase and the classification phase. The weights from the input layer to the Kohonen layer are updated during the training phase. For this purpose, the distance of the input vector to each neuron in the Kohonen layer is computed and the nearest one is declared the winner. If the winner is in the class of the input pattern, then it is moved toward the input vector (attraction); otherwise, the winner is moved away from the input pattern (repulsion). During the training process, the neurons assigned to a class migrate to the region associated with their class. In the classification mode, the distance of an input vector to each neuron in the Kohonen layer is computed and the winner is determined. The class of the winner is assigned to the applied input pattern.

The training steps of LVQ are as follows:

1. Assign small random values to the weights $\mathbf{w}_{(k,j)} = [\, w_{1(k,j)}, w_{2(k,j)}, \ldots w_{N(k,j)}]$, $k = 1..M, j = 1..K$;
2. Choose a vector $\mathbf{x}$ from the training set and apply it as input;
3. Find the winning Kohonen node d_{win} by the following criterion:

$$d_{win} = \arg \min_{(k,j)} \{\|\mathbf{x} - \mathbf{w}_{(k,j)}\|\} \tag{47}$$

where $\|\cdot\|$ denotes the Euclidean norm and $\mathbf{w}_{(k,j)}$ is the weight vector connecting input nodes to the Kohonen node (k,j)

4. Let node (k,j) be the winner. Adjust the weight vector $\mathbf{w}_{(k,j)}$ according to the following update formula:

$$\mathbf{w}_{(k,j)}(t+1) = \begin{cases} \mathbf{w}_{(k,j)}(t) + \alpha(\mathbf{x} - \mathbf{w}_{(k,j)}) & if \quad \mathbf{x} \in class\ k \\ \mathbf{w}_{(k,j)}(t) - \beta(\mathbf{x} - \mathbf{w}_{(k,j)}) & if \quad \mathbf{x} \notin class\ k \end{cases} \tag{48}$$

where α and β are the learning rates for attraction and repulsion, respectively.

5. Repeat Steps 2 to 4 until no significant changes occur in the weights.

The LVQ suffers from the defect that some nodes in Kohonen layer sometimes win too often, while others win too little. This happens when the Kohonen node weights are far from the training vectors. In this case some nodes are initially drawn close, and the others permanently remain far away. To overcome this defect, a variant of LVQ is proposed in [27]. In this approach a bias, which is proportional to the difference between the win frequency of the node and the average win frequency, is calculated and added to the Euclidean distance found in Step 2. The bias term should be well tuned. Too large a bias can simply dominate the Euclidian distance and cause the winning node to depend only upon the observed node win frequencies, while too small a bias will have no effect in equalizing the win frequencies. In practice, the bias term is decreased as training progresses.

Multilayer Perceptron and Back-Propagation Training Algorithm (MLP/BP)

The back-propagation algorithm [58, 72] is a learning algorithm used on multilayer feedforward networks consisting of nonlinear units. Figure 7 illustrates a typical MLP network.

The activation function for a unit j in layer ℓ denoted by a_j^ℓ is

$$a_j^\ell = \sum_i w_{i,j}^\ell y_i^{\ell-1}, \quad \ell \geq 1 \tag{49}$$

where $w^{\ell}_{i,j}$ represents the weight of the connection from the ith unit in the $(\ell-1)^{th}$ layer to the jth unit in the layer ℓ. $\ell = 0$ corresponds to the input layer in which $y^0_i = x_i$.

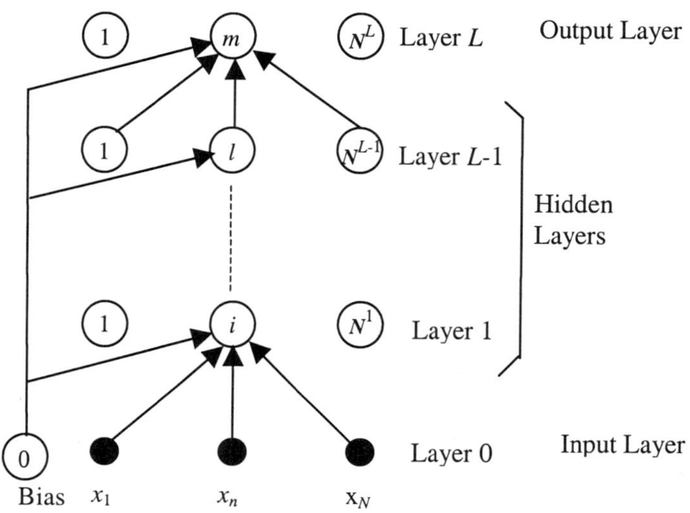

Figure 7. MLP network

The output of each neuron is determined by a shifted sigmoid function:

$$y^{\ell}_j = f(a^{\ell}_j) = \frac{1}{1+e^{-a^{\ell}_j}} - 0.5 \quad \ell \geq 0 \tag{50}$$

The training session consists of the presentation of randomly selected samples in the training set and an update of the weights using the desired output value for the presented sample. An optimum set of weights is obtained after a number of passes over the training set. Weight update equations can be summarized as follows:

$$\Delta w^{\ell}_{j,k} = \varepsilon \delta^{\ell}_k y^{\ell-1}_j \tag{51}$$

where $0 < \varepsilon < 1$ is the learning rate. δ^{ℓ}_k is called the error derivative and given by

$$\delta_k^\ell = -f'(a_k^\ell)e_k^\ell \quad \ell \geq 1 \tag{52}$$

where e_k^ℓ denotes the error for the kth neuron at the ℓth layer, and f' is the derivative of f. For the output layer, the error is calculated using

$$e_k^\ell = d_k - y_k^\ell \quad \ell = L \tag{53}$$

where L is the index of the output layer and d_k is the kth component of the desired output vector.   For hidden layers we have

$$e_k^\ell = \sum_k ä_k^{\ell+1} w_{j,k}^{\ell+1} \quad 1 \leq \ell \leq L \tag{54}$$

Usually, the training is terminated when the global error

$$GE = \frac{1}{2}\sum_{k=1}^{N_L}(e_k^L)^2 \tag{55}$$

for each pattern in the training set becomes less than a predetermined value.

In practical applications the algorithm needs many passes over the training set, and the algorithm is complemented with techniques that minimize the number of training cycles. A way to improve the performance is to impose a momentum term into the weight update equation as

$$\Delta w_{j,k}^\ell = å ä_k^\ell y_j^{\ell-1} + \alpha(w_{j,k}^\ell - (w_{j,k}^\ell)_{prev}) \tag{56}$$

where $(w_{j,k}^\ell)_{prev}$ is the previous value of the weight $w_{j,k}^\ell$, and $0 < \alpha < 1$ is the momentum coefficient.

4. Intelligent diagnostic systems in maternal-fetal medicine

The aim of maternal and fetal medicine is to reduce perinatal morbidity and mortality to a minimum and thus ensure optimum fetal conception and growth. This target can be achieved by diagnosing genetic disorders and fetal health problems as early as possible [7, 11]. The availability of high-capacity microcomputers has facilitated the development of intelligent diagnostic systems [5-7, 9-11]. In the meantime, new computer methodologies based on simulation of the human brain (neural networks) and human thinking (fuzzy systems) have been developed in order to overcome problems arising from the application of low level decision-making systems depending on conventional bio-statistics for the management of nonmodeled, complex biological phenomena.

Intelligent medical diagnostic systems are composed of various methodologies for data acquisition, feature extraction, pattern classification/ recognition, and decision making [9, 11]. As described previously in Section 2, the structures of medical data used to develop such systems in prenatal diagnosis are complicated and different in various problems [7, 11]. One of the systems that we developed is an intelligent preconceptive diagnosis system, which predicts the ovulation day. We developed two intelligent diagnostic systems that bring objective solutions to two different areas of prenatal diagnosis studies. One of them is the hybrid intelligent diagnostic system based on image analysis techniques and ANNs in the field of automated cytogenetics [11, 30]. The second one is again an intelligent screening system with ANNs for determining genetical disorders by using maternal serum markers [7]. These two applications can be integrated within the framework of a general prenatal diagnosis database or can be used separately. A general-purpose expert system that covers these systems will be realized in the future. We have also developed different types of intelligent diagnostic systems in the field of perinatal surveillance methodologies [5, 9, 16]. These systems will be explained in the following subsections.

4.1. Preconceptive and prenatal diagnosis

4.1.1. Prediction of the hCG administration day in hMG

Ovulation induction is used in the management of infertility cases with unovulatory cycles. There are various ovulation induction methodologies for different ovulation disorders. Human menopausal gonadotropin (hMG) and human chorionic gonadotropin (hCG) protocols are widely used in routine practice in such cases [1, 50].

hMG use has been universal for recruitment of multiple follicles in infertile women being treated with assisted reproductive technologies. Protocols that use hMG vary greatly, some using a combination Luteinizing Hormone (LH) and Follicle Stimulating Hormone (FSH), and some including extra FSH in addition to the FSH/LH protocols. Some women undergo ovarian suppression with gonadotropin-releasing hormone analogs (GnRH-a) prior to stimulation with hMG to achieve better results. The bioactivity of hMG may vary as well as the hMG response of patients from cycle to cycle. The critical issue in these controlled hyperstimulated cycles is to use optimum dose in order to have promising folliculogenesis. The response to hMG is best monitored by a combination of ultrasound folliculometry and 17β-estradiol (E2) determinations. In general serial ultrasounds are very helpful in timing the hCG administration to induce ovulation, and E2 levels indicate when it is unsafe to give hCG.

In intelligent diagnostic systems, decision-making processes need careful modeling, especially when the medical information is incomplete, imprecise, and possibly inconsistent. At this point, the theory of "belief functions" introduces many advantages in constructing a suitable structure for solving the prediction problem (Section 3.2).

In this subsection we provide in detail our developed intelligent system that predicts the day of hCG administration in LH/FSH and/or FSH induced cycles in order to provide a detailed illustrative example for the use of fuzzy measures, in particular, belief functions surveyed in Section 3.2.2.

Patients and treatment modality

The method developed in this study was applied to 67 successful ovulation induction cycles, 33 of which resulted in pregnancies. Average age was 32.8 years with a range 24 to 40 years. Women underwent ovarian stimulation with Pergonal (Serono Laboratories, Norwell, Mass.) and/or Metrodin (Serono Laboratories, Norwell, Mass.) following an induced or

 Beksac et al: **Intelligent systems in fetal medicine**

spontaneous menstrual flow. Some patients had been given Lupron (Tap Pharmaceuticals, Deerfield, IL) starting from mid-luteal phase until early follicular phase for down regulation. The treatment with Pergonal was started with 2 ampules daily on day 2 of menses and adjusted to the ovarion response. For the patients who did not stimulate well with Pergonal alone in previous cycles, Metrodin was added for the first 4 days of stimulation to increase folliculogenesis. All cycles were monitored by E2 determinations and folliculometry; our system prompts ultrasonographists to determine the number of follicles in left and right ovaries and the maximum follicle sizes of both ovaries. Table 3 shows a typical ovulation induction protocol and "ovarian response" follow-up chart from which necessary parameters were extracted for the computerized analysis. Ovulation "day 0" in cycle day (column 2) was induced by injection of 10,000 IU hCG (Profasi, Serono Laboratories, Norwell, MA) when the follicles reached a mean diameter of 16-18 mm and the E2 concentrations were between 1000-1500 pg/ml. The last four columns in Table 3 display follicle size in mm in each left and right ovary. The double column in some cases shows two measurements done at different hours of the same day and how uncertainty is an inherent characteristic of the acquired data in this study.

Table 3. An example of ovulation induction follow-up chart

Regimen Index Day	Cycle Day	Medications		E2	Left Ovary	Left Ovary	Right Ovary	Right Ovary
		Pergonal	Metrodin					
1	2	0	0	86				
2	3	0	2					
3	4	0	2					
4	5	2	0					
5	6	2	0	387	10.0 8.4		9.0 8.6	
6	7	2	0		10.0 9.0	7.3	10.2 9.0	8.0
7	8	1	0	972	11.0 9.0	4.3	13.0 12.0	10.0 9.0
8	9	1	0	1257	14.0 12.2	11.2 6.4	14.0 13.0	11.2 7.3
9	10 [¥]	0	0	2033	15.2 12.2	11.0 6.0	14.3 12.3	7.0
10	11 [¥¥]	0	0	-	-	-	-	-

[¥] hCG administered on Cycle Day 10
[¥¥] IUI performed on Cycle Day 11

Our computer program does not permit data entry before having at least one follicle 10 mm in diameter. Once a 10-mm sized follicle has been achieved, follicles over 8 mm are taken into consideration for data recording. The doses of hMG and FSH used in this study were recorded in ampules.

Modeling of medical prognosis

We used "belief functions" in order to describe the specifications of successful stimulated cycles leading to pregnancy. Hence we have selected 33 cycles ending with pregnancy to derive the clinical attitudes and biological facts in developing our belief model. The remaining 34 successful stimulated cycles without pregnancy were only kept for testing the predictive value of the artificial diagnostic system. Belief functions were used to overcome the subtlety of the problem and for the modeling of this inexact medical reasoning.

The concept of belief function theory is mainly based on regarding any data set about a certain event as a set of hierarchical evidences called a frame discernment. Table 4 shows the frame of discernment of our study. Each element of the superset of the frame discernment is named a focal element to be taken as the unit evidence if and only if a nonzero belief is assigned to it. The belief degree and combined belief degree of focal elements are then determined as individual and combined effects of focal elements, respectively, on the related event. Finally the variation of these values with respect to any discrete variable (in this study, this is cycle day) is taken as the simple support function, which is a belief function with an individual focal element. The propagation of this simple support function by being summed by the Dempster-Shafer rule [61] of combination from one cycle day to the next represents the cumulative effect of any focal element on the resulting event, which is that of maturation of follicles.

Table 4. Parameters used to develop the system (frame of discernment)

LABEL	DESCRIPTION
P	Number of Pergonal used daily
M	Number of Metrodin used daily
E2	Estradiol value
LO#	Number of follicles in left ovary
LOMAX	Maximum follicle size in left ovary
RO#	Number of follicles in right ovary
ROMAX	Maximum follicle size in right ovary

The steps of determination of belief functions can be summarized as follows:

1. "Normalized value" of each focal element is calculated

$$\text{norm}(A_{ij}^1) = \frac{A_{ij}^1}{\max(A_{ij}^1)} \tag{57}$$

$$\text{norm}(A_{ij}^1, A_{ij}^2) = \frac{A_{ij}^1 + A_{ij}^2}{\max(A_i^1) + \max(A_i^2)} \tag{58}$$

where

A^1_{ij} and A^2_{ij} are elements of the data set for i^{th} day and j^{th} patient,
(A^1_{ij}) and (A^1_{ij}, A^2_{ij}) are focal elements that are obtained from subsets of data set for i^{th} day and j^{th} patient,
$\max(A^1_i)$ and $\max(A^2_i)$ are the maximum values that belongs to elements A^1 and A^2 for i^{th} day.

2. "Degree of belief" for each focal element is calculated as follows using the normalized values:

$$b(A_{ij}^1) = \frac{\text{norm}(A_{ij}^1)}{\sum \max(all\ focal\ elements\ for\ i^{th}\ day)} \tag{59}$$

$$b(A_{ij}^1 A_{ij}^2) = \frac{\text{norm}(A_{ij}^1, A_{ij}^2)}{\sum \max(all\ focal\ elements\ for\ i^{th}\ day)} \tag{60}$$

where $b(A^1_{ij})$ and $b(A^1_{ij}, A^2_{ij})$ are values of corresponding focal elements for the ith day and the jth patient.

3. Belief functions Bel(A) calculated for each day are combined for each patient. Bel(A) may be represented as

$$\text{Bel(A)}=[A^1, A^2, A^3, A^1 A^2, ..; b(A^1), b(A^2), b(A^3), b(A^1 A^2), ...] \tag{61}$$

where A^i is the ith focal element and $b(A^i)$ is the corresponding basic probability assignments called belief.

A combination of Bel(A) and Bel(B) can be formulated as an orthogonal sum as follows:

$$\mathrm{Bel}(A_{i+1}) \oplus \mathrm{Bel}(B_i) = \mathrm{Bel}(A_{i+1}/B_i)$$

$$= \frac{\mathrm{Bel}\,(A_{i+1} \cup \overline{B_i}) - \mathrm{Bel}(\overline{B_i})}{1 - \mathrm{Bel}\,(\overline{B_i})} \quad i=1..(m\text{-}1), \tag{62}$$

for n observation days, where Bel(B$_i$) specifies the total belief from early days to day i.

This combination from day 1 to day 2 represents the conditioning of day 1 measurements on day 2. If such a combination is done forward from day 1 to day 2, to day 3.. to day n, belief function is propagated from day 1 to day n conditioned upon all past values. Therefore, the output belief function from such a propagation represents not only the last day's measurement but rather the conditioned cumulative effects of all coupled data from day 1 to last day.

4. The time variations of data is modeled as a propagation of belief which, in turn, provides us with predictive values of data for the following days.

Structuring the intelligent diagnostic system

Our data set is composed of seven parameters (Table 4) derived from treatment regimen as shown in Table 3. The number of focal elements (Fs) is equal to $2^7(128)$. In this study we selected 7 highly predictive belief functions out of 128 to construct the decision-making module of the system (Table 5). The cumulative integral ranges obtained from 33 patients whose cycles yielded pregnancy are also shown in Table 5. Here the detected ovulation day when hCG is administrated is designated as "day-0" in the first column. LOMAX means existence of left ovary maximum size follicle; similar argument holds for ROMAX for right ovary. (E2, LOMAX, LO#) is a focal element that represents the existence of serum E2 administrated, left ovary maximum size follicles, and sufficient number of follicles (LO#) in left ovary. The belief function curves for 7 different focal elements used in the decision-making process are given in Figure 8. The hCG administration day is designated "day 0" in this study.

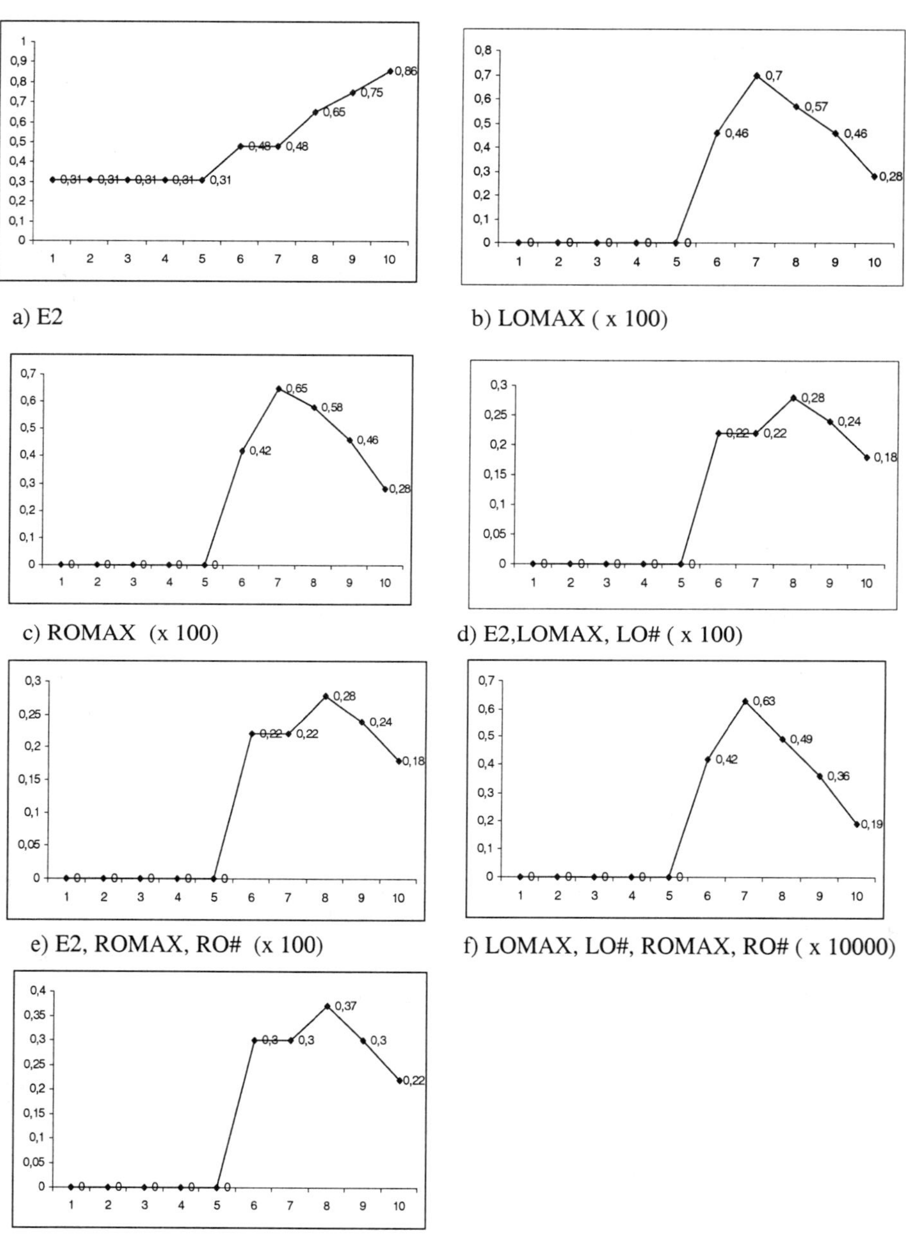

Figure 8. The "belief function" curves about 7 different focal elements. The variations of belief degrees are plotted with respect to consecutive cycle days.

Table 5. Cumulative integral ranges about belief functions of 7 focal elements for different cycle days

CYCLE DAY	FOCAL ELEMENTS						
	E2	LOMAX	ROMAX	E2, LOMAX, LO#	E2, ROMAX, RO#	LOMAX, LO#, ROMAX, RO#	E2, LOMAX, LO#, ROMAX, RO#
	(x1000)	(x1000)	(x1000)	(x1000)	(x1000)	(x1000)	(x1000)
-4	17.3-20.4						
-3	20.4-22.7	<5.0	<5.0	<19.5	<18.7	<15.8	<24.5
-2	22.7-23.2	5.0- 6.5	5.0-6.3	19.5-22.8	18.7-21.7	15.8-17.5	24.5-26.8
-1	23.2-24.7	6.5- 8.7	6.3-7.2	22.8-24.3	21.7-23.6	17.5-18.3	26.8-28.7
0	24.7-25.0	8.7- 9.6	7.2-8.4	24.3-25.6	23.6-24.2	18.3-20.1	28.7-30.1
1	25.0-25.3	9.6-10.2	8.4-8.9	25.6-26.7	24.2-25.1	20.1-20.7	30.1-30.6
2	25.3-30.0	10.2-10.9	8.9-9.7	26.7-28.3	25.1-26.3	20.7-21.5	30.6-31.7

Clinical results

The main program, named *Cesme/Baby-call*, includes a database system for the clinical laboratory findings related to the patient. The program is written in Turbo Pascal version 6.0. The main menu facilitates several functions such as the entrance of data, correction of recorded data, and decision making. At the beginning of the stimulated cycle, the system asks the operator to enter serum E2 level in pg/ml to the program. The analysis program does not permit the system operator to enter folliculometric data before at least one follicle reaches 10 mm in diameter. The system prompts the operator to enter folliculometric measurements every day, preferably with E2 values after this critical day.

The Cesme system was tested with both successfully stimulated cycles ending with pregnancy (n = 33) and nonpregnancy (n = 34). Table 6 shows the computerized diagnoses results assigning cycle days for hCG-administration (0 day) and pre-hCG (-1 day) days, which are important in order to invite the patient for a clinical try.

Table 7 shows the confusion matrix for comparing similarities and dissimilarities among the decisions of the medical experts and the artificial diagnostic system for successfully stimulated cycles ending with and without pregnancy, respectively. The difference is statistically significant ($p < 0.05$).

Table 6. Testing Results of Intelligent Diagnostic System for hCG-administration (0th day) and pre-h-CG (-1st day) days

	PREGNANCY GROUP (n=33)								NONPREGNANCY GROUP (n=34)						
Pno	L	M	P	Rx	CD	0th DAY	-1st day	Pno	L	M	P	Rx	CD	0th day	-1st day
1	N	Y	Y	9	10	0th day	-1st day	1	N	N	Y	7	8	0th day	-2nd day
2	N	N	Y	7	9	-1st day	-2nd day	2	N	N	Y	7	8	-1st day	-2nd day
3	N	N	Y	8	9	0th day	0th day	3	Y	N	Y	8	10	-1st day	-3rd day
4	Y	N	Y	11	12	1st day	1st day	4	N	N	Y	7	8	0th day	-2nd day
5	Y	N	Y	13	22	-2nd day	-2nd day	5	N	Y	Y	8	9	-3rd day	WARNING
6	N	Y	Y	7	9	-2nd day	WARNING	6	N	Y	Y	8	9	-3rd day	WARNING
7	N	N	Y	7	8	0th day	WARNING	7	N	N	Y	9	10	0th day	-1st day
8	N	N	Y	9	10	0th day	0th day	8	N	N	Y	9	10	0th day	0th day
9	N	N	Y	7	9	-1st day	-2nd day	9	N	N	Y	7	9	-1st day	-2nd day
10	Y	Y	Y	10	11	0th day	-1st day	10	N	N	Y	9	10	0th day	0th day
11	N	N	Y	8	10	-1st day	-1st day	11	N	Y	Y	6	8	WARNING	WARNING
12	N	N	Y	10	11	WARNING	0th day	12	N	N	Y	9	10	-2nd day	WARNING
13	Y	Y	Y	8	10	-1st day	-1st day	13	N	N	Y	8	9	1st day	0th day
14	N	N	Y	8	9	1st day	0th day	14	N	N	Y	9	10	1st day	WARNING
15	Y	N	Y	10	11	-2nd day	-3rd day	15	N	N	Y	8	9	0th day	-2nd day
16	Y	N	Y	12	12	-4th day	WARNING	16	Y	Y	Y	10	12	-1st day	-1st day
17	N	Y	Y	12	13	0th day	-1st day	17	N	N	Y	7	8	0th day	-2nd day
18	N	Y	Y	12	14	-1st day	-2nd day	18	N	N	Y	8	9	-1st day	WARNING
19	N	Y	Y	8	9	0th day	-1st day	19	N	N	Y	8	9	0th day	-1st day
20	Y	N	Y	9	19	WARNING	WARNING	20	N	N	Y	10	11	1st day	0th day
21	N	Y	Y	8	9	0th day	-1st day	21	N	N	Y	9	10	0th day	1st day
22	N	N	Y	8	9	0th day	0th day	22	N	N	Y	9	41	-2nd day	-3rd day
23	N	N	Y	9	10	0th day	-1st day	23	N	N	Y	10	12	-2nd day	-2nd day
24	N	N	Y	8	9	0th day	-1st day	24	N	N	Y	8	9	1st day	0th day
25	N	N	Y	9	10	0th day	NO DATA	25	N	Y	Y	10	12	-2nd day	-2nd day
26	Y	Y	Y	14	19	1st day	NO DATA	26	N	N	Y	8	9	1st day	0th day
27	N	Y	Y	9	10	1st day	0th day	27	N	N	Y	10	11	WARNING	WARNING
28	Y	N	Y	10	12	-1st day	-2nd day	28	Y	N	Y	7	10	WARNING	NO DATA
29	Y	Y	Y	12	30	WARNING	NO DATA	29	Y	Y	Y	8	16	-4th day	WARNING
30	Y	N	Y	11	41	WARNING	WARNING	30	N	N	Y	8	10	-1st day	WARNING
31	Y	Y	Y	11	12	0th day	0th day	31	Y	N	Y	12	28	WARNING	WARNING
32	N	Y	Y	7	8	-2nd day	WARNING	32	N	N	Y	9	11	-1st day	-2nd day
33	Y	Y	Y	10	12	-1st day	-2nd day	33	N	N	Y	7	10	-1st day	-2nd day
								34	N	N	Y	8	10	-2nd day	WARNING

Pno = Patient number; L = Loupron; M = Metrodin; P = Pergonal; Rx = Regimen Index; CD = Cycle Day

This system warns the medical expert when something is wrong in folliculogenesis. The warning rates were found to be 15.9% (10 out of 67 *Cesme* measurements) and 22.4 % (15 out of 67) on 0th and -1st days for pregnancy and nonpregnancy groups respectively.

Tables 6 and 7 show that post-hCG administration day ($+1^{st}$ day) is described in 5 (7.9%) and 6 (9.0%) occasions in pregnancy and nonpregnancy groups, respectively. The system mostly estimates 0th and -1st days as -3rd and -2nd and -1st days. This type of minor variation in decision making is observed in 41.3% and 50.7% of calculations in pregnancy and nonpregnancy groups, respectively.

Table 7. The confusion matrix comparing the similarities and dissimilarities among the decisions of the Medical Expert System related to pre- and post-hCG days together with other comments in hMG-induced cycles ending with and without pregnancy

MEDICAL EXPERT	INTELLIGENT DIAGNOSTIC SYSTEM							
	-4th day	-3rd day	-2nd day	-1st day	0th day	1st day	WARNING	NO DATA
STIMULATED CYCLES ENDED WITH PREGNANCY (n = 33)								
-1st day [¥]	0	1	6	9	7	1	6	3
0th date [¥¥]	1	0	4	7	13	1	4	0
STIMULATED CYCLES ENDED WITHOUT PREGNANCY (n = 34)								
-1st day [¥]	0	2	10	3	6	1	11	1
0th date [¥¥]	1	2	5	8	9	5	4	0

[¥] 1 day before hCG-administration; [¥¥] hCG-administration day

The system is tested with successfully induced cycles ending with and without pregnancy. It has been demonstrated that the concordance rates of the test are 34.9% and 17.9% in detecting the hCG-day (0th day) and pre-hCG day (-1st day) in pregnancy and nonpregnancy cycles, respectively. In 7 cases of pregnancy cycles (21.2%), both hCG-administration and pre-hCG days are determined correctly in the same patient. This rate is 5.9% in nonpregnancy (2 cases) cycles.

In this study, the presence of ovulation is validated by progesterone determination in both groups. Our results demonstrate that ovulation itself is not enough for pregnancy. Here, the concept of ovulation quality comes in.

We showed in our work that there is a criterion representing ovulation quality behind E2 determinations and folliculometric measurements. Various biological mechanisms are involved in successful ovulation induction and it is the aim of this work to find a kind of parametric representation for this problem. Our results demonstrate that our computerized system is good enough to overcome problems arising from low-quality ovulation. Such failures may be due to immature ooccyte-II, premature ovulation, or impaired intragonadal mechanisms.

4.1.2. Automated cytogenetics

Automated cytogenetic analysis of chromosomes has become an important and efficient tool in the diagnosis of chromosomal abnormalities. Computerized image processing and analysis techniques and rule-based classification algorithms for karyotyping have been in world-wide use since the 70s, replacing the manual cutting up of chromosome photography with scissors and their human-based arrangement [11, 30]. Since most of the systems are rule based, they are very sensitive to information losses. A very limited number of studies are based on the application of ANN [6, 11].

We developed one of the first intelligent diagnostic systems for automated cytogenetics, called the *Cankaya System.* Our system provides medical decision making as well as automated karyotyping [11]. The hardware configuration of the *Cankaya System* consists of a Nikon Microphot-fxa fluorescence microscope, a Hitachi CCTV camera, and a PC including an Image Processing Unit (IPU IAS25-IV 25) as a frame grabber, whose outputs are digital image files. The block diagram of this hardware structure is shown in Figure 9. The *Cankaya data set* is used in training and testing of our expert systems. Features of the chromosomes are obtained directly from the digital chromosome images as explained in detail later in this section.

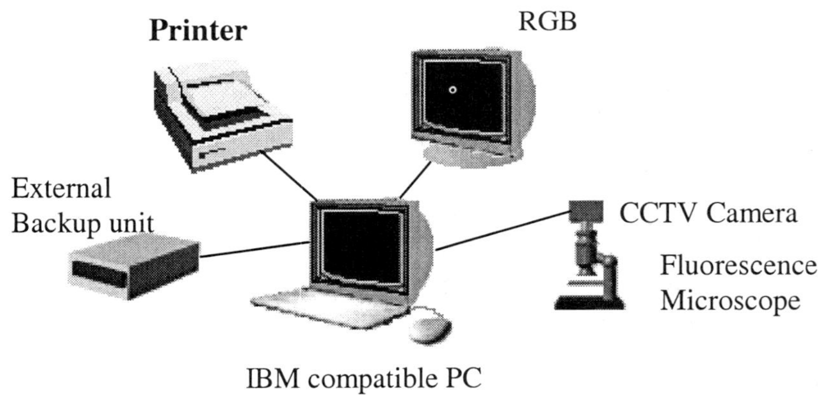

Figure 9: The hardware set-up used in the *Çankaya System*

In the first version of the *Cankaya System*, we used a SOM network and an original rule-based classification algorithm to find a karyotyped form of randomly distributed chromosomes over a complete metaphase [11]. Furthermore, we used a wavelet transform to obtain features from the gray level profiles (i.e., band patterns) of the chromosomes. In the second version, a hybrid intelligent karyotyping system based on SOM and MLP has been developed [30]. Figure 10 shows the output of the *Cankaya System* [11].

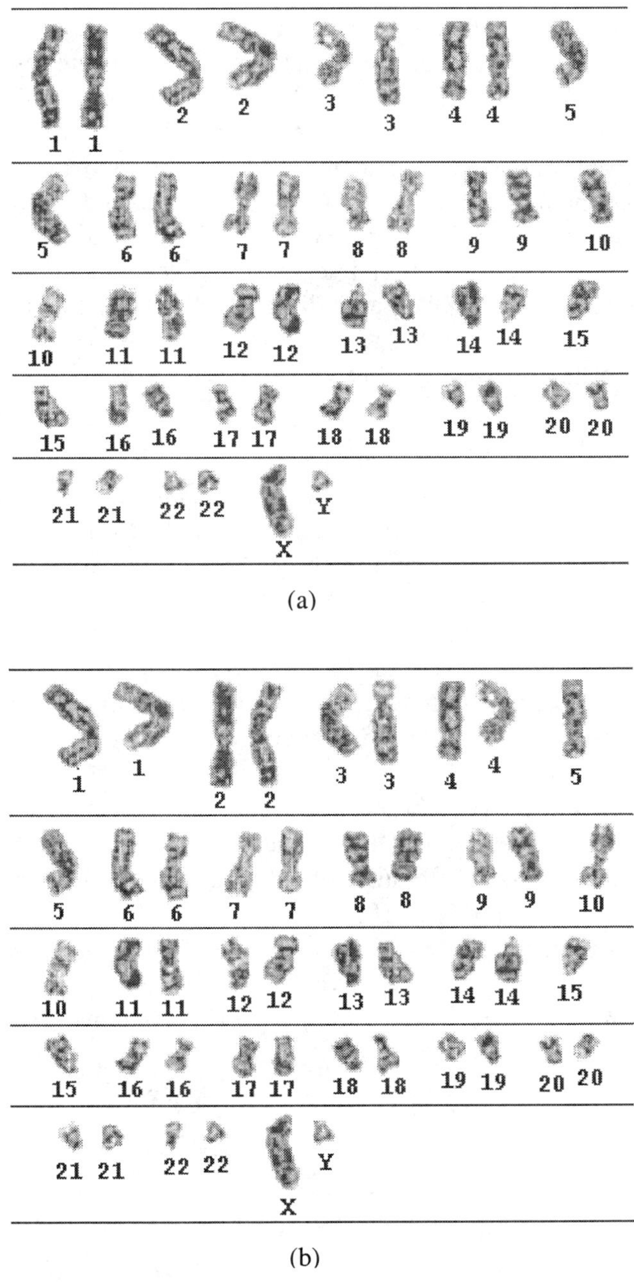

(a)

(b)

Figure 10. Karyotyping results obtained by the current state of the *Çankaya System*. a) the output obtained by rule-based classification algorithm, b) the output of the system based on hybrid ANN structure.

We will provide details of our approach for the sake of completeness in illustrating the applications of the methods given in the survey carried out in Sections 3.1, 3.2.1, and 3.2.3. The block diagram of the overall system in our approach is given in Figure 11. From the automated cytogenetics point of view, the separation of touching chromosomes and the decomposition of overlapping ones are the main problems, which should be solved before the pattern recognition and classification steps. With the objective of these problems, we allowed the user to draw a thin line of one pixel width between touching surfaces, so that they are taken as individual objects in the automatic object detection stage, and to mark the four cut points on the overlapping regions by means of a user interface, thus allowing the handling of all cases.

Feature extraction

The feature extraction phase is the most important process in developing intelligent systems using neural networks. Indeed, the system learning performance mainly depends on the characteristics and combination of inputs and on the way they represent the properties of the patterns. Feature vector components, which can be obtained by our system and their meanings are listed in Table 8. In our case, this phase consists of 1) individually handling all chromosomes, and 2) computing the measurements of these chromosomes in order to obtain feature vector components used as inputs to the hybrid ANN structure of the system. For these purposes, we have used two recently developed algorithms. The chromosomes are first detected by the automatic object detection algorithm (AODA), and then feature vector components, being inputs to the ANNs, are automatically calculated by means of an object skeletonizing algorithm (OSA) [10].

The measurement labeled GLPV is often called a chromosome band pattern and is an array of gray level values of a one-dimensional pattern formed by projecting the chromosome's gray level density profile onto its skeleton.

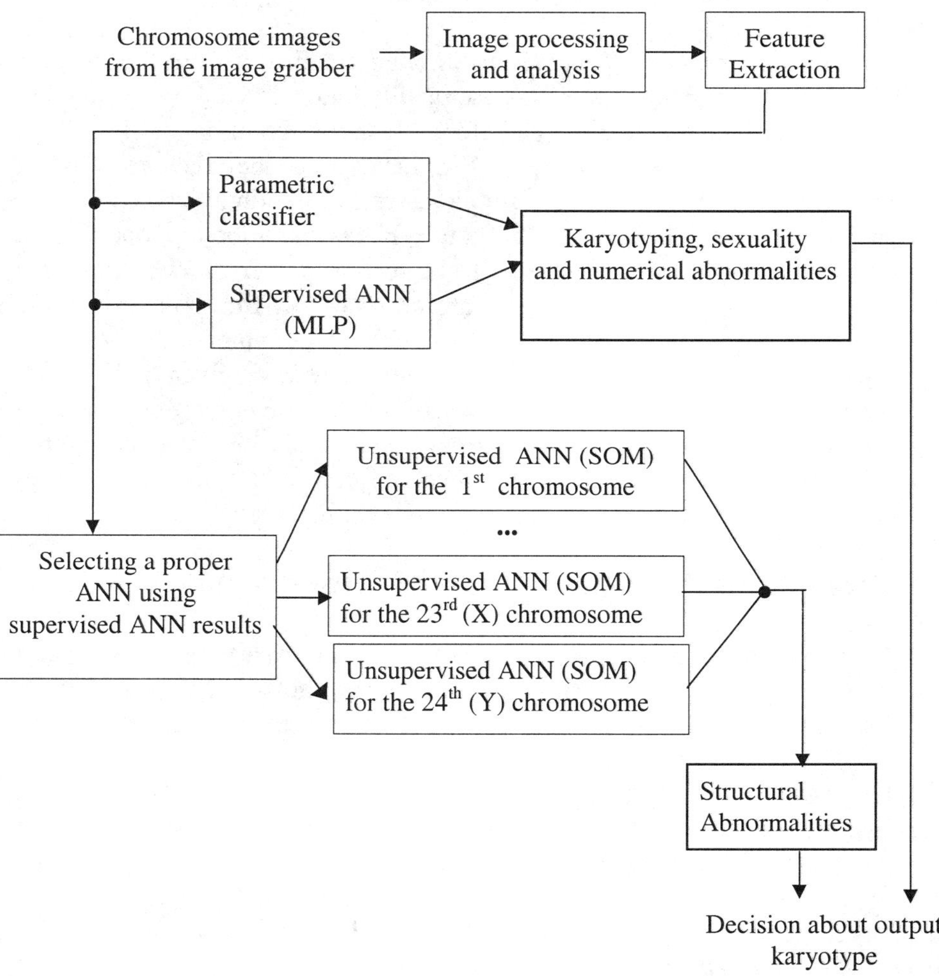

Figure 11. Block diagram of hybrid intelligent karyotyping architecture.

Table 8. Feature vector components (measurements list)

LABEL	DESCRIPTION
NP	Detected area of chromosome (number of pixels)
GLMN	Gray level mean of chromosomes
LC	Length of chromosome
CL	Centromere location
GLPV	Gray level profile values

Band patterns with wavelet transform

The band patterns of chromosomes differ dramatically from the banding quality, which is referred to as metaphase quality index defined by the number of bands per metaphase image. Therefore, the representation of the whole pattern (GLPV) becomes important. We have used the discrete wavelet transformation (DWT) instead of a simple discrete sampling method in order to overcome this problem [24]. DWT is a fast, linear operation that operates on a data vector whose length must be a fixed integer power of two. Since the chromosome length varies in different chromosomes, we first transformed the original GLPV signal to a standardized form with a fixed number of entries for each chromosome, i.e., $2^{10}=1024$. We used the wavelet basis given by Equation (7), for which discrete wavelet transformation of a function f is given by Equation (9). We then tried the reconstruction process with different number of entries of the DWT array. We obtained the optimum result with the 10 highest entries and their respective position indexes in the array.

Chromosome classification by neural networks

A rule-based classification process for obtaining a karyotyped form in a conventional fashion is also allowed as an optional path. This is provided for use either as an alternative to the hybrid ANN structure or for comparing the ANN results (Figure 11).

The supervised part of our hybrid structure is an MLP consisting of two hidden layers trained by the backpropagation algorithm explained in Section 3.2.3. Although different values of algorithm parameters alter considerably the learning performance, there is still no reliable mathematical way to determine them with respect to a specific problem. Therefore, we tried many cases which will be described in the illustrative results section.

As seen from Figure 11, the unsupervised part of our hybrid ANN structure consists of 24 unsupervised ANN modules, which are assigned to each class of chromosomes representing one of the enhancements to the previous version of the system. This part of the system is mainly used to determine different chromosome classes (i.e., the types of first chromosomes, the types of second chromosomes, etc.) in order to allow more reliable information about the structural specifications of chromosomes. The common network topology is a two-dimensional network which is designed to be trained by SOM, explained in Section 3.2.3.

Intelligent karyotyping

When a digital metaphase image is placed in the analyzing process, initially the feature vector components for each chromosome are automatically calculated. Then the trained supervised ANN takes these feature vectors as inputs and determines the group numbers from 1 to 24 for each chromosome. The results of this ANN module are then used to determine whether or not there is numerical abnormality. Meanwhile the same vectors are transmitted to the unsupervised ANN part of the hybrid system. The group numbers assigned by the supervised ANN classifier are used to select the corresponding unsupervised module as seen in Figure 11. At this stage a chromosome which cannot be mapped with any group or can be mapped with more than one group is considered as structurally abnormal.

Illustrative results

We processed 178 normal metaphase images to construct a digital chromosome database containing physical measurements of 8188 (46x178) chromosomes, listed in Table 8. The chromosome data set was divided into two parts as training and unseen sets having measurements of 96 and 82 digital metaphase images, respectively. The classification performance was measured using only the unseen data set.

Training and test of Supervised ANN module: During all training trials, we used networks with a bias node in layers except the output layer, because of their effects on diminishing the training time. The convergence criterion, in other words, the stopping criterion of the training process was chosen as 0.008 for the value of the global error formulated in Equation (55) for each training pattern. After many trials we found that the effects of learning rate and momentum term depend on the combination of inputs, in other words, the structure of the input space. Therefore, we performed three experiments with a fixed network topology with two hidden layers each having 50 nodes. The results are given in Table 9. In the first configuration, the inputs consist of only physical measurements NP, LC, CL. In the second configuration, the inputs consist of NP, LC, CL, and 10 highest discrete wavelet coefficients and the position indexes of these maximums. In the third configuration, the inputs consist of NP, LC, CL, and 10 highest discrete wavelet coefficients. In order to optimize the number of nodes in the hidden layers, we trained our supervised ANN with various numbers of nodes in successive hidden layers; Table 10 summarizes the results obtained in these experiments.

Table 9. Variations in the average classification error (%) of supervised ANN (MLP) with three different input configurations

Learning Rate	Momentum Term	Classification Error (%)		
		1st configuration	2nd configuration	3rd configuration
0.3	0.8	31.6	23.2	18.1
0.4	0.8	24.6	22.1	19.3
0.6	0.8	20.9	18.7	12.3
0.6	0.7	30.6	21.8	18.3
0.7	0.7	26.1	28.5	16.0

Table 10. Variations in the average classification error (%) of supervised ANN with different network topologies. Inputs are the same as the 3rd configuration of Table 9. The learning rate and momentum term are 0.6 and 0.8, respectively

NUMBER OF NODES		CLASSIFICATION ERROR RATES (%)
Hidden layer 1	Hidden layer 2	
55	25	19.8
60	25	21.2
65	25	33.9
70	25	38.7
75	25	31.0
55	28	19.9
55	30	23.2
55	35	15.4
55	38	11.3
55	40	12.8
55	45	25.7

Training and testing of unsupervised ANN modules: In order to reach a best learning performance in unsupervised ANN modules of the hybrid system, we investigated different structures (SOM) by conducting two experiments.

1) Measuring total average classification errors for different output nodes configuration with fixed training time as 150 cycles. The results obtained for the even numbered unsupervised ANNs are reported in Table 11. The number of classes observed on the output nodes is indicated in parentheses at each trial.

2) Measuring total average errors at different discrete training times with fixed output node configurations (13 by 13). The results obtained for even numbered unsupervised ANNs are given in Table 12.

Table 11. Variation in the average training error of even-numbered unsupervised ANN modules with different sizes of the output combinations at fixed training time (150 cycles)

| SOM | AVERAGE CLASSIFICATION ERROR (NUMBER OF CLASSES) | | | | | | | | | | | |
SIZE	1st	3rd	5th	7th	9th	11th	13th	15th	17th	19th	21st	23rd
7 by 7	23.4 (4)	24.5 (4)	32.5 (3)	34.2 (3)	26.3 (3)	19.7 (3)	31.6 (3)	26.2 (4)	18.9 (3)	25.7 (4)	22.4 (4)	26.1 (5)
11 by 11	28.6 (3)	16.2 (3)	29.3 (5)	26.4 (3)	31.2 (2)	23.2 (3)	32.7 (4)	21.5 (3)	15.1 (3)	26.7 (3)	34.3 (3)	21.3 (3)
13 by 13	13.2 (3)	17.2 (3)	10.9 (3)	15.8 (5)	8.5 (3)	12.3 (2)	12.9 (3)	11.2 (4)	13.5 (3)	15.3 (3)	9.1 (4)	14.4 (4)
15 by 15	27.8 (3)	22.3 (3)	20.1 (3)	14.1 (6)	11.5 (3)	23.4 (3)	15.9 (4)	20.1 (3)	18.3 (3)	18.0 (4)	18.4 (3)	17.0 (6)
20 by 20	18.4 (5)	21.8 (3)	16.8 (3)	16.3 (5)	14.6 (4)	16.8 (3)	16.8 (4)	14.4 (4)	27.9 (4)	17.1 (5)	16.2 (3)	32.1 (3)

Table 12. Variation in the classification error (%) of even-numbered unsupervised ANN modules with the increasing training time at fixed output planar combination (13 by 13)

| CYLE | AVERAGE CLASSIFICATION ERROR RATE (%) | | | | | | | | | | | |
	1st	3rd	5th	7th	9th	11th	13th	15th	17th	19th	21st	23rd
50	41.7	29.3	28.3	28.0	39.1	19.8	21.4	32.2	25.3	33.5	22.7	15.7
100	30.3	29.2	21.6	26.7	34.4	14.5	19.2	11.5	17.3	21.7	19.5	15.1
150	13.2	17.2	10.9	15.8	8.5	12.3	12.9	9.8	13.5	15.3	9.1	14.4
200	13.0	17.1	10.8	15.6	8.2	12.3	12.7	9.8	13.2	15.3	9.0	14.2

Finally we measured average classification errors of the hybrid ANN architecture in comparison with rule-based classifier for different Denver classes of chromosomes. The results are reported in Table 13. The resulting karyotypes (conventional/intelligent) obtained by the current version of the system from a sample digital metaphase image belonging to the unseen data set are given in Figure 10.

The most important characteristic of this intelligent system is the ability to detect chromosome aberrations (structural abnormalities) due to its hybrid structure including 24 unsupervised ANNs assigned to the different classes of chromosomes (Denver groups). The current version of the system can determine whether or not the encountered chromosome is normal.

Table 13. Comparison of classification performance of rule-based classifier and hybrid ANN structures for different class of chromosomes. RBE: Rule-based error rate, HANNE: Hybrid ANN error rate

	AVERAGE CLASSIFICATION ERROR RATE (%)											
	1st	2nd	3rd	4th	5th	6th	7th	8th	9th	10th	11th	12th
RBE	20.8	21.7	21.9	34.5	36.7	19.8	20.1	17.8	15.1	21.3	16.8	18.4
HANNE	32.2	30.4	33.1	30.6	20.2	13.7	4.5	5.2	1.7	5.3	2.4	3.5
	13th	14th	15th	16th	17th	18th	19th	20th	21st	22nd	X	Y
RBE	10.8	9.5	11.7	25.4	13.2	8.1	5.5	8.4	23.4	22.2	15.4	3.4
HANNE	9.7	12.5	10.1	18.7	15.3	4.2	6.9	2.3	4.9	8.7	27	2.5

Therefore, a study comprising the training of this hybrid system with different data sets and the comparison of obtained results is a feature work. Finally, the use of new digital texture analysis or transformation techniques may enhance the number and characteristics of feature vector components, thus decreasing the convergence time and increasing the learning performance of the ANNs.

4.1.3. Triple test

Various investigators reported a link between Down's syndrome and low levels of maternal serum α-fetoprotein (AFP), high levels of human chorionic gonadotropin (hCG), and low levels of unconjugated estriol (E3) [7]. It has also been reported that the use of these three biochemical measurements ("Triple Test") together with maternal age could substantially improve the prenatal diagnosis of Down's Syndrome [7]. Maternal serum screening is also very important for detecting certain other genetic disorders such as neural tube defects, Turner syndrome, and 18-trisomy. However, the biological rationale for the altered concentrations of AFP, hCG, and E3 has yet to be clarified. The integrated function of fetal and maternal endocrine systems and the interaction of the placenta in these processes make prenatal screening more complex and difficult to understand. We believe that the application of ANNs to maternal serum screening will bring objectivity in decision making and will prevent speculative discussions concerning the exact biological rationale for the altered "Triple Test" results [7].

We used a MLP network trained by a modified BP to develop the intelligent diagnostic system that is called the *Hacettepe System* [7]. The input parameters of the *Hacettepe System* are maternal age, gestational week, AFP, hCG, and unconjugated E3 values. After data acquisition, the MLP network having one hidden layer is used for classification. The *Hacettepe System* consists of two different MLP networks whose decision-making functions are different. One is designed to search for genetic disorders, while the other detects mid-pregnancy fetal well-being [7].

4.2. Perinatal surveillance

4.2.1. Antepartum fetal heart rate testing (nonstress testing)

Antepartum (AP) fetal heart rate (FHR) testing has gained widespread popularity as a screening test for perinatal surveillance [10, 16]. Various investigators have reported studies of the computerized systems for AP-FHR testing, in order to prevent the problems arising from visual analysis. We have previously developed a rule-based expert system (*Ankara System*, version 2.29 and 2.34) for the interpretation of the AP-FHR tracings [13, 18, 19]. A Doppler ultrasound heart rate monitor with autocorrelation was used to detect fetal pulse [16]. Perceived fetal movements were recorded by the patients. The fetal monitor was connected to a PC by means of a frame grabber. Early versions of the *Ankara System* were all rule based, and various algorithms were used to obtain the classical parameters such as FHR variability, baseline, acceleration, and deceleration. Recently we developed an automated intelligent diagnostic system based on automated signal processing and ANN [9]. After data acquisition, AP-FHR testing is handled as a pattern recognition (feature extraction and classification) and decision-making problem. Wavelet transformation is used for feature extraction [29]. Parameters obtained by feature extraction are fed as input to the MLP that classifies fetal heart rate waveforms into three groups (clinical decisions such as: Assuring FHR; Non-assuring FHR; and Difficulty in Decision-Making, Repeat the Test). This recent version of the *Ankara System* (Version 4.50) will be further extended into a hybrid structure combining ANNs and FDM [10].

4.2.2. Doppler velocimetry

Adequate blood flow through the umbilical circulation is essential for providing the fetus with oxygen and nutrients; therefore, umbilical cord haemo-dynamics should be a priority in perinatal surveillance [9]. There has been increasing interest in the application of Doppler ultrasound velocimetry as a fetal diagnostic tool. However, there is serious debate as to how and when to use umbilical artery Doppler velocimetry. The pathophysiologic background of waveform changes is multifactorial and the biological rationales behind the

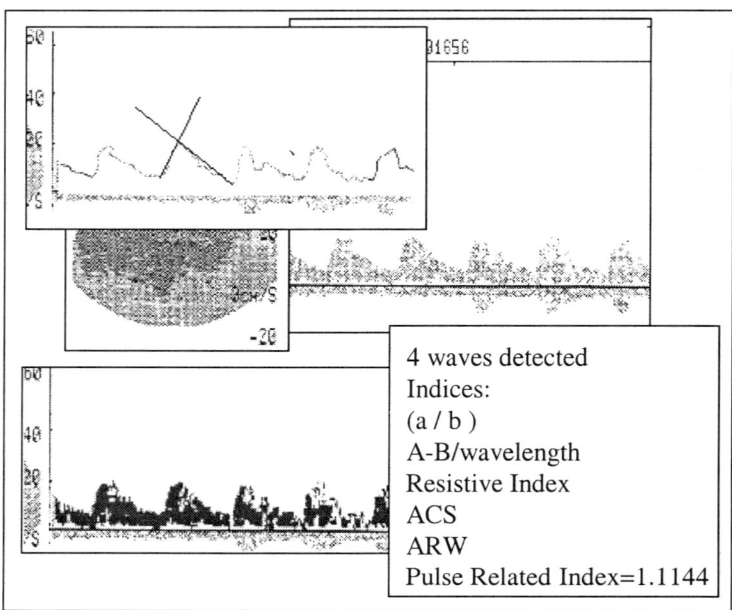

Figure 12. Output sheet with various image processing steps used in the *Bolu System*. a) edge detection, b) enhancement and c) thresholding and smoothing. The analysis results are given in the lower window located on the right-hand side of the image.

conventional indices are ill-defined. We have developed an intelligent diagnostic system, which is called the *Bolu System*, for the interpretation of blood flow velocity waveforms.

A Doppler ultrasound instrument (Radius HR, General Electric CGR, France/USA) is connected to a PC by means of a frame grabber (IRIS DT 2853, Data Translation Inc., 100 Locke Drive, Marlboro, MA 01752-1192, USA) with special data acquisition software [12]. A 3.75 MHz duplex pulsed-wave ultrasound transducer (Radius HR, General Electric CGR, France/USA) is used. Automated image processing is initiated after blood flow velocity waveform (BFVW) images are transferred from the ultrasound monitor to the computer as digital image files [3]. In the first version of the *Bolu System*, various algorithms were used to obtain the A/B ratio, the resistance index (RI), the pulse-related index (PRI), the area ratio of wave (ARW), and the angle between coincident slopes (ACS) [5]. Figure 12 shows the result of image processing and analysis procedures. All these features are used as input parameters to the classification tool of the *Bolu System* (Figure 13). In this first version, we used a MLP for classification [5].

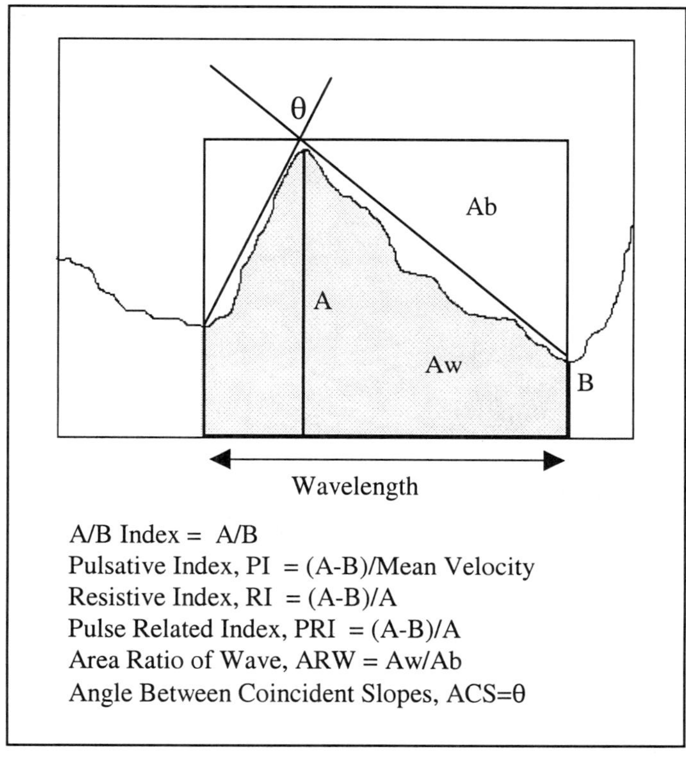

Figure 13. Demonstration of six velocity waveform indices calculated by image processing and analysis in the *Bolu System.*

Recently we developed a new automated intelligent diagnostic system, in which an LVQ network is used for pattern recognition. Several image processing techniques such as enhancement, smoothing/thresholding and edge detection, and image analysis are applied for feature extraction [8]. Six waveform indices obtained by feature extraction (Figure 13) are used as the inputs to the LVQ network, which classifies waveforms into six groups. A clinical decision is assigned to each group by the medical expert [9]. In another version we used a hybrid structure based on SOM and MLP for classification [4]. Figure 14 shows the procedure used in the development of the automated classification system [4].

4.2.3. Fetal ultrasonography

Recent progress in biomedical engineering enabled automated analysis of medical images and the development of intelligent diagnostic systems [14]. Ultrasound examination is now potentially available to all pregnant women. Recently we developed an intelligent diagnostic system that determines the gestational age using ultra-sonographic fetal head images. Sonographic parameters such as biparietal diameter (BPD) and head circumference (HC) are obtained by automated image processing and analysis. A MLP network is used for classification and decision making. We believe that progress in texture analysis and other image analysis techniques will bring new dimensions to medicine [14].

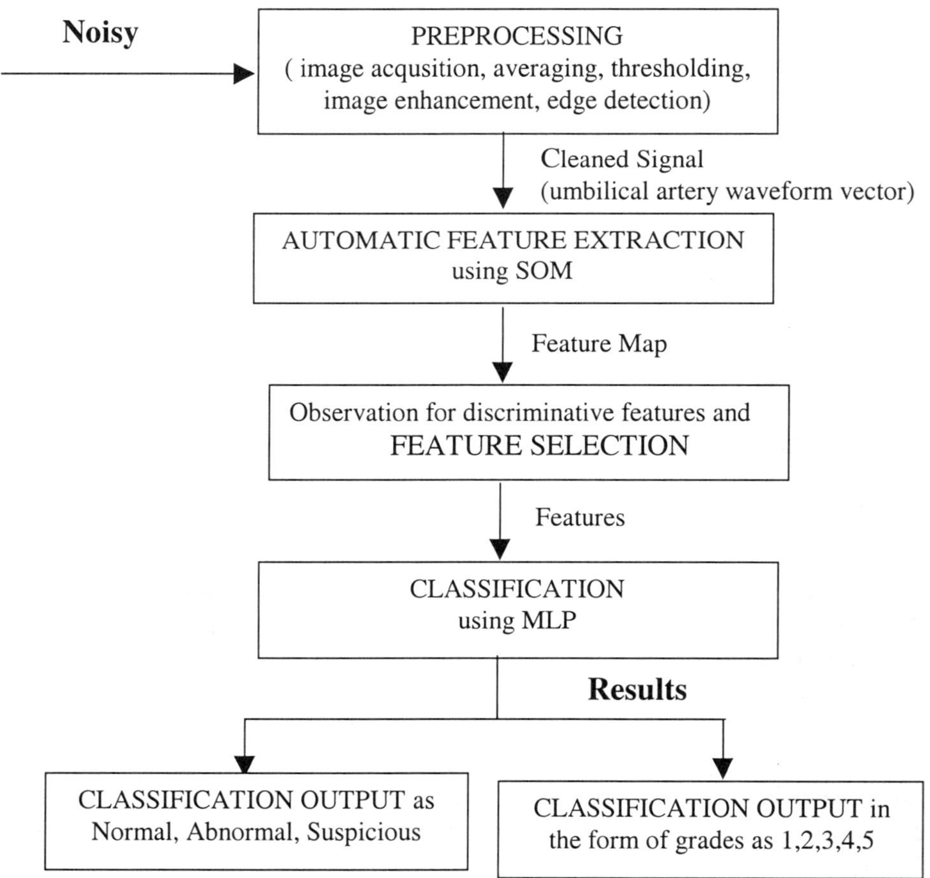

Figure 14. The procedure used in the development of the *Bolu System* for Doppler velocimetry

5. Conclusions

Biomedical technology is in rapid development, especially in the last decade in which many diagnostic or therapeutic procedures that could not be envisaged before are now becoming possible. Accomplishment of these procedures requires increased interdisciplinary studies with engineers. Obstetrics is one of the areas of medicine that makes extensive use of technological advances. As a result of these developments, imaging of fetal chromosomes and the fetus in his/her environment is routinely being accomplished while intrauterine sensory access to the fetus is also possible. This results in intrauterine detection of congenital or genetic abnormalities that provide the parents with important information concerning possible decisions toward abortion.

A major goal of perinatal medicine is to reduce perinatal morbidity and mortality. Various noninvasive technologies have been developed in this context and we review the leading ones in this chapter. The ANN-based automated cytogenetic analysis is the first of its kind in automated Karyotyping, and involves the two basic steps of chromosome image processing/analysis and the classification of numerical/structural abnormalities in detected and sorted chromosomes. The motivation behind the use of ANNs instead of rule-based approaches is in the uncertainties in the rules of Denver's nomenclature and their imprecise definitions.

In all ANN applications, and more precisely those in medicine, the main difficulty lies in the feature extraction phase for the generation of the input components leading to good performances in the learning phase. An optimum feature extraction of medical signals has been found to be the wavelet transform. In our automated karyotyping system, the wavelet transform of the chromosome band patterns is used to overcome the problems arising due to metaphase quality index. In the Antepartum FHR testing, such a transformation is used to avoid the problems inherent to the determination of classical FHR parameters such as baseline, acceleration, deceleration, and variability. We have also shown, through reconstruction of original signal from wavelet coefficients, that the wavelet transformation is a valuable method in characterizing the raw signal with a small number of features (wavelet coefficients). This objective approach may also provide standardization in test protocols. The wavelet coefficients have been proven to carry all critical information without any loss of sharp variation features such as those that exist in the fetal blood flow Doppler images of Doppler velocimetry, or in any fetal ultrasonography.

In the approaches reported in this chapter, diagnostic classes/clusters of these features are automatically obtained at the output of a system based on MLP, SOM, or LVQ according to the data processed. Ambiguity and vagueness are frequently major characteristics of uncertainty that are faced in the design of automated biomedical interpretation and decision systems. Fuzzy parameters, fuzzy measures such as belief functions, and fuzzy neural networks (not excluding belief networks) are crucial extensions to diagnostic techniques in objectively handling and efficiently compressing the vagueness and ambiguity in sensory or training data fed to diagnostic systems. We have presented a system that we developed using belief functions to describe specification of successful stimulated cycles leading to pregnancy.

Engineering in biotechnologies, as reported in this chapter, aims to enhance human quality of life right from the beginning, which encompasses healthy conception and fetal well being and growth.

Acknowledgments
This research is supported by the Turkish State Planning Institute Project Numbers 90K120540 and 96K120950, and Turkish Scientific and Technical Research Institute. We are grateful to Prof. Dr. A. Nur Cakar and Prof. Dr. Selma Yörükan for their support in preparing this manuscript.

References and further readings

[1] Aksel, S., (1993), Amenorrhea, anovulation induction, *Reproductive Endocrinology and Infertility*, (Aksel, S., Beksac, M.S. Eds.), Ankara, AL: Medical Network; 78-90.

[2] Antsaklis, P.J. and Passin, K.M., (eds.), (1983), *An Introduction to Intelligent and Autonomous Control*, Norwell, MA, Kluwer Academic Publishers, 1983.

[3] Basaran, F., Beksac, M.S., and Erkmen, A.M., (1993), An automated system for the evaluation of antepartum blood flow velocity waveforms: feature extraction, *Trends in the Journal of Medical Science*, 18: 227-232.

[4] Baykal, N., Reggia, J.A., Yalabik, N., Erkmen, A., Beksac, M.S., (1996) Feature discovery and classification of Doppler umbilical artery blood flow velocity waveforms, *Comput Biol Med*; 26: 451-462.

[5] Beksac, M.S., Basaran, F., Eskiizmirliler, S., Erkmen, A.M., and Yorukan, S., (1996), A computerized diagnostic system for the interpretation of umbilical artery blood flow velocity waveforms, *Eur J Obstet Gynecol Reprod Biol*; 64: 37-42.

[6] Beksac, M., Beksac, M.S., Tipi, V.B., Duru, H.A., Karakas, M.U., and Cakar, A.N., (1997), An artificial intelligent diagnostic system on differential recognition of hematopoietic cells from microscopic images, *Cytometry (Communications in Clinical Cytometry)*, 30: 145-150.

[7]　Beksac, M.S., Durak, B., Ozkan, O., Cakar, A.N., Balci, S., Karakas, U., and Laleli, Y., (1995), An artificial intelligent diagnostic system with neural networks to determine genetical disorders and fetal health by using maternal serum markers, *Eur J Obstet Gynecol Reprod Biol*; 59: 131-136.

[8]　Beksac, M.S., Egemen, A., Erkmen, A.M., and Di Renzo, G.C., (1997), Automated image processing and analysis of umbilical artery Doppler velocity waveforms, *Prenat Neonat Med*; 1: 131-136.

[9]　Beksac, M.S., Egemen, A., • zzetoglu, K., Ergun, G., and Erkmen, A.M., (1996), An automated intelligent diagnostic system for the interpretation of umbilical artery Doppler velocimetry, *Eur J Radiol*; 23: 162-167.

[10] Beksac, M.S., Ergun, G., and Erkmen, A.M., (1997), Antepartum fetal kalp atim hizi testi: Ankara Systemi (Version 4.50), *Klinik Bilimler ve Doktor*; 3: 894-899.

[11] Beksac, M.S., Eskiizmirliler, S., Cakar, A.N., Erkmen, A.M., Dagdeviren, A., and Lundsteen, C., (1996), An expert diagnostic system based on neural networks and image analysis techniques in the field of automated cytogenetics, *Technology Health and Care*; 3: 217-229.

[12] Beksac, M.S., Goren, C., Kartal, G., and Erkmen, A.M., (1992), An image processing for umbilical artery blood flow velocity waveforms, *Tur J Med Res*; 10: 298-300.

[13] Beksac, M.S., Karakas, U., Yalcin, S., Ozdemir, K., and Sanliturk, E., (1990), Computerized analysis of antepartum fetal heart rate tracings in normal pregnancies (version 88/2.29), *Eur J Obstet Gynecol Reprod Biol*; 37: 121-132.

[14] Beksac, M.S., Odcikin, Z., Egemen, A., and Karakas, U., (1996), An intelligent diagnostic system for the assessment of gestational age based on ultrasonic fetal head measurements, *Technology Health Care*; 4: 223-231.

[15] Beksac, M.S., Onderoglu, L.S., Atac, B., Karakas, U., and Karaagaoglu, E., (1991), Comparison of two different versions of a knowledge-based system for the interpretation of fetal heart rate tracings (Version 88/2.29 and 89/2.34), *Doga-Tr J Med Sci*; 15: 454-8.

[16] Beksac, M.S., Onderoglu, L.S., Ozdemir, K., and Karakas, U., (1991), The validation of a computerized system for the interpretation of the antepartum fetal heart rate tracings (version 89/2.34), *Eur J Obstet Gynecol Reprod Biol*; 42: 9-14.

[17] Beksac, M.S., Ozdemir, K., Erkmen, A., and Karakas, U., (1994), Assessment of antepartum fetal heart rate tracings using neural networks, *A Critical Appraisal of Fetal Surveillance*, (Van Geizn, H.P. and Copray, F.J.A., Eds.), Elsevier Science BV; 354-62.

[18] Beksac, M.S., Ozdemir, K., Karakas, U., Yalcin, S., and Karaagaoglu, E., (1990), Development and application of a simple expert system for the interpretation of the antepartum fetal heart rate tracings (version 88/2.29), *Eur J Obstet Gynecol Reprod Biol*; 37: 133-141.

[19] Beksac, M.S., Ozdemir, K., Onderoglu, L.S., Karakas, U., Chew, R., and Atac, B., (1989), The validation of a simple expert system for the interpretation of the antepartum fetal heart rate tracings (Ankara System, version 88/2.25), *Acta Reprod Turc*; 10: 69-74.

[20] Brownston, L., Farrel, R., Kant, E., and Martin, N., (1986*), Programming Expert Systems in OPS5,* Reading, MA, Addison-Wesley.

[21] Buchanan, B. and Shartliffe, E.H., (1984), *Rule-Based Expert System, MYCIN*, Reading, MA, Addison-Wesley.

[22] Chui, C.K., (1992), *An Introduction to Wavelets*, Academic Press, Boston MA.

[23] Cohen, L., (1995), *Time Frequency Analysis,* Prentice Hall, Signal Processing Series, Englewood Cliffs, NJ.

[24] Daubechies, I., (1992), *10 Lectures on Wavelets*, CBMS-NSF Series in Applied Math, SIAM, PA.

[25] Dawes, G.S., Moulden, N., and Redman, C.W.G., (1991), System 8000: computerized fetal heart rate analysis, *J Perinat Med*; 19: 47-51.

[26] Dawes, G.S., Redman, C.W.G., and Smith, J.L., (1985), Improvements in the registration and analysis of fetal heart rate records at the bedside, *Br J Obstet Gynecol*; 92: 317-325.

[27] DeSieno, D., (1988), Adding a conscience to competitive learning, *Proceedings of the Second IEEE International Conference on Neural Networks.*

[28] DiRenzo, G.C., Copray, F.J.A., O'Herlihy, C., and Van Geizn, H.P., (1994), Maternal-fetal surveillance within the European community, *A Critical Appraisal of Fetal Surveillance*, Van Geizn, H.P. and Copray, F.Z.A. (Eds), Elsevier BV; 11-15.

[29] Ergun,, G., Erkmen, M.A., Beksac, M.S., Ozzetoglu, K., and Karakas, U., (1995), Evaluation of fetal heart rate tracings based on feature extraction by wavelet transformation, *Gynecol Obstet Reprod Med*; 1: 5-7.

[30] Eskiizmirliler, S., Erkmen, A.M., Basaran, F., Beksac, M.S,, and Cakar, A.N., (1996), "A hybrid intelligent diagnostic system based on neural networks and image analysis techniques in the field of automated cytogenetics", *Proceedings of IEEE International Conference on Image Processing;* 1:315-318.

[31] Fahlman, S.E., (1988), *An Empirical Study of Learning Speed in Back-propagation Networks*, Carnegie Mellon University Computer Science Department, CMU-CS-88-162.

[32] Friedman, J.H. and Turkey, J.W., (1974), A projection pursuit algorithm for exploratory data analysis, *IEEE Trans. on Comput.*, C-23: 881-890.

[33] Fourier, J., (1922), *The Analytical Theory of Heat*, translated by Freeman, A., (1878), Cambridge University Press, London.

[34] Gabor, D., (1946), Theory of communication, *Journal of Inst. Electrical Engineering*, London; 93: 111; 429-457.

[35] Godo, L., Copex de Mantaras, R., Sierra, C., and Verdaguer, A., (1988), Managing linguistically expressed uncertainty in MILORD: Application to medical diagnosis, *Artic. Intell. Commun.*; 1: 14-31.

[36] Haar, A., (1910), Zur theorrie der orthogonalen functionen systeme, *Mathematische Annalen 69*; 331-271.

[37] Halici, U. and Gelenbe, E., (1996), *Neural Networks*, Lecture Notes, Middle East Technical University.

[38] Hayas-Roth, F., et-al., (1985), *Building Expert Systems*, Reading, MA, Addison-Wesley.

[39] Haykin, S., (1994), *Neural Networks: A Comprehensive Foundation*, McMillan.

[40] Ince, T., Leblebicioglu, K., Sayan, G.T., (1996), Target classification by a time-frequency analysis, *IEEE APS Int. Symp. and URSI Radio Science Meeting, Proc of URSI*, Maryland; 2:20.

[41] Jain, L.C., (Ed.), (1997), *Soft Computing Techniques in Knowledge-Based Intelligent Engineering Systems*, Springer Verlag, Germany.

[42] Klir, G.J. and Yuan, B., (1995), *Fuzzy Seta and Fuzzy Logic: Theory and Applications*, Prentice Hall PTR; Upper Saddle River, NJ

[43] Kohonen, T. et al., (1988), Statistical pattern recognition with neural networks: benchmark studies, *Proc. Second IEEE International Conference on Neural Networks*.

[44] Kohonen, T., (1989), *Self Organisation and Associative Memory*, Springer Verlag, NY.

[45] Kung, S.Y., (1993), *Digital Neural Networks*, PTR Prentice Hall, Englewood Cliffs, New Jersey.

[46] Lippmann, R.P., (1993), Neural networks, bayesian a posteriori probabilities, and pattern classification, *Proc. of the NATO Advanced Studies Institute on Statistics and Neural Networks, Theory and Pattern Recognition Applications*, Les Arcs, Bourg Saint Maurice, France, pp. 83-104.

[47] Lin, C.T. and George Lee, C.S., (1996), *Neural Fuzzy System: A Neuro-Fuzzy Synergism to Intelligent System*, Prentice Hall PTR, NJ.

[48] Mallat, S., (1987), A compact multiresolution representation: the wavelet model, *Proc. IEEE Workshop Comput. Vision*, Miami, FL.

[49] Mamdani, E.H., (1974), Application of fuzzy algorithm for control of simple dynamic plant, *Proc. IEEE*, 121: 12: 1585-1588.

[50] March, C.M., (1993), Ovulation induction, *J. Reprod. Med.*; 38: 335-46.

[51] Mao, J. and Jain, A.K., (1995), Artificial neural networks for feature extraction and multivariate data projection, *IEEE Trans on Neural Networks*; 6-2: 296-317.

[52] Meyer, Y., (1985), Principe d'incertitutde, bases hilbertiennes et algebres d'opérateurs, *Séminaire Bourbaki*, 209-223.

[53] McCulloch, W.S. and Pitts, W., (1943), A logical calculus of ideas immanent in nervous activity, *Bulletin of Mathematical Biophysics*; 5:115-133; reprinted in Anderson and Rosenberg, (1988).

[54] Morlet, J., Arens, G., Fourgeau, and Girard D., (1982), Wave propagation and sampling theory, part II, *Geophysics*; 47: 203-236.

[55] Munakata, T. and Jani, Y., (1994), Fuzzy systems: an overview, *Commun. ACM*; 37(3): 69-76.

[56] Riss, P.A., Koebl, H., Reinthaller, A., and Deutinger, J., (1988), Development and application of simple expert system in obstetrics and gynecology, *J Perinat Med*; 16:287.

[57] Rubner, J. and Schulten, K., (1990), Development of feature detectors by self organisation, *Biol. Cyber.* 62: 193-199.

[58] Rumelhart, D.E., Hinton, G.E., and Williams, R.J., (1986), Learning internal representations by error propagation, *Parallel Distributed Processing: Explorations in the Microstructure of Cognition*, Rumelhart, D.E., McClelland, J.L. (Eds.), Vol. 1, Chapter 8, Cambridge, MA: MIT Press.

[59] Sabourin, M. and Mitiche, A., (1993), Modeling and classification of shape using a kohonen associative memory with selective multi-resolution, *Neural Networks*; 6: 275-283.

[60] Sayan, G.T. and Leblebicioglu, K., (1997), Electromagnetic Target Classification by Self Organizing Maps, *Proc. Int. Conf. on Engineering Applications of Neural Networks,* Stockholm, Sweden; 295-298.

[61] Shaffer, G., (1976), *A Mathematical Theory of Evidence*, Princeton University Press, NJ.

[62] Schweitzer, B. and Sklar, A., (1961), Associative functions and statistical triangle inequalities, *Publicationes Mathematicae Debrecen*; 8:169-186.

[63] Schweitzer, B. and Sklar, A., (1963), Associative functions and abstract semigroups, *Publicationes Mathematicae Debrece*, 10: 69-81.

[64] Searle, J.R., Devoe, L.D., Philips, M.C., and Seale, N.S., (1988), Computerized analysis of resting fetal heart rate tracings, *Obstet Gynecol*; 71: 407-411.

[65] Shalkof, R.J., (1992), *Pattern Recognition: Statistical, Structural and Neural Approaches*, John Wiley & Sons, NY.

[66] Shortliffe, E.H., (1976), *Computer-Based Medical Consultation: MYCIN*, Elsevier, NY.

[67] Smith, M.J.T. and Barnwell, T.P., (1986), Exact reconstruction techniques for tree-structured subband coders, *IEEE Trans. Acoust. Signal Speech Process*; 34: 434-441.

[68] Sokol, R.J. and Chik, L., (1988), A prototype system for perinatal knowledge engineering using an artificial intelligence tool, *J Perinat Med*; 16: 273-281.

[69] Webb, A.R. and Lowe, D., (1990), The optimized internal representation of multilayer classifier networks performs nonlinear discriminant analysis, *Neural Networks*; 3: 367-375.

[70] Weiss, S.M. and Kulihowski, C.A., (1984), *A Principal Guide to Designing Expert Systems*, Rowman and Allehald, NJ.

[71] Weker, S., (1983), A general concept of fuzzy connectives, negations and implications based an t-norms and t-co-norms, *Fuzzy Sets and Systems*, 11: 115-134.

[72] Werbos, P., (1974), *Beyond Regression: New Tools for Prediction and Analysis in the Behavioral Sciences*, Ph.D. Thesis, Harvard, MA.

[73] Zadeh, L.A., (1965), Fuzzy sets, *Information and Control*, 8: 338-353.

Chapter 7

Wavelet network with convex wavelets: applications to nonlinear system modeling and feature extraction in vectorcardiography

Eiji Uchino, Takashi Samatsu, and Takeshi Yamakawa

This chapter describes several applications of wavelet networks in biomedical signal processing. A specific wavelet network with convex wavelets is introduced and its distinctive features are presented. The main characteristics of the network are good designability (the number of network connection weights can be determined by the designer) and improved generalization capability.

Three applications of the wavelet networks with convex wavelets are presented, namely, modeling of the nonlinear dynamical systems, feature extraction from vectorcardiograms, and data compression. We demonstrate how the extracted features can be used for visualization for medical diagnoses. The network is then used in data compression for electrocardiograms (ECGs). We introduce an improved (faster) learning algorithm for data compression, based on wavelets. Conclusions regarding the use of wavelet networks with convex wavelets in cardiography and in other medical applications are presented in the final section of the chapter.

For the basic theory of wavelet transform and for other applications in the field of medicine, the reader is referred to the textbooks in the *Reference* list and to the titles in the *Further reading* section at the end of the chapter.

1. Introduction

Many researchers have recently contributed to the wavelet theory and its applications, for example, [1-7]. Wavelet functions are "local" functions. In applications, wavelet basis functions are placed over the fluctuation range of the analyzed signal and allow a local analysis of the signal. An arbitrary nonlinear function can be represented by a wavelet series expansion [4]. The wavelet coefficients can be determined analytically – for some classes of wavelet basis functions and several classes of signals – or by computation (approximation). Computation by classic methods may be time consuming. From the practical application viewpoint, the amount of calculation should be reduced as much as possible. One solution is to employ learning [5, 6]. Toward this purpose we introduce a "wavelet network" to benefit from the advantages of employing learning and adaptability.

The wavelet network is a kind of functional link net [7]. Its basis functions are wavelets. Under some circumstances the wavelet network can also be regarded as a fuzzy system with the wavelets as membership functions in the antecedent and singletons in the consequent.

We describe a convex wavelet [8, 9], which is a piecewise cosine function. Based on it, the analysis becomes simpler; furthermore, the generalization capability is improved, as will be exemplified for some case studies. The proof of the convergence of this wavelet expansion is given in Appendix A.

A simple wavelet network model with one input and one output is applied to function approximation and to modeling nonlinear dynamical systems in Section 4. Then, the presented wavelet network is applied to the analysis of vectorcardiograms and electrocardiograms (ECGs). Vectorcardiography [10], [11] measures the strength of an electromotive force, in addition to its direction, while normal electrocardiography only measures the strength of the electromotive force. The features of a vectorcardiogram are extracted by using the presented wavelet network. Furthermore, the data compression of an electrocardiogram by this wavelet network and a faster learning algorithm are also presented.

2. Wavelet network and its learning algorithm

2.1. Desirable features of the wavelet function for the wavelet network

We first introduce briefly the wavelet function and show its features. Let $\psi(t)$ be a mother wavelet with $\psi(t) = 0$ at $t = \pm\infty$. A wavelet basis function is generally defined as

$$\psi_{a,b}(t) = \frac{1}{\sqrt{a}} \psi\left(\frac{t-b}{a}\right) \tag{1}$$

Here, a is called a scaling parameter and it represents the spreading ("dilation") of the basis function; b is called shifting parameter and it represents the position of the basis function. An arbitrary function $f(t)$ is generally expressed with use of the wavelet basis functions [4],

$$f(t) = \sum_a \sum_b W_{a,b} \psi_{a,b}(t) \tag{2}$$

where $W_{a,b}$ denotes the wavelet coefficients.

For wavelet analysis, an ideal wavelet function must conform to the admissibility condition [12], orthogonality, compactness, and smoothness. (The definition of the admissibility condition and the explanation of the orthogonality are given in the Appendix A.) However, all these conditions are not always needed for wavelet networks (from the engineering viewpoint). In this section, we discuss the wavelet function features that are useful for the wavelet network.

First we consider the admissibility condition. For ordinary wavelet theory, the admissibility condition is needed for an inverse transformation. Nevertheless, for a wavelet network, the admissibility condition is not necessary, because the wavelet coefficients in Equation (2-2) are adjusted by learning; therefore, the conditions imposed to the wavelet functions for the wavelet network will become looser.

Let us consider the orthogonality property. Wavelet coefficients can be obtained analytically when the wavelet functions are orthogonal. However, the orthogonality condition is not needed when we determine the coefficients by learning.

In the third place, the compactness property is considered. The amount of calculation for the wavelet coefficients is generally much greater than that needed by the other series expansions. However, if a wavelet is compactly supported (finitely supported), the amount of calculation is reduced. Thus, the condition of "compact support" is important for wavelets used in the wavelet networks.

Finally we consider the smoothness property. For wavelet networks, the output signal $f(t)$ is (re)constructed as a weighted sum of wavelet bases. Theoretically, the sum is infinite. When the sum is truncated, i.e., if the reconstructed signal is represented by a finite series, the shape of the wavelet bases significantly influences the reconstruction error. The reconstructed signal does not have "ripples", and to increase the generalization capability of a wavelet network, the wavelet function used in the wavelet network should be carefully chosen.

2.2. Several types of wavelet networks

In this section several types of wavelet networks are introduced. Figure 1 shows a simple wavelet network, where the input signal X_k is supplied (as usual) to each basis function. The output of this network is represented by a weighted sum of the basis functions

$$f_k(X_k) = \sum_{i=1}^{n} W_i \psi_i(X_k) \tag{3}$$

This network represents a single-input, single-output nonlinear system.

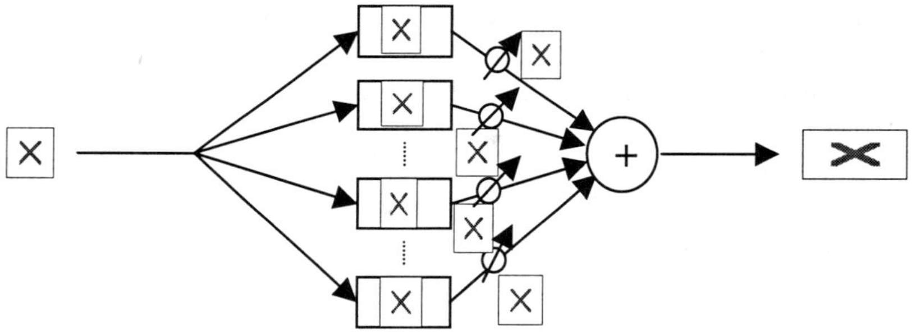

Figure 1. A simple wavelet network.

Figure 2 shows an input-noncorrelated wavelet network. This network consists of a combination of simple wavelet networks as presented in Figure 1. The output Y is represented by

$$Y = \sum_{k=1}^{s} f_k(X_k) = \sum_{k=1}^{s}\sum_{i=1}^{n} W_i^k \psi_i(X_k) . \tag{4}$$

The relation between the input X_k $(k = 1, 2, \cdots, s)$ and the output Y is embedded in the functions f_k $(k = 1, 2, \cdots, s)$ by learning. The output Y is dependent on all the weights W_i^k. Therefore, if we use the squared error criterion to compute the weights, local minimums do not exist. Indeed, the error criterion is based on a quadratic form with respect to the weights, and thus the optimal weights can be found.

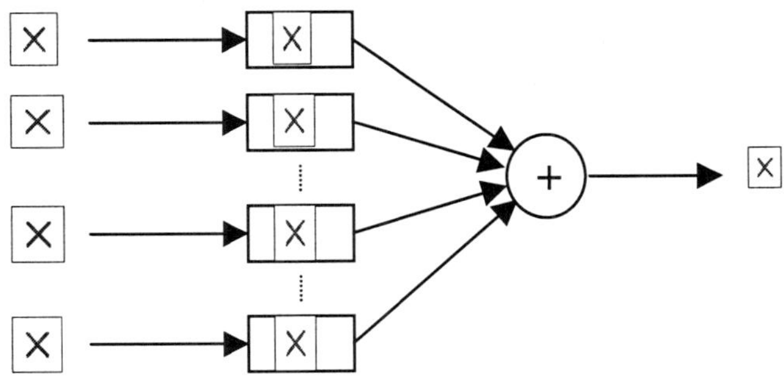

Figure 2. An input-noncorrelated wavelet network.

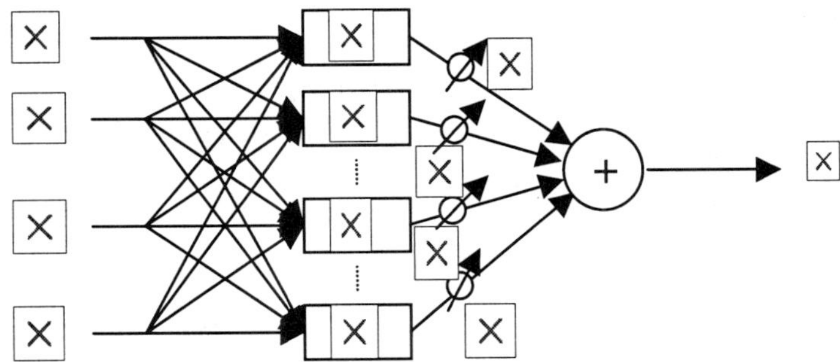

Figure 3. An input-correlated wavelet network.

Figure 3 shows an input-correlated wavelet network. In this case, the output Y is

$$Y = \sum_{i=1}^{n} W_i \psi_i (X_1, X_2, \cdots, X_k, \cdots, X_s).$$ (5)

This network can be used to model complicated multidimensional nonlinear systems.

2.3. Learning algorithms

The network weights W_i of the wavelet network are determined by using a modified steepest-descend method. In the traditional steepest-descend method, the learning rate has a constant value, determined by a trial-and-error procedure. This may cause slow learning, oscillatory learning, or divergent learning. To solve this problem we present a modified steepest-descend method. The method is then used to train the wavelet network.

The renewal of weights in the traditional steepest-descend method is given by the formula

$$\Delta W_i = -G \frac{\partial E}{\partial W_i} \tag{6}$$

with

$$E = \frac{1}{2} \cdot \sum_{j=1}^{m} \left(f_j - \hat{f}_j \right)^2 \tag{7}$$

Here, G denotes the learning rate, f_j is an actual output of the network, and $\hat{f}_j$ is its training data. The weights are adapted as

$$\Delta W_i = -G(l) \cdot \mathrm{sgn}\left(\frac{\partial E}{\partial W_i} \right) \tag{8}$$

where

$$\mathrm{sgn}(x) = \begin{cases} 1 & (x \geq 0) \\ -1 & (x < 0). \end{cases} \tag{9}$$

In this learning procedure, the learning rate $G(l)$ $(l = 1, 2, \cdots)$ is variable, and it is initialized for each weight, in every iteration. The initial value $G(0)$ is assigned to be unity. A tentative value $G'(l+1)$, that is assigned to be equal to $G(l)$, is adopted first to calculate the weight $W_i'(l+1)$ and the error tentative $E'(l+1)$. If this tentative error $E'(l+1)$ is less than the error $E(l)$ at the previous step, the value $G(l+1)$ is retained; otherwise, it is assigned to be half of the previous value $G(l)$,

$$G(l+1) = \begin{cases} G(l) & (E'(l+1) < E(l)) \\ \dfrac{1}{2}G(l) & (otherwise). \end{cases} \tag{10}$$

This iteration is repeated until the condition $|E(l+1) - E(l)| \leq \delta$ is satisfied, where δ is given in advance.

3. Convex wavelet and its assignment

The mother wavelet $\psi(t)$ is adopted to be a convex wavelet [8, 9]

$$\psi(t) = \begin{cases} \cos \pi t & (-0.5 \leq t \leq 0.5) \\ 0 & (\textit{otherwise}). \end{cases} \tag{11}$$

The shape of this function is illustrated in Figure 4. This convex wavelet is compactly supported, and thus the learning speed is increased. Furthermore, because this convex wavelet has only one extreme value over the support, a signal reconstructed with these wavelets is not oscillatory. The generalization capability is improved by employing this type of convex wavelet [8, 9].

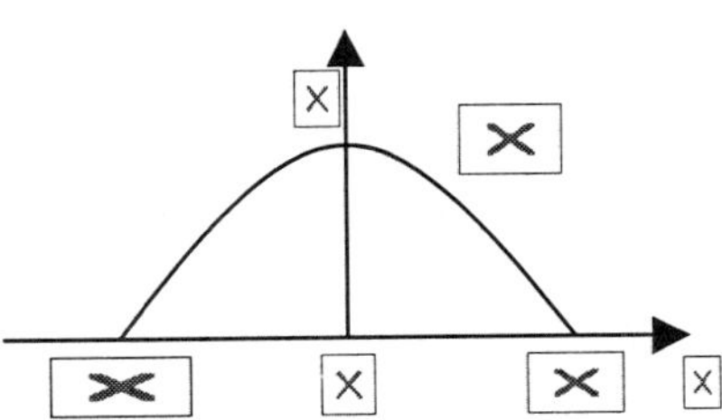

Figure 4. The convex wavelet.

The mother wavelet $\psi(t)$ generates the basis functions

$$\psi_{a,b}(t) = \psi(at - b), \tag{12}$$

where a $(= 0, 1, \ldots, M)$ is a scaling parameter and b $(= 0, 1, \ldots, a)$ is a shifting parameter.

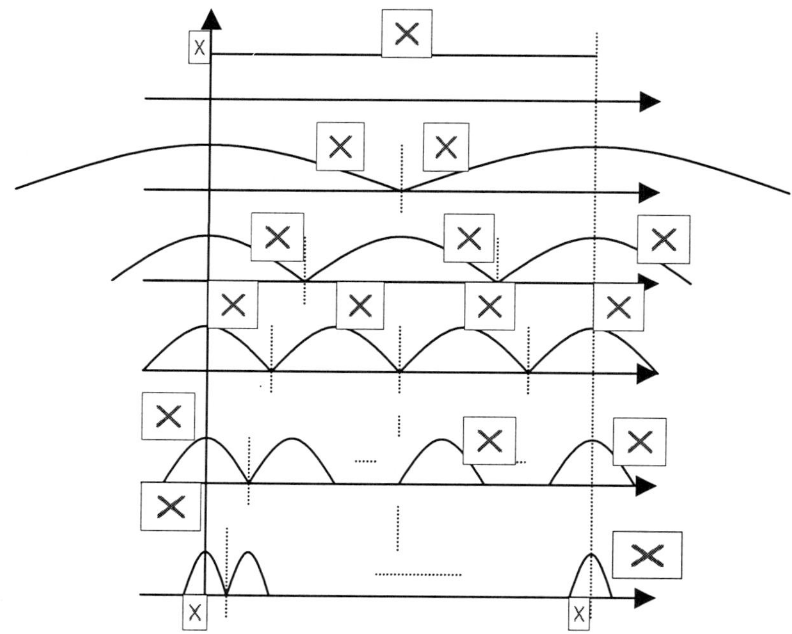

Figure 5. The assignment of convex wavelets.

These basis wavelets are assigned over the normalized fluctuation range as shown in Figure 5. The numbers of wavelet bases are $1, 2, \cdots, M+1$ for the scaling parameter $a = 0, 1, \ldots, M$, respectively. The proof of convergence of this wavelet series is given in Appendix B.

4. Performance of the wavelet network

In this section, we discuss the generalization capability of the presented wavelet network. First the network is applied to function approximation. We consider a function having both piecewise linear and smooth parts. Then, the network is used to model a nonlinear dynamical system.

4.1. Function approximation

The simple wavelet network in Figure 1 is used to approximate a function having both piecewise linear and smooth parts. The experimental results are shown in Figure 6. Learning is performed over 100 iterations. (One iteration feeds a whole data set of a target function to the network.) In this simulation,

101 points of the target function are supplied to the network. Figure 7 shows the R.M.S. (root-mean-squared) learning error versus machine time (basic 80386 16 MHz CPU with a co-processor).

To demonstrate the ability of the convex wavelet, another type of wavelet shown in Figure 8 is employed for comparison. This wavelet is compactly supported, but has three extreme values. Learning is accomplished for 100 iterations. The results are shown in Figure 9. Notice that the approximated curve obtained using this wavelet is more oscillatory than in the case of the convex wavelet. The influence of the shape of the basis function can be better seen in Figure 9 near the value $x = 0.5$.

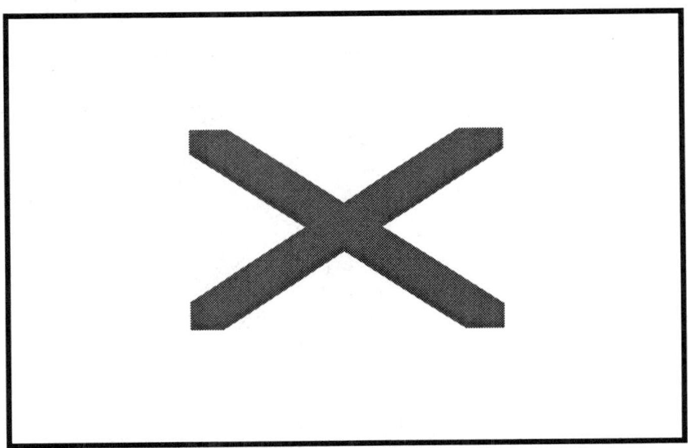

Figure 6. Function approximation. Solid line: approximation (output of the network, 1001 points); dotted line: original function (101 points).

Figure 10 shows the R.M.S. error at 1001 points versus the number of wavelet bases of the present convex wavelet. The approximation result obtained using a wavelet is shown in Figure 8, and the result for Harr wavelets [13] are shown in Figure 10. These results demonstrate that the convex wavelet has higher generalization capability than other wavelets.

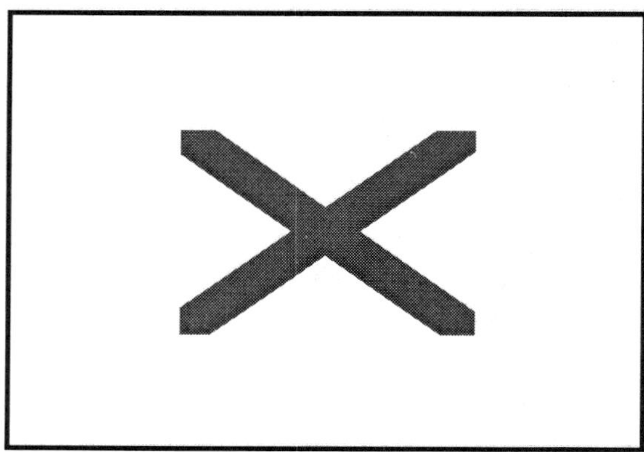

Figure 7. R.M.S. error versus machine time.

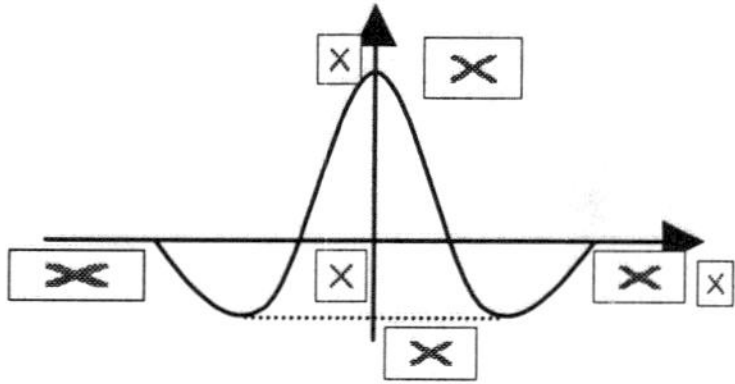

Figure 8. A wavelet which has three extreme values.

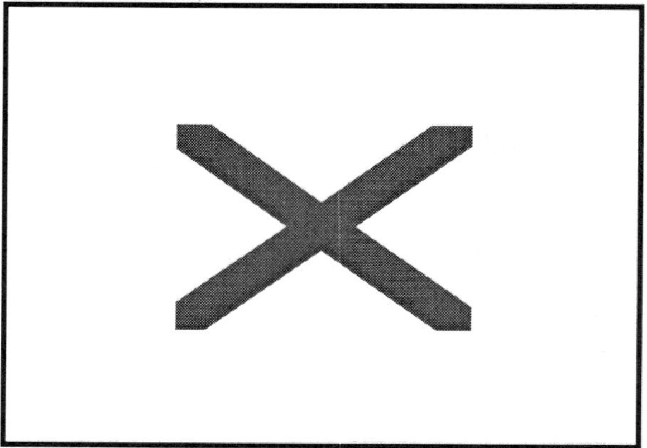

Figure 9. Function approximation using the wavelets shown in Figure 8. Solid line: approximation (output of the network, 1001 points). Dotted line: original function (101 points).

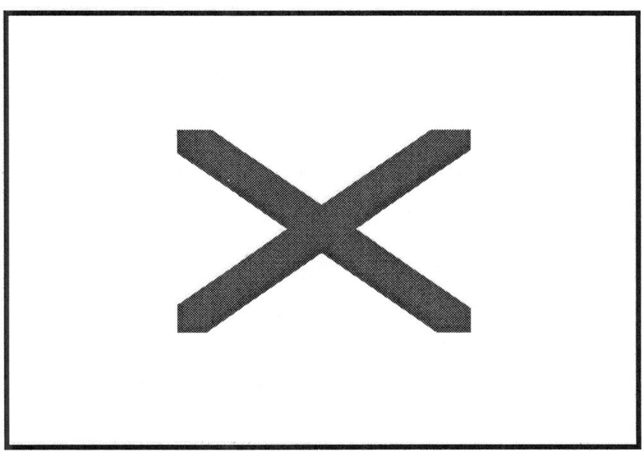

Figure 10. R.M.S. error (between the original function and the output of the network at 1001 points) versus the number of wavelet bases. (a) The convex wavelet, (b) a wavelet shown in Figure 8, and (c) the Harr wavelet.

4.2. Modeling nonlinear dynamical systems

The presented wavelet network is applied to model the nonlinear dynamical system described by the equation

$$X_{p+1} = \frac{5X_p}{1 + X_p^{\,2}} - 0.5X_p - 0.5X_{p-1} + 0.5X_{p-2} \tag{13}$$

The initial values are $X_0 = 0.2$, $X_1 = 0.3$, and $X_2 = 1.0$. Figure 11 shows the wavelet network used for this modeling. The output of the network is

$$\hat{X}_{p+1} = \sum_{k=1}^{s} f_k(X_{p-k+1}) = \sum_{k=1}^{s}\sum_{a=0}^{M}\sum_{b=0}^{a} W_{a,b}^{k}\,\psi_{a,b}(X_{p-k+1}) \tag{14}$$

The connection weights $W_{a,b}^{k}$ are tuned using the learning algorithm presented in Section 2.3. $\hat{X}_{p+1}$ represents the output of the network. After learning, the relation between $X_p, X_{p-1}, \cdots, X_{p-s+1}$ and X_{p+1} is embedded into $f_1, f_2, \cdots, f_s$ by means of the set of connection weights.

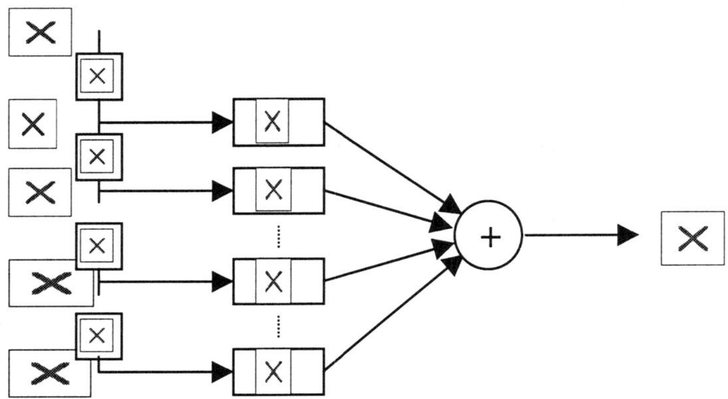

Figure 11. The structure of a wavelet network for modeling the nonlinear dynamical system. D denotes the unitary delay elements.

The signal generated by Equation (13) is chaotic and thus it is difficult to predict by using classic methods. Figure 12 shows the time series of this signal. The samples $X_0, X_1, \cdots, X_{100}$ are used for learning and the sequence $X_{101}, X_{102}, \cdots, X_{150}$ is used for the evaluation of the prediction capability of this wavelet network.

We adopt the Euclidean one-step-ahead prediction error to determine the order of the dynamical system. The learning aims to decrease the error function

$$E = \frac{1}{2} \sum_{p=s}^{100} (\hat{X}_p - X_p)^2 \tag{15}$$

Here, s is the number of the inputs of this wavelet network and corresponds to the order of a dynamical system.

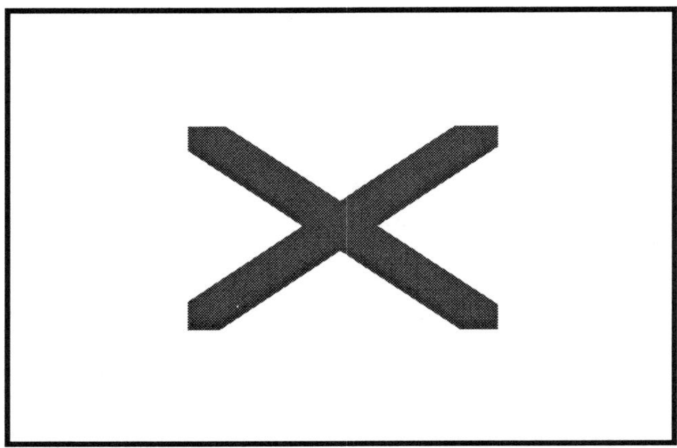

Figure 12. Sample path of a signal generated by Equation (13).

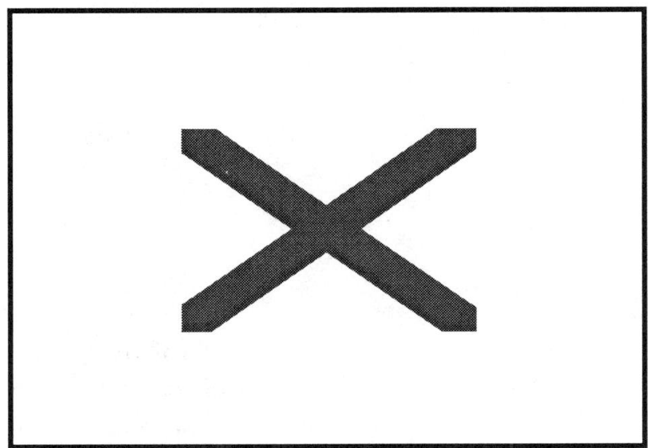

Figure 13. Prediction error: (a) noise free system, (b) noisy system.

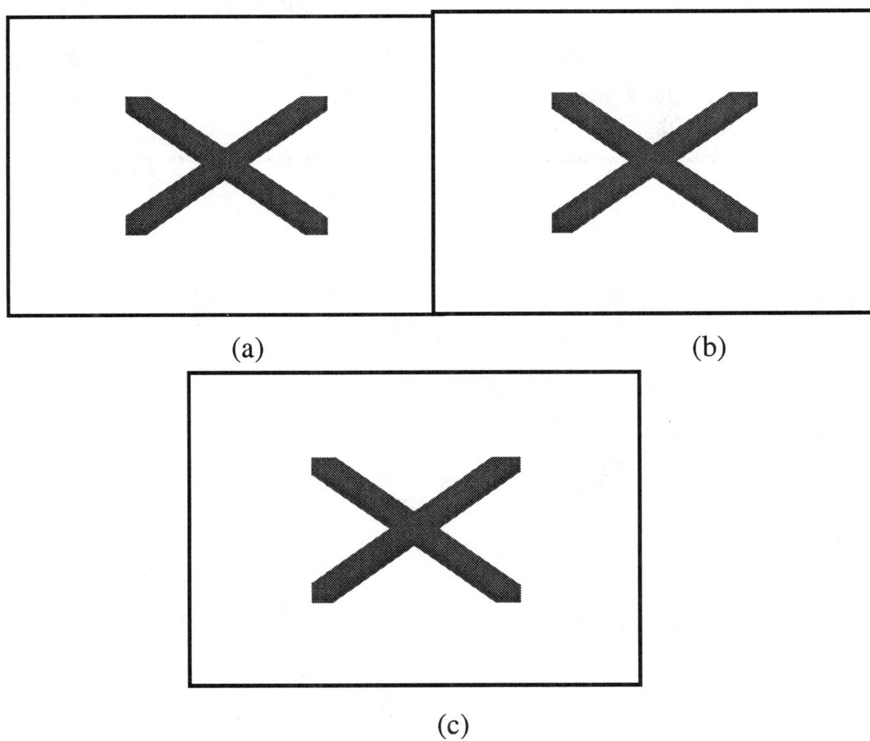

(a)   (b)

(c)

Figure 14. Identified nonlinear mapping functions: (a) f_1, (b) f_2, (c) f_3.
(Solid line: identified; dotted line: true curve.)

After learning, the sequence $X_p, X_{p-1}, \cdots, X_{p-s+1}$ is applied to the inputs and to obtain $\hat{X}_{p+1}$ at the output terminal, which is called a one-step-ahead prediction. The R.M.S. error is

$$RMSE = \sqrt{\frac{1}{50} \sum_{p=101}^{150} (\hat{X}_p - X_p)^2} \tag{16}$$

is shown in Figure 13 for (a) noise free system when $s = 2, 3, 4, 5$. Uniform random numbers in the interval [-0.3, 0.3] are added to the signal in Figure 12 as an observation noise. The number of iterations of the learning phase is 100. The minimum prediction error is obtained for $s = 3$; therefore, we may estimate that the order of this dynamical system is three.

The outputs of the mapping functions f_1, f_2, and f_3 after learning are shown in Figure 14. Once the learning is accomplished, the last three data X_p, X_{p-1}, and X_{p-2} are applied to the inputs. We then obtain the one-step-ahead prediction of the signal at the output terminal.

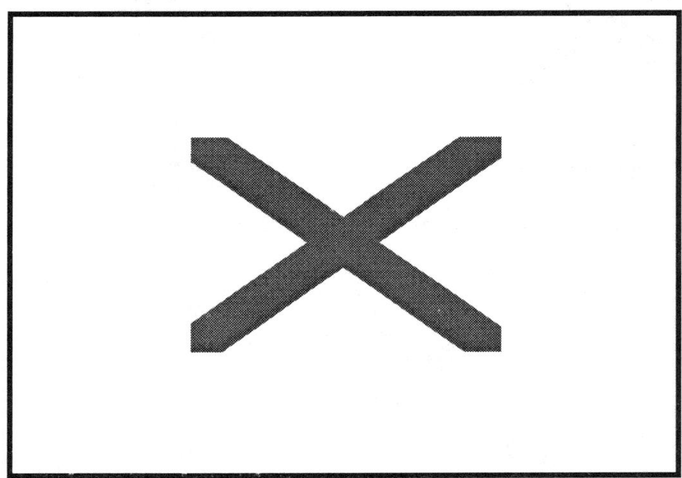

Figure 15. Prediction by the wavelet network.
Solid line: predicted; dotted line: true signal.

Repeatedly feeding this output signal back to the input terminal, we can predict the future behavior of the dynamical system. Figure 15 shows the prediction results. The wavelet network satisfactorily predicts the behavior of the dynamical system up to about seven steps ahead.

5. Applications to electrocardiography

5.1. Vectorcardiogram feature extraction

Vectorcardiography [10, 11] can measure both the strength of the electromotive force and its direction, while classic electrocardiography in current use only measures the strength of an electromotive force. Vectorcardiography is not yet popular in spite of its high accuracy for diagnosis. The main reason for this situation is that the vectorcardiogram is a 3-D signal and thus its classification is very difficult in comparison with 1-D electrocardiogram. Therefore, the feature extraction from a vectorcardiogram and its visualization is important. We address the use of the wavelet network with convex wavelets to features extraction. We shall also indicate a method to visualize the extracted.

5.1.1. Lead systems for vectorcardiography

There are two main types of lead systems for vectorcardiography. One is a noncorrected orthogonal lead system with orthogonal axes along the main directions of the body of human subject (one vertical and two horizontal axes). The other main lead system is a corrected orthogonal lead system [14, 15] that compensates electric distortion. The most popular system is the so-called Frank lead system [15], which is a type of corrected orthogonal lead system.

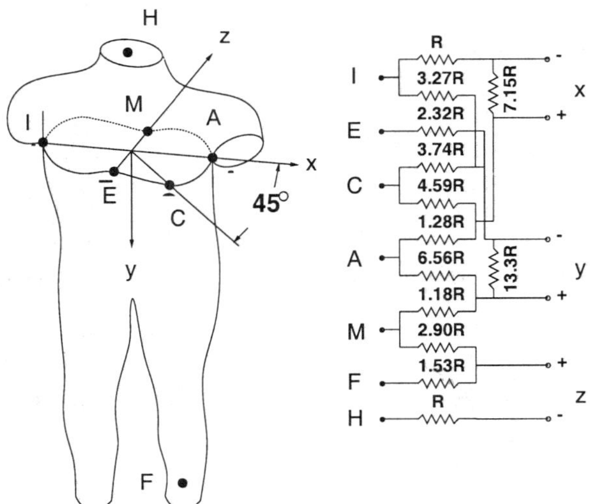

Figure 16. Position of electrodes and its compensating network for Frank lead system.

Figure 16 shows the position of electrodes and the compensating network in the Frank lead system. Five electrodes A, C, E, I, and M are placed on a transverse plane. H is placed on the back of the neck, and F is placed on the left leg. This lead system can produce a vectorcardiogram free of any electric deformation, despite the differences in individual position of the heart dipole and body shapes. The signals shown in the examples discussed in this chapter were acquired using the Frank lead system.

5.1.2. Wavelet network for vectorcardiogram

We address the vectorcardiogram modeling using the presented wavelet network. The vectorcardiogram is regarded as a three-dimensional dynamical system. Figure 17 shows the wavelet network employed, with the corresponding delay elements. The mapping functions f_x, f_y, and f_z are obtained by three-input, one-output wavelet networks, as shown in Figure 3.

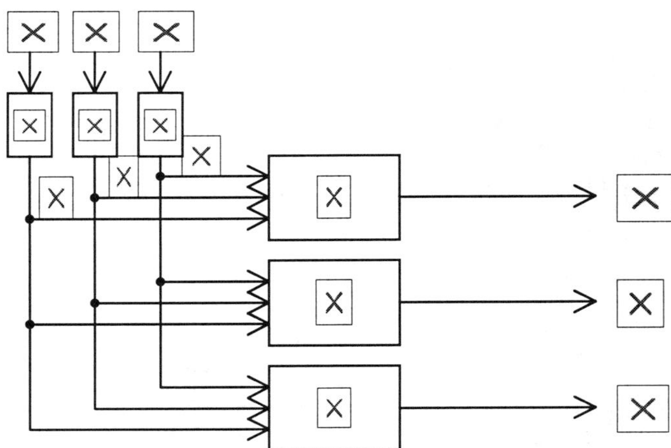

Figure 17. Wavelet network for modeling a vectorcardiogram. f_x, f_y, and f_z are realized by three-input, one-output wavelet networks shown in Figure 3. D: Delay element.

The following mother convex wavelet employed here is the same as in Section 3.

$$\psi(x) = \begin{cases} \cos \pi x & (-0.5 \le x \le 0.5) \\ 0 & (\textit{otherwise}). \end{cases} \tag{17}$$

The one-dimensional wavelet bases of the network are then constructed as follows:

$$\psi_{a,b}(x) = \psi(ax - b) \tag{18}$$

where $a(= 0, 1, \cdots, M)$ is a scaling parameter and $b(= 0, 1, \cdots, a)$ is a shifting parameter. If the resolution of the model is specified, the value of M is automatically determined and the number of connection weights is thus determined. That is, the network structure is automatically determined according to the resolution, and furthermore this network has a high designability in contrast with usual sigmoidal neural networks or RBF networks.

A three-dimensional base $\psi_{a,b,c,d}(x_t, y_t, z_t)$ is obtained as a product of three one-dimensional bases, as follows:

$$\Psi_{a,b,c,d}(x_t, y_t, z_t) = \psi(ax_t - b)\,\psi(ay_t - c)\,\psi(az_t - d) \tag{19}$$

where a is a scaling parameter, and b, c, and d are shifting parameters for x, y, and z, respectively. Then the output of each wavelet network is described as

$$\hat{x}_{t+1} = \sum_{a=0}^{M}\sum_{b=0}^{a}\sum_{c=0}^{a}\sum_{d=0}^{a} W^{x}_{a,b,c,d}\,\Psi_{a,b,c,d}(x_t, y_t, z_t) \tag{20}$$

$$\hat{y}_{t+1} = \sum_{a=0}^{M}\sum_{b=0}^{a}\sum_{c=0}^{a}\sum_{d=0}^{a} W^{y}_{a,b,c,d}\,\Psi_{a,b,c,d}(x_t, y_t, z_t) \tag{21}$$

$$\hat{z}_{t+1} = \sum_{a=0}^{M}\sum_{b=0}^{a}\sum_{c=0}^{a}\sum_{d=0}^{a} W^{z}_{a,b,c,d}\,\Psi_{a,b,c,d}(x_t, y_t, z_t), \tag{22}$$

where $W^{x}_{a,b,c,d}$, $W^{y}_{a,b,c,d}$, and $W^{z}_{a,b,c,d}$ are connection weights of the network for f_x, f_y, and f_z. These weights show the features of a vectorcardiogram, and they can be used for diagnosis purposes.

5.1.3. Vectorcardiogram modeling

In this subsection we show an application of the wavelet network to the modeling of the vectorcardiographic signals. The signals x, y, and z shown in Figure 18 represent the three components of a vectorcardiogram. The vectorcardiographic signal is obtained by sampling (sampling period 10 msec) through the compensating network shown in Figure 5.1. These three components (signals) are normalized to the interval [0, 1] and then are used for training the network. The connection weights $W^x_{a,b,c,d}$ (or $W^y_{a,b,c,d}$, $W^z_{a,b,c,d}$) of f_x (or f_y, f_z) are determined by using the training data x, y, z, and x_{t+1} (or y_{t+1}, z_{t+1}).

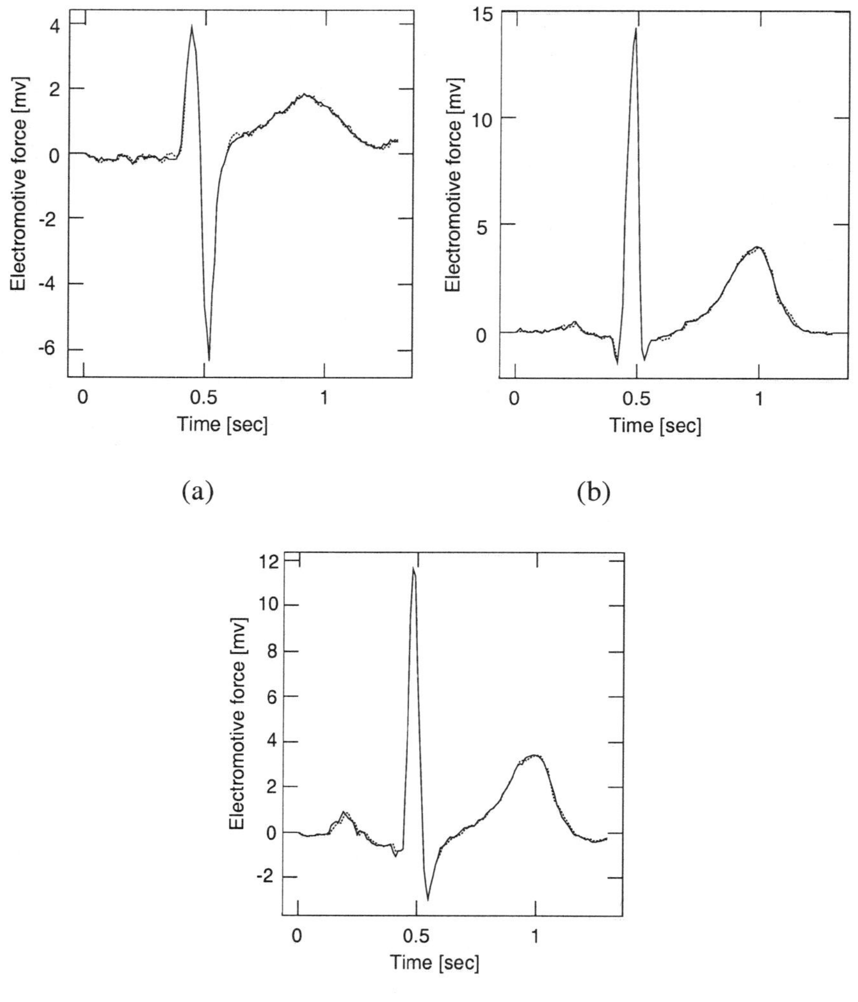

(a) (b)

(c)

Figure 18. A vectorcardiogram decomposed into three components and output of the wavelet network: (a) x_t, (b) y_t, (c) z_t. Solid line: original signal (for each of the components of the vectorcardiogram); dotted line: output of the corresponding wavelet network.

After learning, the wavelet network shown in Figure 5.2 generates the outputs $\hat{x}_{t+1}$, $\hat{y}_{t+1}$ and $\hat{z}_{t+1}$. For learning, the number of iterations is 100, and $M = 6$ for Equations (5-4), (5-5), and (5-6). The modeling R.M.S. error is less than 5% for each component (x_t, y_t and z_t) of the original vectorcardiographic signal.

5.1.4. Feature visualization

A vectorcardiogram records the dynamics of the electric dipole of the heart. This means that the dynamic characteristics of the electrical activity of the heart appear in the vectorcardiogram. The proposed wavelet network is suitable to grasp the local change of the signal [8], and it does not overlook even small changes of the signal. The features of a vectorcardiogram are embedded in the network weights. Therefore, if we monitor the change of the network weights, we can detect the changes of the dynamics of a heart. Consequently, even small abnormalities of the heart function can be detected.

We explain the relation between the connection weights and the signal shape by using an example of a 1-D mapping function shown in Figure 5.4 (a). Recall that the wavelet network can approximate the mapping function.

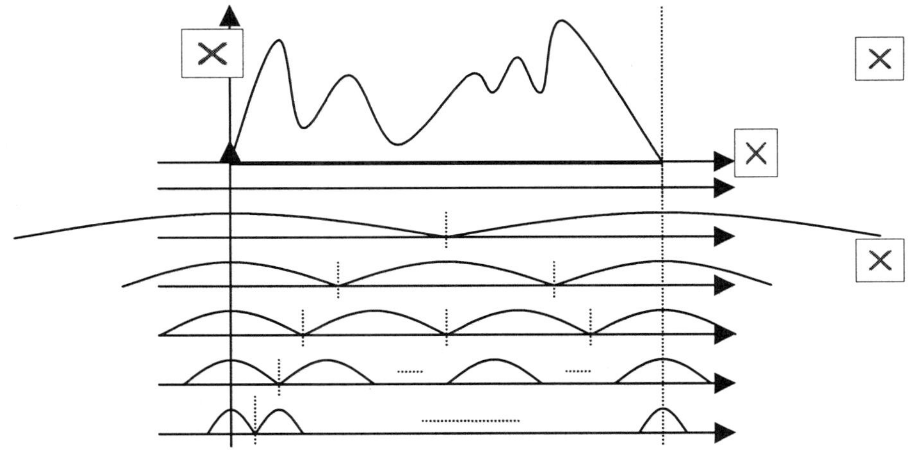

Figure 19. (a) An example of 1-D mapping function and
(b) an assignment of 1-D convex wavelets.

A mapping function is expressed by a weighted sum of the basis functions (Figure 19 (b)). The features of a mapping function are embedded in the connection weights (after the learning phase). The connection weights can be viewed as the amount of influence to the next step, i.e.,, from x_t to x_{t+1}. Because a shifting parameter b shows the position of a base, a change of b indicates the position of the fluctuation of the mapping function. The scaling parameter a shows the size of a base; therefore, a change of a indicates the sharpness of the change of the signal at position b. If a is small, the width of the base is wide; therefore, this base strongly affects the result of the next step of the computation. If a is large, the width of the base is narrow; consequently, this base only locally affects the next step. This is valid in case of 3-D signals too.

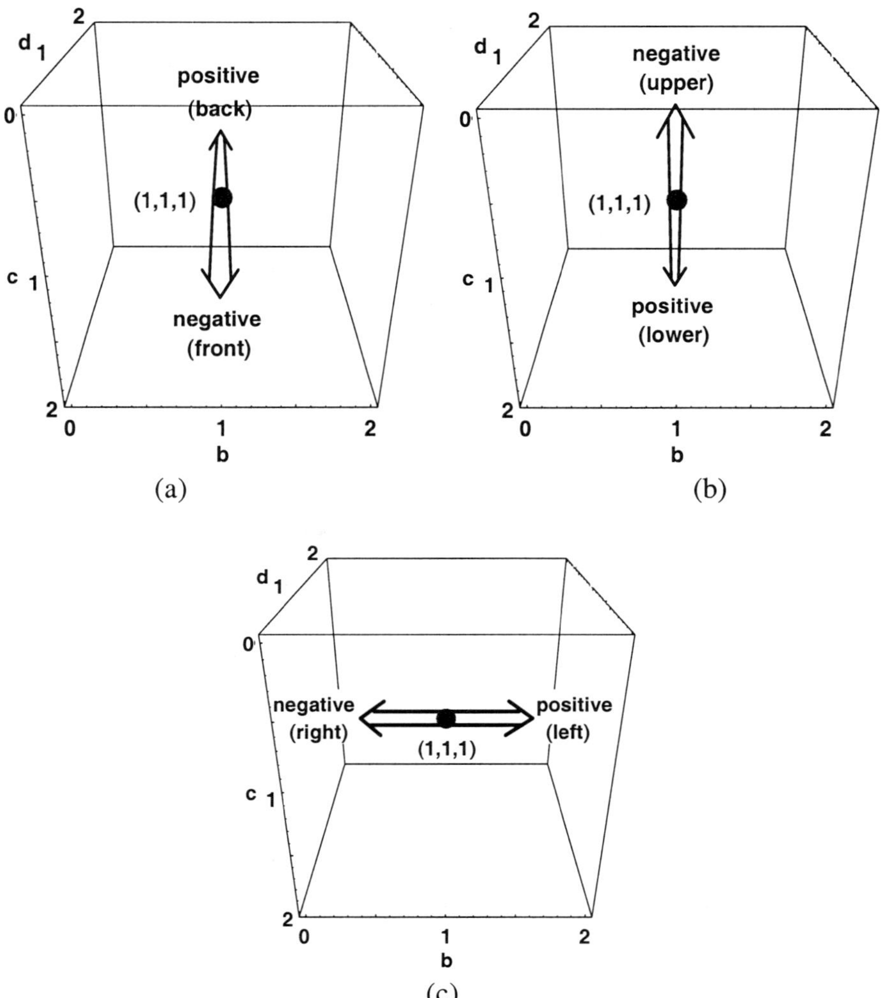

Figure 20. The direction of the influence to the next step: (a) x_t, (b) y_t, and (c) z_t.

In order to explain the representation (and displaying) method for the connection weights, we consider an example, namely, $a = 2$, $b = c = d = 1$. For a mapping function f_x, the center of the base $\psi_{2,1,1,1}$ is located at $(1, 1, 1)$. This base affects the value of x_{t+1} in the direction of the arrow as shown in Figure 20 (a) at the next time step. If the connection weight $W^x_{2,1,1,1}$ is positive, the base $\psi_{2,1,1,1}$ affects x_{t+1} so that x_{t+1} may increase (to the left-hand side of the human subject) by the amount $W^x_{2,1,1,1}$. The base $\psi_{2,1,1,1}$ also affects y_{t+1} and z_{t+1} in the direction of the arrow, as shown in Figures 20 (b) and (c).

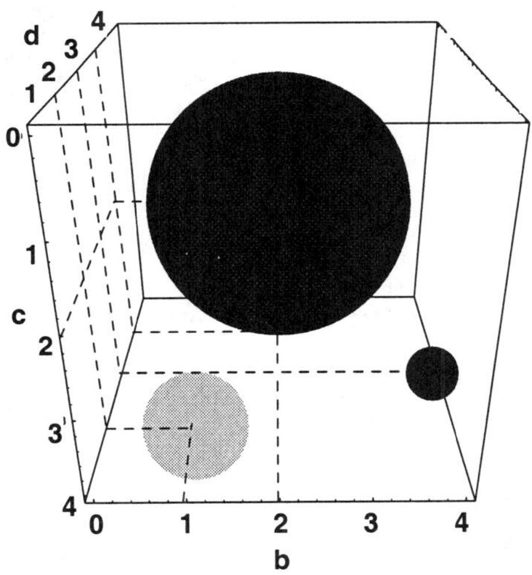

Figure 21. Example of a feature visualization.

In order to display all the weights with the same scaling parameter a, we use spheres to show the magnitude and the sign of connection weights. For example, the connection weights $W^x_{4,2,2,3} = 100$, $W^x_{4,1,4,1} = -40$, and $W^x_{4,4,4,2} = 20$ are shown in Figure 21.

The radii of spheres represent magnitude of weights, and "black" and "gray" represent positive and negative sign of weights, respectively. The location of the center of a sphere corresponds to the shifting parameter (b, c, d).

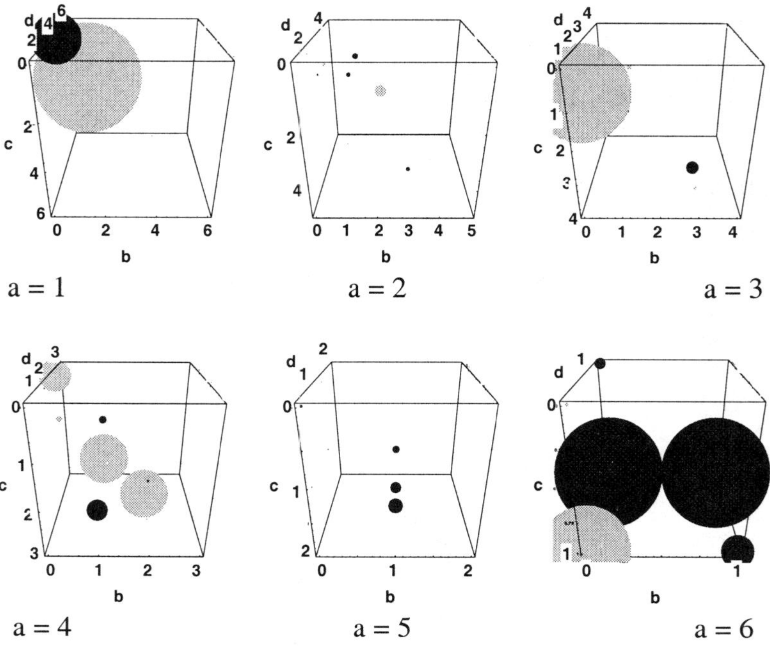

Figure 22. Features of the mapping function f_x.

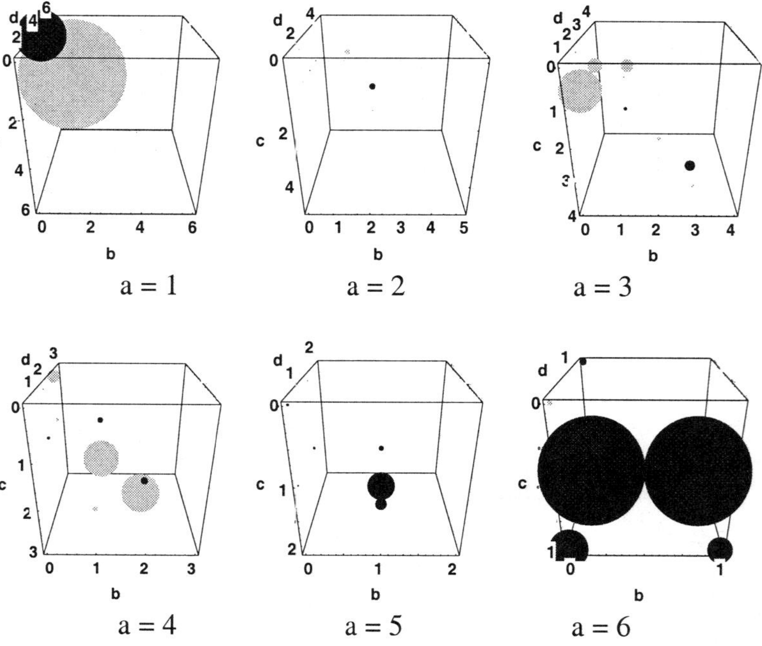

Figure 23. Features of the mapping function f_y.

Examples of visualization of the connection weights are shown in Figures 22, 23, and 24. These figures are obtained by modeling the vectorcardiogram presented in Section 5.1.3. The vector, which constructs "T loop" defined as a small loop in the 3-D vectorcardiogram on the transverse plane ($x - z$ plane), rotates clockwise in case of heart abnormalities, while it rotates counterclockwise in case of normal hearts [10]. The scale and direction of the T loop corresponds to the magnitude and the sign of the weights. Therefore, a heart abnormality can be detected by watching the size of the spheres and by the color of the spheres (whether these spheres are black or gray). This visualization method is still in an early stage of development. Tests for usability of this method in experimental settings were not yet performed.

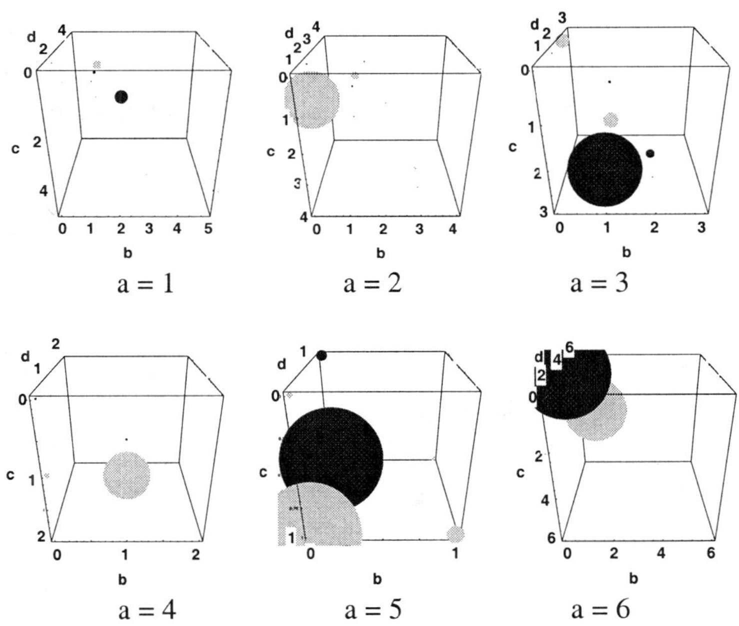

Figure 24. Features of the mapping function f_z.

5.2. Data compression of electrocardiograms

In this section the wavelet network shown in Figure 3 is applied to data compression for electrocardiograms. The compression is based on the fact that the relevant information needed to reconstruct the signal is stored in the weights of the network that models the signal, after learning. The number of weights is much lower than the number of samples in the original signal.

Consequently, by determining the weights, we also perform significant data compression. We also describe a modified learning scheme for fast learning.

5.2.1. High speed learning algorithm

The output $y(t)$ of the wavelet network with convex wavelet is given by a weighted sum of each basis function.

$$y(t) = \sum_{a=0}^{M} \sum_{b=0}^{a} W_{a,b} \Psi_{a,b}(t) \tag{23}$$

where $W_{a,b}$ is a connection weight, a is a scaling parameter, and b is a shifting parameter. $\Psi_{a,b}(t)$ is a wavelet base as in Equation (12). In the learning algorithm of the wavelet network, the renewal of weights is performed for all weights from $W_{0,0}$ to $W_{M,M}$. Now we consider the following situation:

$$\int_{\frac{2b-1}{2a}}^{\frac{2b+1}{2a}} (\hat{y}(t) - y_a(t))dt \approx 0 \tag{24}$$

where $y_a(t)$ is an output of a wavelet network after an adjustment of $W_{a,a}$ and $\hat{y}(t)$ is an original signal (see Figure 25).

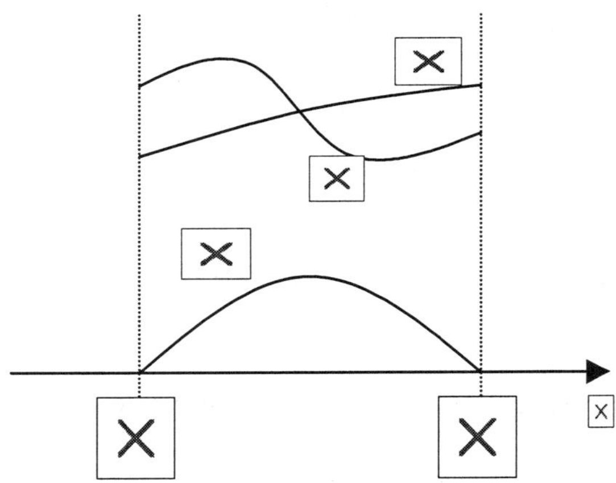

Figure 25. A situation after adjustment of $W_{a,a}$.

In this situation, the connection weight $W_{a+1,\,b}$ is not changed by the iteration. Consequently, we may omit the adjustment of $W_{a+1,\,b}$. This results in an increase of the learning speed.

5.2.2. Application to electrocardiograms

In general, signals of similar shapes appear in an electrocardiogram in a sequence of similar shapes, due to the almost-periodicity of the ECG signal. We divide an electrocardiogram in signals of similar shapes. The first period is approximated by the simple wavelet network shown in Figure 2-1. At the next period, we check the number of weights that were changed by learning. After learning for every period, an original signal and restored signal are shown in Figure 5.11. Notice the good modeling capability.

Table 6-1 shows the number of changed weights in comparison with the first period. The results show that the weights are not frequently changed in each period. If we store only the changed weights after the second period, then this procedure allows the data compression of an electrocardiogram. The data compression is useful for detecting a heart disease whereby a long-term record is necessary, for example, an uneven heartbeat.

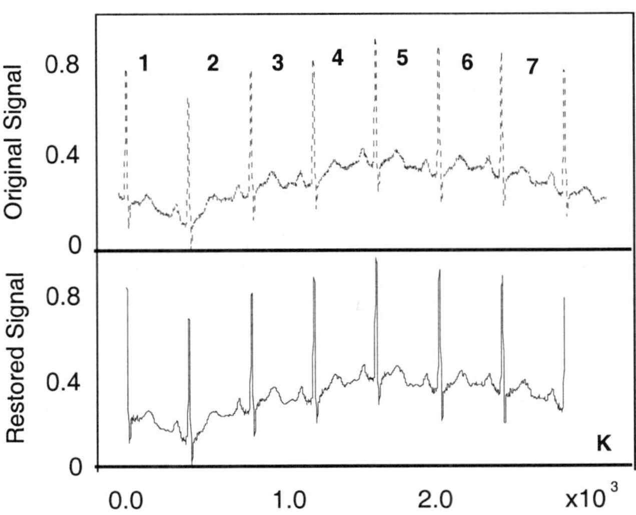

Figure 26. Restored signals of an electrocardiogram ($M = 45$).

Table 1. Number of changed weights

Number of weights not equal to 0 in the first period: 404	
Period	Number of weights changed
2	73
3	9
4	12
5	4
6	10
7	17

6. Conclusions

In this chapter we described a wavelet network which has convex wavelets as basis functions and several applications of this network. The convex wavelet improves the capability of generalization. Furthermore, this wavelet is compactly supported, so that the learning speed is increased.

To demonstrate the usefulness of the method, the simple wavelet network was first applied to function approximation problems. The network was shown to approximate complex curves with good accuracy. Moreover, a wavelet network with delay elements was applied to modeling nonlinear dynamical systems. We demonstrated that this wavelet network also has a good performance in modeling.

Furthermore, the network has been applied for modeling electrocardiograms. First, the vectorcardiogram was modeled by a wavelet network with three-dimensional convex wavelet. The modeling R.M.S. errors were low enough. We introduced a method to visualize the features of vectorcardiogram, extracted by the wavelet network. Second, we demonstrated the possibility that the wavelet networks are applied to data compression of electrocardiograms. Further research is needed to investigate the relationship between various diseases and the features extracted by the presented wavelet network.

Appendix A

Admissibility condition and orthogonality for wavelet functions

A.1. Admissibility condition

The wavelet transformation is defined as

$$W_{a,b} = \frac{1}{\sqrt{c_\psi}} \int_{-\infty}^{\infty} \psi_{a,b}(t) f(t) dt \, . \tag{A-1}$$

If the mother wavelet $\psi(t)$ (see Equation (1)) satisfies the following admissibility condition [12]:

$$c_\psi \equiv \int_{-\infty}^{\infty} \frac{|\hat{\psi}(\omega)|^2}{\omega} d\omega \;<\; \infty \, , \tag{A-2}$$

where $\hat{\psi}(\omega)$ is a Fourier transform of $\psi(t)$ defined by

$$\hat{\psi}(\omega) = \int_{-\infty}^{\infty} \exp(-i\omega t) \, \psi(t) dt \, , \tag{A-3}$$

then there exists an inverse transform of Equation (A-1):

$$f(t) = \frac{1}{\sqrt{c_\psi}} \int_{-\infty}^{\infty} \int_{-\infty}^{\infty} W_{a,b} \psi_{a,b}(t) \frac{dadb}{a^2} \, . \tag{A-4}$$

The following condition is the same as the admissibility condition in Equation (A-2), if $\psi(t)$ has a sufficient decay.

$$\int_{-\infty}^{\infty} \psi(t) dt = 0 \, . \tag{A-5}$$

A.2. Orthogonality

Meyer's wavelet [16] and Doubechies's wavelet [17] are well-known orthogonal wavelets. For orthogonal wavelets, the scaling parameter a and the shifting parameter b are frequently expressed as

$$(a, b) = \left(\frac{1}{2^j}, \frac{k}{2^j} \right). \tag{A-6}$$

In this case, the wavelet series expansion becomes

$$f(t) = \sum_{j=-\infty}^{\infty} \sum_{k=-\infty}^{\infty} W_{j,k} \Psi_{j,k}(t). \tag{A-7}$$

Appendix B

Proof of the convergence of the wavelet series with convex wavelets

This appendix gives proof of the convergence of the presented wavelet series with convex wavelets. In this appendix, the superscript F denotes the Fourier series and W denotes the wavelet series, respectively.

Let $S_M^F(x)$ and $S_M^W(x)$ be a finite cosine Fourier series and a finite wavelet series for an arbitrary target function, $f(x)$, in [0, 1] as follows:

$$S_M^F(x) = \sum_{a=0}^{M} V_a \cos a\pi x, \tag{B-1}$$

$$S_M^W(x) = \sum_{a=0}^{M} \sum_{b=0}^{a} W_{a,b} \Psi_{a,b}(x), \tag{B-2}$$

where V_a and $W_{a,b}$ are Fourier and wavelet coefficients, respectively. $\Psi_{a,b}(x)$ is the wavelet basis function introduced in Equation (12), a is a scaling parameter that corresponds to frequency, and b is a shifting parameter. Here we define the R.M.S. errors as

$$E^F = \int_0^1 \left\{ f(x) - S_M^F(x) \right\}^2 dx \tag{B-3}$$

$$E^W = \int_0^1 \left\{ f(x) - S_M^W(x) \right\}^2 dx \tag{B-4}$$

We shall prove that

$$\lim_{M \to \infty} E^W = 0. \tag{B-5}$$

Let $f_a(x)$ be a component of the Fourier series

$$f_a(x) = V_a \cos a\pi x \tag{B-6}$$

and $\varepsilon_a(x)$ be the corresponding error. Then, $f(x)$ can be written as

$$f(x) = \sum_{a=0}^M f_a(x) + \sum_{a=0}^M \varepsilon_a(x) = \sum_{a=0}^M \left\{ f_a(x) + \varepsilon_a(x) \right\} \tag{B-7}$$

We define $h_a^F(x)$ and $h_a^W(x)$ for each a as follows:

$$h_a^F(x) = V_a \cos a\pi x \quad (= f_a(x)) \tag{B-8}$$

$$h_a^W(x) = \sum_{b=0}^a W_{a,b} \Psi_{a,b}(x). \tag{B-9}$$

By letting $g_a(x) \equiv f_a(x) + \varepsilon_a(x)$, we define E_a^F and E_a^W:

$$E_a^F = \int_0^1 \left\{ g_a(x) - V_a \cos a\pi x \right\}^2 dx, \tag{B-10}$$

$$E_a^W = \int_0^1 \left\{ g_a(x) - h_a^W(x) \right\}^2 dx, \tag{B-11}$$

E_a^F is the R.M.S. error between $g_a(x)$ and $h_a^F(x)$; E_a^W is the R.M.S. error between $g_a(x)$ and $h_a^W(x)$.

In the following, we prove the relation $E_a^F \geq E_a^W$. In the specific case $a = 0$, the relation (B-12) is obtained as

$$E_0^F = E_0^W .$$

(B-12)

If $a \neq 0$, the proof is proceeded for the following three cases.

(i) Case $b \neq 0$ and $b \neq a$.

$W_{a,b}$, which minimizes Equation (B-11), is obtained by solving $\partial E_a^W / \partial W_{a,b} = 0$ as follows:

$$W_{a,b} = 2a \int_0^1 g_a(x) \psi_{a,b}(x) dx$$

(B-13)

or

$$W_{a,b} = \pm 2a \cdot \int_{\frac{2b-1}{2a}}^{\frac{2b+1}{2a}} g_a(x) \cos a\pi x \, dx$$

(B-14)

The positive or negative sign comes from the property of the presented convex wavelet, which is produced to turn the negative part of the cosine function into positive values.

We define the R.M.S. error between $g_a(x)$ and $h_a^F(x)$ or $h_a^W(x)$ on $[(2b-1)/2a, (2b+1)/2a]$ $(b = 1, 2, \cdots, a-1)$, for each series,

$$e_{a,b}^F = \left(\frac{2b+1}{2a} - \frac{2b-1}{2a} \right)^{-1} \cdot \int_{\frac{2b-1}{2a}}^{\frac{2b+1}{2a}} \left\{ g_a(x) - h_a^F(x) \right\}^2 dx =$$

(B-15)

$$= a \cdot \int_{\frac{2b-1}{2a}}^{\frac{2b+1}{2a}} \left\{ g_a(x) \right\}^2 dx \mp V_a W_{a,b} + \frac{V_a^2}{2}$$

and

$$e_{a,b}^{W} = \left(\frac{2b+1}{2a} - \frac{2b-1}{2a}\right)^{-1} \cdot \int_{\frac{2b-1}{2a}}^{\frac{2b+1}{2a}} \left\{g_a(x) - h_a^{W}(x)\right\}^2 dx =$$

$$\text{(B-16)}$$

$$= a \int_{\frac{2b-1}{2a}}^{\frac{2b+1}{2a}} \left\{g_a(x)\right\}^2 dx - \frac{W_{a,b}^{2}}{2}$$

Then, we obtain the relation

$$e_{a,b}^{F} - e_{a,b}^{W} = \frac{1}{2}\left(V_a \mp W_{a,b}\right)^2 \geq 0 \qquad \text{(B-17)}$$

Therefore, we obtain

$$e_{a,b}^{F} \geq e_{a,b}^{W} \qquad \text{(B-18)}$$

(ii) Case b = 0.

In the same manner as we derived Equation (B-14), we obtain

$$W_{a,0} = 4a\int_{0}^{\frac{1}{2a}} g_a(x)\cos a\pi x\,dx \qquad \text{(B-19)}$$

From Equation (B-19), we derive

$$e_{a,0}^{F} = 2a\int_{0}^{\frac{1}{2a}} \left\{g_a(x)\right\}^2 dx - V_a W_{a,0} + \frac{V_a^{2}}{2} \qquad \text{(B-20)}$$

$$e_{a,0}^{W} = 2a\int_{0}^{\frac{1}{2a}} \left\{g_a(x)\right\}^2 dx - \frac{W_{a,0}^{2}}{2} \qquad \text{(B-21)}$$

and the following relation is then obtained:

$$e_{a,0}^{F} - e_{a,0}^{W} = \frac{1}{2}\left(V_a - W_{a,0}\right)^2 \geq 0. \qquad \text{(B-22)}$$

Thus,

$$e_{a,0}^{F} \geq e_{a,0}^{W}.$$

(B-23)

(iii) Case b = a.

In the same manner as we obtained Equation (B-14), we derive

$$W_{a,a} = \pm 4a \cdot \int_{\frac{2a-1}{2a}}^{1} g_a(x) \cos a\pi x \, dx.$$

(B-24)

Based on Equation (B-24), we derive

$$e_{a,a}^{F} = 2a \int_{\frac{2a-1}{2a}}^{1} \{g_a(x)\}^2 \, dx \mp V_a W_{a,a} + \frac{V_a^2}{2}$$

(B-25)

$$e_{a,a}^{W} = 2a \int_{\frac{2a-1}{2a}}^{1} \{g_a(x)\}^2 \, dx - \frac{W_{a,a}^2}{2}.$$

(B-26)

The following relation is obtained:

$$e_{a,a}^{F} - e_{a,a}^{W} = \frac{1}{2}\left(V_a \mp W_{a,a}\right)^2 \geq 0.$$

(B-27)

Therefore,

$$e_{a,a}^{F} \geq e_{a,a}^{W}.$$

(B-28)

By summing up the error for each interval $[(2b-1)/2a,(2b+1)/2a]$, we obtain

$$E_a^{F} = \frac{1}{a}\sum_{b=1}^{a-1} e_{a,b}^{F} + \frac{1}{2a}\left(e_{a,0}^{F} + e_{a,a}^{F}\right)$$

(B-29)

$$E_a^{W} = \frac{1}{a}\sum_{b=1}^{a-1} e_{a,b}^{W} + \frac{1}{2a}\left(e_{a,0}^{W} + e_{a,a}^{W}\right).$$

(B-30)

Based on the results for the cases (i), (ii), and (iii), we get

$$E_a^F \geq E_a^W.$$

(B-31)

Hence, the following inequality is finally obtained:

$$E^F \geq E^w \geq 0.$$

(B-32)

On the other hand, for the Fourier series, the following convergence is well known:

$$\lim_{M \to \infty} E^F = 0$$

(B-33)

Therefore, we obtain

$$\lim_{M \to \infty} E^w = 0$$

(B-34)

because $E^F \geq E^w \geq 0$. This concludes the proof.

References

[1]   Morlet, J., Arens, G., Fourgeau, E., and Giard, D., Wave propagation and sampling theory. part 1: complex signal and scattering in multilayered media, *Geophysics*, Vol. 47, No. 2, pp. 203-221, 1982.

[2]   Morlet, J., Arens, G., Fourgeau, E., and Giard, D., Wave propagation and sampling theory. part 2: sampling theory and complex waves. *Geophysics*, Vol. 47, No. 2, pp. 222-236, 1982.

[3]   Benedetto, J.J. and Frazier, M.W., *Wavelet: Mathematics and Applications*, CRC Press, 1994.

[4]   Chui, C.K., *An Introduction to Wavelets*, Academic Press, Inc., 1992.

[5]   Szu, H.H. and Kadambe, S., Neural network adaptive wavelets for signal representation and classification, *Optical Engineering*, Vol. 31, No. 9, pp. 1907-1916, 1992.

[6]   Zhang, Q. and Benveniste, A., Wavelet networks, *IEEE Trans. Neural Networks*, Vol. 3, No. 6, pp. 889-898, 1992.

[7]   Pao, Y., *Adaptive Pattern Recognition and Neural Networks*, Addison-Wesley Publishing Company, 1989.

[8]   Yamakawa, T., Uchino, E., and Samatsu, T., Wavelet neural networks employing over-complete number of compactly supported non-orthogonal wavelets and their applications, *Proc. 1994 IEEE Int. Conf. Neural Networks*, pp. 1391-1396, 1994.

[9] Yamakawa, T. and Samatsu, T., Wavelet neural networks realizing high speed learning, *Proc. Int. Conf. Neural Information Processing*, Seoul, Korea, pp. 1571-1576, 1994.

[10] Friedman, H.H., *Diagnostic Electrocardiography and Vectorcardiography*, McGraw-Hill, 1971.

[11] Mori, H., et al., *Actual Diagnosis for Vectorcardiography*, Igaku-Shuppan-Sha Co., Japan, 1978 (in Japanese).

[12] Grossmann, A. and Morlet, J., Decomposition of hardy functions into square integrable wavelets of constant shape, *SIAM J. Math. Anal.*, Vol. 15, No. 4, pp. 723-736, 1984.

[13] Harr, A., Zur theorie der orthogonalen funktionensysteme, *Math. Ann.*, 69, 1910.

[14] Schmitt, O.H. and Simonson, E., The present status of vector-cardiography, *Arch. Int. Med.*, 96, pp. 574-590, 1995.

[15] Frank, E., *The Image Surface of a Homogeneous Torso. Circulation*, pp. 757-768, 1953.

[16] Meyer, Y., *Wavelets and Operators*, Cambridge University Press, 1992.

[17] Daubechies, I.., Orthonormal bases of compactly supported wavelets, *Communication of Pure and Applied Mathematics*, XLI, pp. 909-996, 1988.

[18] Deco, G. and Schurmann, B., Neural learning of chaotic dynamics, *Neural Processing Letters*, Vol. 2, No. 2, pp. 23-26, March 1995.

[19] Rape, R., Fefer, D., and Drnovsek, J., Time series prediction with neural networks: a case study of two examples, *1994 IEEE Instrumentation & Measurement Technology Conference*. IEEE, New York, NY, USA, pp. 145-148, 1994.

[20] Pethel, S.D., Bowden, C.M., and Scalora, M., Characterization of optical instabilities and chaos using fast multilayer perceptron training algorithms, *Proceedings of the SPIE*, Vol. 2039, pp. 129-140, 1993.

[21] Adachi, M. and Aihara, K., Nonlinear prediction by neural networks, *Journal of the Institute of Electrical Engineers of Japan*, Vol. 113, pp. 533-536, 1993.

[22] Hsu, W., Hsu, L.S., and Tenorio, M.F., The ClusNet algorithm and time series prediction, *International Journal of Neural Systems*, Vol. 4, No. 3, pp. 247-255, Sept. 1993.

[23] Grabec, I., Prediction of chaos in non-autonomous systems by a neural network, *Proc., 1992 International Conference on Artificial Neural Network*, Elsevier, Amsterdam, Netherlands, pp. 379-382, 1992.

[24] Principe, J.C., Rathie, A., and Jyh-Ming, K., Prediction of chaotic time series with neural networks and the issue of dynamic modeling, *International Journal of Bifurcation and Chaos in Applied Sciences and Engineering*, Vol. 2, No. 4, pp. 989-996, 1992.

[25] Werbos, P.J., *The Roots of Backpropagations*, John Wiley & Sons, Inc, New York, NY, USA, 1994.

[26] Rumelhart, D.E., Hinton, G.E., and Williams, R.J., Learning internal representations by error propagation, *Parallel Distributed Processing: Explorations in the Microstructure of Cognition*, Vol. 1, MIT Press, Cambridge, MA, USA, pp. 318-362, 1986.

Further reading on wavelet decompositions
Horia-Nicolai Teodorescu

Readers are referred to Chapter 6, *Intelligent Diagnostic Systems in Maternal and Fetal Medicine*, and to Chapter 8, *Features-Oriented Filtering of Biological Signals,* in this volume, for applications of wavelet applications and for other types of function decomposition.

For more information on the use of wavelets in combination to fuzzy clustering in the field of medicine, the reader is also referred to

Amir B. Geva and Dan H. Kerem: Brain state identification and forecasting of acute pathology using unsupervised fuzzy clustering of EEG temporal patterns. Chapter 3, pp. 57-91, H.N. Teodorescu, A. Kandel, L.C. Jain (Eds.): *Fuzzy and Neuro-Fuzzy Systems in Medicine.* CRC Press, FL, 1998.

For other types of wavelet networks used in medicine, namely, in image processing, see

Luis Patino, André Constantinesco, and Ernest Hirsch: Contouring blood pool myocardial gated SPECT images with a sequence of three techniques based on wavelets, neural networks, and fuzzy logic. Chapter 4, pp. 95-134, H.N. Teodorescu, A. Kandel, L.C. Jain (Eds.): *Fuzzy and Neuro-Fuzzy Systems in Medicine.* CRC Press, FL, 1998.

A textbook on wavelet is

M. Vetterli, J. Kovacevic, *Wavelets and Subband Coding*, Prentice Hall, 1995, New Jersey, USA.

A review paper on applications of wavelets in medicine is

M. Akay, Wavelet Applications in Medicine, *IEEE Spectrum*, 1997, Vol. 34, 5, pp. 50-56.

F. Yang, W. Liao, Modeling and Decomposition of HRV Signals with Wavelet Transforms, *IEEE Engineering in Medicine and Biology*, 1997, Vol. 16, 4, pp. 17-22.

P.C. Ivanov, M.G. Rosenblum, C.K. Peng, J. Mietus, S. Havlin, H.E. Stanley, A.L. Goldberger, Scaling Behavior of Heartbeat Intervals Obtained by Wavelet-Based Time-Series Analysis, *Nature*, 1996, Vol. 383, 26, pp. 323-327.

S. Blanco, S. Kochen, O.A. Rosso, P. Saldado, Applying Tone-Frequency Analysis to Seizure EEG Activity, *IEEE Trans. Engineering in Medicine and Biology*, 1997, Vol. 16, 1, pp. 64-71.

C.D. Haagensen, *Diseases of the Breast*, Third Edition, Saunders Company, 1986.

Institute of Medicine, *Report of a Study. Breast Cancer: Setting Priorities of Effectiveness in Research*, National Academy Press, 1990.

L.P. Clarke, M. Kallergi, W. Qian, H.D. Li, R.A. Clark, M.L. Sibiger, Tree-Structured Nonlinear Filter and Wavelet Transform for Microcalcification Segmentation in Digital Mammography, *Cancer Letters*, 1994, 77, pp. 173-181.

M. Antonini, M. Barlaud, P. Mathieu, I. Daubechies, Image Coding Using Wavelet Transform, *IEEE Transactions on Image Processing*, 1992, Vol. 1, 2, pp. 205-220.

Chapter 8

Features-oriented filtering of biological signals

Horia-Nicolai Teodorescu and Cristian Bonciu

This chapter is focused on neural signal processing, specifically on merging classic neural filtering processes with the neural features extraction methods. Neural signal filtering, pattern recognition and control are still viewed as subsequent, completely separate stages in these types of tasks. Modalities of merging these subfields and methods are investigated. The objective of this chapter is to show how hybrid techniques can handle merging the signal filtering and conditioning level with the recognition level, as well as possibly the control level.

The merging technique concerns mainly the design of an intelligent link between the neural filter and the features extractor. The emphasis is on the associated learning systems, which are able to form a useful semantic link, and to the degree of generality of the presented methods.

The basic concepts related to features space filtering are introduced in the first two sections of this chapter. In the following sections, two different neural network features extractors are described: the Principal Component Analysis (PCA) network and the Radial Basis Functions (RBF) network. These features extractors are used for filtering applications in hybrid neural systems in the fifth section. Several results of ECG signal filtering in feature spaces are presented in the sixth section. Concluding remarks and an appendix end the chapter.

1. Signal processing as a task-oriented process

Computational intelligence methods [1] are widely used today in complex signal processing, pattern recognition, identification, and control of dynamic systems. Hybrid computational intelligence methods combine neural networks, fuzzy systems, and evolutionary computing with classic data processing and symbolic artificial intelligence methods and are thus able to handle problems that are more complex. The challenge is to obtain flexible abstract concepts and intelligent systems from rough and noisy data sets using simple and consistent basic rules.

The main features of computational intelligence methods emerge from their intrinsically adaptive nature, which accounts for the capacity to learn a desired or an optimal behavior in the environment context. Combining intelligent techniques to solve complex problems generally involves coupling fundamentally different systems, which are driven by various adaptation laws. This combination increases the system complexity, which must be offset by improved performance of the new system.

Functional and *hierarchical* decompositions are the main procedures employed to partition the tasks, reduce complexity, and increase control over the data processing systems. The former functionally separates different stages in order to design chains of cascaded processing systems. The latter organizes the subtasks as levels in a hierarchy, and designs qualitatively different processing stages, each of them ensuring the global synchronization and convergence for the subordinate stage.

Whatever the structuring concept and the combination between the structuring procedures, the ability of such hybrid system to solve the problem at hand depends not only on the quality of each component, but also on the effectiveness of the links between the components. The hierarchical decomposition assures the intelligent link between processing stages using global information flows from subordinate stages, for the decision making, and drives the subordinate stages by means of local information flows, for synchronization and correction. Without a supervisory integrating level, it is often difficult to obtain better overall results in a single chain of coupled data processors, compared with the processing quality of each component apart. One way to overcome this drawback is to design bidirectional local data paths between system components which carry mutual information. Tracking, understanding, and driving the interdependencies between the hybrid system chain components may play a crucial role in the quality of overall system response.

The need for hierarchical task organization is well perceived in many neural hybrid system realizations [2-5] and effectively increases the quality of the system response. Unfortunately, the interdependencies between hybrid system chain components at the same processing level are not sufficiently investigated yet. *A priori* functional assignment principle is largely used in practice. Each data processor has a predetermined function and its processing capabilities are measured based only on its intrinsic characteristics at the system design stage. A decisive factor in increasing the quality of hybrid systems response is the design of efficient interlinks between system components, based on particular component mechanisms for acquiring data about its neighbors' functions and evolution.

The connectionist paradigm employed in neural systems [6] states that the information is stored by an adaptation procedure in the links between elementary processing cells. The inward and outward data flows in connectionist systems provide an efficient way to use this kind of information. However, this type of implicit information encoding in neural systems remains obscure or equivocal in many respects. The need to control the artificial neural system behavior and the internal data coding schemes was determinant in the effort to limit the size of neural networks and to restrict the type of processing elements which contribute to the internal network representation of a given environment.

It is generally accepted today that complex neural processing systems must be well structured on functional ensembles. Moreover, the learning environment for each ensemble must be carefully selected. Quantitative accumulation of artificial neural masses performs poorly without clearly defined functionality, that is, without specific learning paradigms and representation restrictions. This is due to the lack of modularity and, more important, to the lack of direct and appropriate information sources for building useful internal representations during learning.

We scrutinize neural signal processing, specifically emphasizing the integration of classic neural filtering processes with the neural features extraction methods. Biomedical applications are demanding due to the complexity of the tasks. Neural signal filtering, pattern recognition, and control are still viewed as subsequent, completely separate stages in these types of tasks. Modalities of merging these subfields and methods are investigated. The results demonstrate the feasibility and advantages of using hybrid techniques that merge the signal filtering, the conditioning level, and the recognition level. The integration of the control level is possible as well.

The applications of these techniques range from classic signal conditioning and enhancement, to optimized pattern recognition in robotics, and, more generally, to optimized control.

We use Pineda's general approach to neural computation [7]. Pineda uses the concept of assembled primitive neural processors to design a general framework for neural networks, coupled dynamics, and learning, keeping the specificity of each neural system component. The presented approach is based on the same principles, but with a different aim: the superior integration between the neural adaptive filter and the features extractor.

2. Features-space filtering systems

The classic features-space filtering systems are designed with two cascaded processing blocks: the filter and the features extractor. The filter performs the initial processing – the noise canceling task – and the features extractor builds the representation of the filtered signal into the features space (Figure 1).

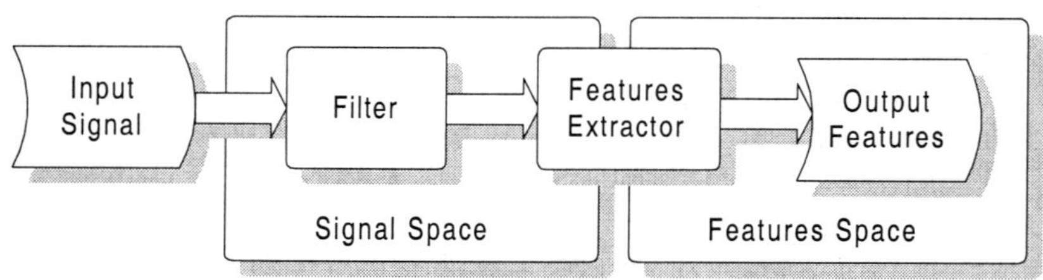

Figure 1. Direct features-space filtering system structure.

Each component of the system is usually designed independently, using different design rules and different performance criteria. This allows a greater flexibility in the overall system design, but the final quality of the processed signal remains dependent on the quality of the link between the system components. Although the performance of each component may fulfill the design requirements, the system may fail to work due to a mismatch between the processing stages. A powerful way to alleviate this type of problem is the use of adaptive components for filtering and features extraction.

The adaptive approach considers, in addition to the component itself, an adaptation mechanism that depends on the input signal and (possibly) on the target signal. This increases the degree of adequacy of the overall system to the characteristics of the signal to be processed, but it may reduce the efficiency of the system when it is fed with other types of signals.

2.1. Adaptive structures

Both the filtering and the features extractor blocks may have an adaptive structure, which must include specific adaptation mechanisms (Figure 2). The adaptive filtering is performed with a supervised adaptation procedure, which considers the adaptation error as a distance in the signal samples' space. We consider here the simplest adaptive filtering technique, in which the samples of the actual output signal are compared with the samples of a reference (model) signal. The resulting distance value feeds the adaptation block, which performs the tuning of the filter parameters.

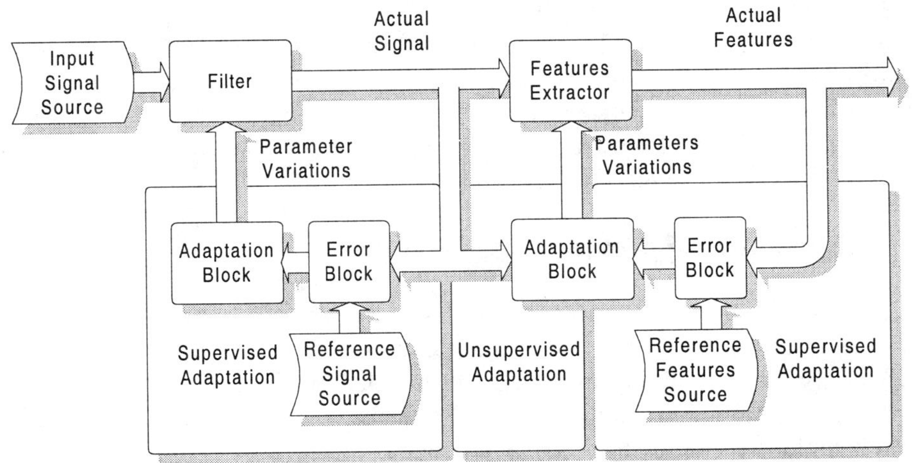

Figure 2. Features-space adaptation system structure.

The features extractor adaptation procedure may follow the same supervised technique, when the reference feature vectors are available in the features-space, or it may follow an unsupervised procedure. In the first case, the adaptation mechanism builds a mapping between a specific features-space representation – supplied by the reference features vectors – and the input signal. This is often called a *constrained* representation. The final error in the features space gives the measure of the similitude between the specified features and the actual features of the signal. This measure is less dependent on the features-space adaptation mechanism because the error is computed following the features-space reference representation. Thus, the degree of generality of constrained representations is directly dependent on the degree of significance of the imposed reference representations.

For the unsupervised procedures, the adaptation is performed using the input and the output signal samples. The adaptation mechanism builds an input-dependent mapping onto the features space. The features extractor parameter tuning is based on an iterative procedure. The unsupervised adaptation mechanism provides an internal measure of the adaptation progress that stops the adaptation when the internal representation is complete. The actual output realization is not compared with a reference. It is dependent only on the input signal characteristics with respect to the features space. The final output signal in features space is called an *unconstrained* representation. The formed features are dependent on the structure of the features extractor and the adaptation mechanism. When the latter ensures a low degree of dependence on the specific feature extractor structure, the unconstrained representation becomes a unique representation during the adaptation process.

Both constrained and unconstrained representations are used in features-oriented processing systems [8]. The system component adaptation for the direct structure (Figure 2) may be performed independently. The filter adaptation does not depend on the features space representation. Conversely, given the reference signal samples, it is possible to build a reference features space (defined in the following section) or one features-space reference when the constrained representation is required.

2.2. Features-spaces for filtering systems

The choice of the features space is a key problem in modern signal processing. In pattern detection and classification systems, the choice is dictated by the separability properties of the space with respect to the class of processed signals. For features-oriented filtering systems, the features space must be able to distinguish signals from noise.

The classic filter design theory makes some strong assumptions about the noise characteristics. These assumptions are general because they are imposed on the noise statistical properties. For mathematical tractability, the noise is often assumed to be a normal distribution of uncorrelated samples. Thus, the classic statistics theory may be applied in the design of the filtering system. However, these assumptions are not realistic and other hypotheses on the noise characteristics must be made. This may be realized using *a priori* information about the noise. Thus, noise-dedicated filtering systems may be designed to cope with specific environmental conditions for a large class of signals.

Conversely, supplemental information about the denoised signal may be used as well. The classic adaptive filtering systems use this kind of information – the reference (target) signal. The filter is signal-dedicated in this case, and no hypotheses about the noise characteristics are needed. However, a careful selection of input signals must be prepared for the adaptation procedure to ensure the "graceful degradation" of the performance when the filter is fed with another type of signal, or when the noise is not stationary. Consequently, in the design process there is always a trade-off between the degree of generality with respect to the type of the input signal or the type of noise and the filtering performance.

The features space may be a known predefined space. In this case, the features extractor realizes the mapping of the input signal to the corresponding features representation explicitly using the samples-features mapping. Fixed features spaces, like the Fourier coefficients space, allow the direct comparison of different decompositions because the features are represented in the same space, which is not data-dependent. Another type of features space is the input-dependent (projection) space, like the PCA and the RBF decomposition spaces. The PCA space is formed with the dominant eigenvectors of the autocorrelation matrix of the input signal. These vectors are not known *a priori*, and the space characteristics are determined using an input signal-dependent procedure. The same applies to the RBF decomposition space, which is also formed using an input signal.

There are two ways to deal with different input signals for input-dependent features spaces. The first approach uses relative values of the measures applied to features in each space and then compares the measure values obtained in several features spaces. The second approach uses a reference signal to construct a reference features space. Then, this space is considered as a predefined space and is used to extract the features from any input signal. The first approach is more elaborate and needs supplemental measures. The measures must be invariant with respect to the space realization and must not degrade the features' specific information. The second approach makes the implicit assumption that the reference space is near to all its actual realizations and this approximation is negligible with respect to the features representation in the reference space.

In the following sections, two different neural network features extractors will be described, namely, the Principal Component Analysis network and the Radial Basis Functions network. These feature extractors are used for filtering applications based on hybrid neural systems, as detailed in the last sections of this chapter.

3. Principal component analysis in features extraction

The Principal Component Analysis (PCA) is a linear transform applied on the input space with the goal of dimensionality reduction. It is also known as the Karhunen-Loéve transform (KLT) in signal analysis [9] and as the Hotteling transform in communications theory [10]. In this case the input space is formed by the last N samples of the input signal (input N-delay space). KLT is closely related to spectral analysis and particularly to discrete cosine transform, which is used mainly in data compression applications. As a dimensionality reduction method, PCA generates a subset of features of the input data matrix. Each row of the data matrix is considered a vector in the input space, and the output features are low-dimensional linear combinations between all vector elements.

3.1. Dimensionality reduction through PCA

Let us consider an *N*-dimensional input vector at the discrete time *n*, $\mathbf{x}(n)=$ $(x_1, x_2, ..., x_N)$ from a sequence of temporal length *P* (Figure 3). This vector may be written as linear combinations of the elements of another vector $\mathbf{y}(n)=$ $(y_1, y_2, ..., y_N)$, obtained from a rotation of the original representation space onto a new space, given by the orthonormal basis $(\mathbf{u}_1, \mathbf{u}_2, ...\mathbf{u}_N)$

$$
\begin{bmatrix} x_1(n) \\ x_2(n) \\ ... \\ x_{N-1}(n) \\ x_N(n) \end{bmatrix} = \sum_{i=1}^{N} y_i(n) \begin{bmatrix} u_{1,i} \\ u_{2,i} \\ ... \\ u_{N-1,i} \\ u_{N,i} \end{bmatrix} \tag{1}
$$

or, in vectorial form,

$$
\mathbf{x}(n) = \sum_{i=1}^{N} y_i(n)\mathbf{u}_i \tag{2}
$$

where $\mathbf{u}_i^T \mathbf{u}_j = 0$ when $i \neq j$ and $\mathbf{u}_i^T \mathbf{u}_j = 1$ when $i = j$, for all $i, j = 1,..., N$. The orthogonality property of the basis $(\mathbf{u}_1, \mathbf{u}_2, ..., \mathbf{u}_N)$ leads to the reverse formula

$$
y_i(n) = \mathbf{u}_i^T \mathbf{x}(n) \tag{3}
$$

To achieve the goal of dimensionality reduction, it is useful to keep only a subset *M*, *M* < *N*, of the basis vectors $\mathbf{u}_i$ and to approximate the $\mathbf{x}(n)$ vector in the subspace of dimension *M*. The relation (1) expands

$$
\mathbf{x}(n) = \sum_{i=1}^{M} y_i(n)\mathbf{u}_i + \sum_{i=M+1}^{N} z_i\mathbf{u}_i = \hat{\mathbf{x}}(n) + \mathbf{e}(n) \tag{4}
$$

where the first sum is the approximation of the original vector and the second sum is the residual error vector of this approximation, expressed in terms of its projections onto the residual subbase of the space.

The data compression operation must preserve a maximum of information from the original signal. Thus, considering in Equation (2) the projection of the rotation basis $(\mathbf{u}_1, \mathbf{u}_2, \ldots, \mathbf{u}_N)$ and the residual coefficients $\mathbf{z} = (z_{M+1}, z_{M+2}, \ldots, z_N)$ as unknown quantities, it is possible to define an information-preserving criterion that these unknown variables must maximize. Conversely, we can define an approximation error that must be minimized by the unknown vector $\mathbf{z}$. The approximation error is usually defined for all the data vectors in the sequence, and has the form

$$E = \frac{1}{2}\sum_{n=1}^{P}\|\mathbf{e}(n)\|^2 = \frac{1}{2}\sum_{n=1}^{P}\|\mathbf{x}(n) - \hat{\mathbf{x}}(n)\|^2 = \frac{1}{2}\cdot\sum_{n=1}^{P}\sum_{i=M+1}^{N}(y_i(n) - z_i)^2 \qquad (5)$$

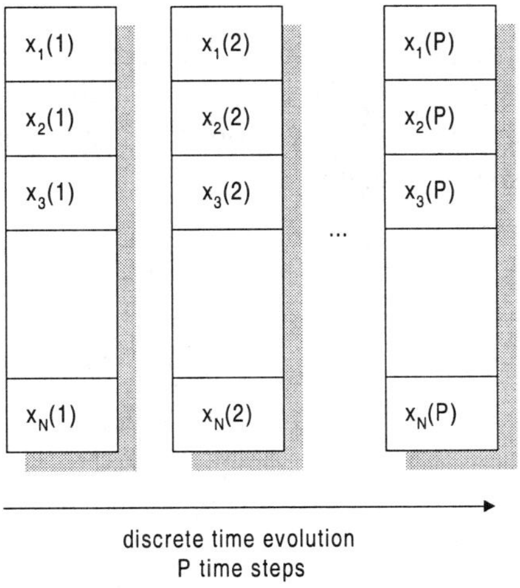

Figure 3. Heterogeneous input data flow.

Solving this system of N-M linear equations with respect to the unknowns, z_i, we obtain

$$z_i = \frac{1}{P}\sum_{n=1}^{P}y_i(n) = \mathbf{u}_i^{T}\mathbf{M}_1(\mathbf{x}), \quad \mathbf{M}_1(\mathbf{x}) = \frac{1}{P}\sum_{n=1}^{P}\mathbf{x}(n) \qquad (6)$$

where the vector $\mathbf{M}_1$ contains the temporal average of each input data vector element.

The error E may be expressed in terms of the data elements $x_i(n)$ and of the unknown orthogonal basis subset $(\mathbf{u}_M, \mathbf{u}_{M+1}, \ldots \mathbf{u}_N)$ by substituting $y_i = \mathbf{u}_i^{T}\mathbf{x}$ in Equation (3)

$$E = \frac{1}{2} \cdot \sum_{n=1}^{P} \sum_{i=M+1}^{N} \left(\mathbf{u}_i^T \left(\mathbf{x}(n) - \mathbf{M}_1(\mathbf{x}) \right) \right)^2$$

$$= \frac{1}{2} \cdot \sum_{i=M+1}^{N} \mathbf{u}_i^T \sum_{n=1}^{P} \left(\mathbf{x}(n) - \mathbf{M}_1(\mathbf{x}) \right) \left(\mathbf{x}(n) - \mathbf{M}_1(\mathbf{x}) \right)^T \mathbf{u}_i^T \tag{7}$$

$$= \frac{1}{2} \cdot \sum_{i=M+1}^{N} \mathbf{u}_i^T \mathbf{C}(\mathbf{x}) \, \mathbf{u}_i^T$$

where $\mathbf{C}(\mathbf{x})$ denotes the covariance matrix of the input variables $x_i(n)$. $\mathbf{C}(\mathbf{x})$ is a symmetric matrix. Minimizing the function E with respect to the basis subset $(\mathbf{u}_M, \mathbf{u}_{M+1}, \dots \mathbf{u}_N)$ means in these conditions [11] that the solution vectors $(\mathbf{u}^*_M, \mathbf{u}^*_{M+1}, \dots \mathbf{u}^*_N)$ satisfy the eigenvalues equation:

$$\mathbf{C}(\mathbf{x}) \, \mathbf{u}^*_i = \lambda_i^* \mathbf{u}_i \tag{8}$$

Substituting Equation (8) into Equation (7), we obtain the expression of the approximation error of the form

$$E = \frac{1}{2} \sum_{i=M+1}^{N} \lambda_i \tag{9}$$

Thus, the minimum error is obtained by leaving apart the projections corresponding to the smallest eigenvalues once the dimension of the projection space was chosen.

The input covariance matrix is diagonal in its corresponding eigenspace (i.e., the space spanned by all the N eigenvectors). The diagonal entries are the eigenvalues. This means that the projection space determined by the eigenvectors $(\mathbf{u}_1, \mathbf{u}_2, \dots, \mathbf{u}_M)$ will produce M uncorrelated components y_j for the input signals x_i. This is an important characteristic of the PCA decomposition, which allows us, in some cases, to directly design finite impulse response (FIR) filters.

3.2. FIR filter design and PCA

In the case of the delay line which feeds a parallel device (Figure 4), the input vector elements are delayed samples of the same signal. Thus, the covariance matrix in Equation (7) becomes the autocorrelation matrix $\mathbf{A}(\mathbf{x})$ of the input signal. Therefore, in this case, the eigenvalues are computed for the $\mathbf{A}(\mathbf{x})$ matrix.

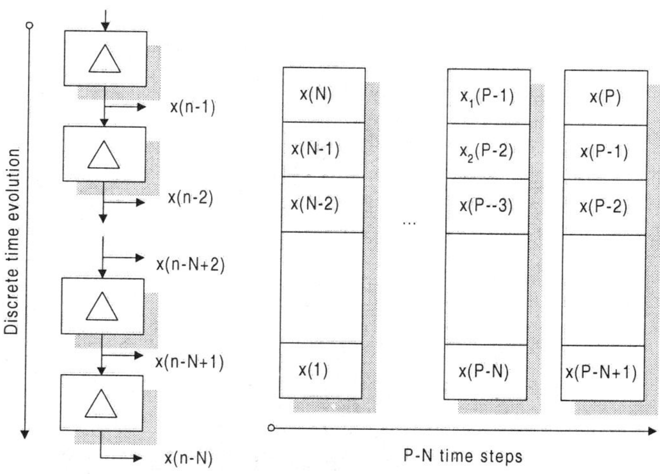

Figure 4. Delay line (homogenous) input data flow.

The autocorrelation matrix is an important tool in digital finite impulse response (FIR) filter design and naturally arises in the analysis of the filtering performance. Considering the FIR filter equation of the form

$$y(n) = \sum_{i=0}^{N-1} w_i x(n-i) = \mathbf{w}^T \mathbf{x}(n) \tag{10}$$

where the $\mathbf{w}^T$ is the vector of the filter unknown parameters and $\mathbf{x}(n)$ denotes the signal N–length window at time n (Figure 5).

The output signal power is

$$E\left[y^2(n)\right] = E\left[\mathbf{w}^T \mathbf{x}_n \mathbf{x}_n^T \mathbf{w}\right] = \mathbf{w}^T \mathbf{A}(\mathbf{x})\,\mathbf{w} \tag{11}$$

The $\mathbf{A}$ matrix is positive semidefinite and doubly symmetric. Moreover, its diagonal entries are identical, i.e., $\mathbf{A}$ is a Toeplitz matrix. When a white noise $e(n)$ of power σ_e^2 is added to the input signal $x(n)$, the signal-to-noise ratio (SNR) at the output of the filter is

$$SNR = \frac{E\left[y^2(n)\right]}{E\left[e^2(n)\right]} = \frac{E\left[y^2(n)\right]}{\mathbf{w}^T \sigma_e^2\, \mathbf{w}} = \frac{\mathbf{w}^T \mathbf{A}\,\mathbf{w}}{\mathbf{w}^T \mathbf{w}\, \sigma_e^2} \tag{12}$$

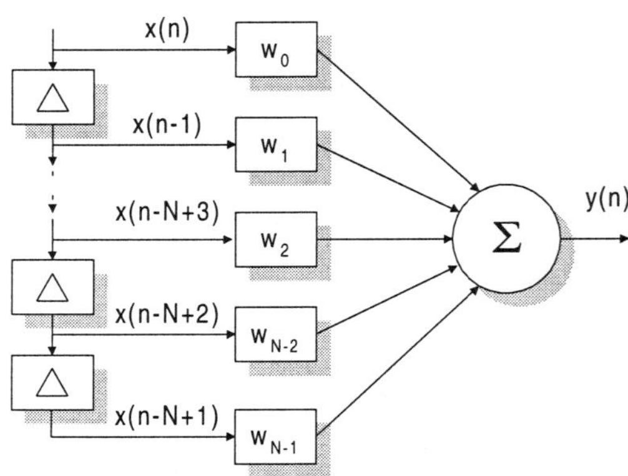

Figure 5. Finite impulse response (FIR) filter in transversal configuration.

The SNR is maximized with respect to the unknown filter coefficient vector when the numerator is maximized subject to the constraint $\mathbf{w}^T\mathbf{w} = 1$ (the unity attenuation is considered in the filtering case). Using a Lagrange multiplier [9], one has to maximize the quantity $\mathbf{w}^T \mathbf{A} \mathbf{w} + \lambda (1 - \mathbf{w}^T\mathbf{w})$ with respect to $\mathbf{w}$. The solution is given by the eigenvalues equation $\mathbf{A} \mathbf{w}^* = \lambda \mathbf{w}^*$. Thus, the optimum filter coefficient vector $\mathbf{w}^*$ is given by the eigenvector of the autocorrelation matrix associated with the largest eigenvalue λ_{max}. The optimum filter ensures the maximum of the signal power at the output, and thus the maximum SNR. Conversely, the eigenvector of the autocorrelation matrix associated with the smallest eigenvalue λ_{min} will give the minimum power signal at the output.

From this point of view, the principal component analysis allows the energy decomposition of the input signal. Its relation to the spectral constituents of the input signal may be directly derived using a definition of the Discrete Fourier Transform (DFT) based on the Finite Fourier Transform (FFT).

$$DFT_x(v) = \lim_{n\to\infty} FFT_x(v) = \lim_{n\to\infty} \frac{1}{\sqrt{2N+1}} \sum_{n=-N}^{N} x(n)\, e^{-2\pi j\, v\, n} \qquad (13)$$

The spectrum of the signal is obtained as the square of the *DFT* modulus and is written as

$$S(v) = \left| DFT_x(v) \right|^2 = DFT_x(v)\overline{DFT_x(v)}$$

$$= \lim_{n \to \infty} \frac{1}{2N+1} \sum_{n=-N}^{N} x(n)\, e^{-2\pi j\, v\, n} \sum_{m=-N}^{N} x(m)\, e^{-2\pi j\, v\, m}$$

$$= \lim_{n \to \infty} \frac{1}{2N+1} \sum_{n=-N}^{N} \sum_{m-N}^{N} x(n)x(m)\; e^{-2\pi j\, v\,(n+m)} \tag{14}$$

$$= \sum_{p=-\infty}^{\infty} a_x(p)\, e^{-2\pi j\, v\, p}$$

where a_x is the autocorrelation function of the signal x, of the form

$$a_x(p) = \lim_{N \to \infty} \frac{1}{2N+1} \sum_{n=-N}^{N} x(n)x(n-p) \tag{15}$$

Consequently, when the statistic of the x signal is known, it is possible to estimate the $S(v)$ spectral constituents using (14). Conversely, the autocorrelation function of a signal may be expressed in terms of the spectral constituents using the reverse formula.

$$a_x(p) = \int_{-\frac{1}{2}}^{\frac{1}{2}} S(v)e^{2\pi j\, v\, p}\, dv \tag{16}$$

when the spectrum $S(v)$ of the x signal is known. For finite sequences, the relation between the autocorrelation matrix of the sequence and the spectral composition obtained by making the sequence periodic leads to the following inequalities:

$$\min_{-1/2 \le v \le 1/2} S(v) \le \lambda_i \le \max_{-1/2 \le v \le 1/2} S(v) \tag{17}$$

where λ_i are the eigenvalues of the autocorrelation matrix. Moreover, using the properties of the Finite Fourier Transform, we obtain [9]

$$\lambda_{\min} \leq \min_{0 \leq k \leq n-1} E\left[\left|\, FFT_x(k)\right|^2\right] \quad ; \quad \lambda_{\max} \geq \max_{0 \leq k \leq n-1} E\left[\left|FFT_x(k)\right|^2\right] \quad (18)$$

Thus the output signal spectral power is bounded by the eigenvalues of the autocorrelation matrix. For large sequences, when N approaches infinity from Equation (17), it results that the inequalities Equation (18) turn into equalities as soon as the Finite Fourier Transform approaches the Discrete Fourier transform.

3.3. PCA neural network

In many contexts, artificial neural networks are considered to be parallel signal processing devices based on simple functional blocks, the processing elements (PEs). The PEs are linked together in a structure of variable strength connections, which defines the network operation. The values of the connection weights are selected following an adaptation procedure. The PCA transform expressed in Equation (1) may be performed using the so-called PCA neural network.

The main idea behind the PCA network is the design of a multi-input multi-output adaptive device able to perform the rotation of the input space following the eigenvectors of the input signal autocorrelation matrix in a very useful form. The same applies to heterogeneous input vectors when the PCA detects the eigenspace of the input covariance matrix. The PCA network sorts the eigenvectors in decreasing order. The sorting criterion is the value of the associated eigenvalue. Thus, after the adaptation, the PCA network outputs correspond to the projections of the input signal on the principal (largest) eigenvectors. The energy of each output signal is smaller than the energy of the output signal generated by the precedent node.

The PCA neural realization meets both biological and engineering requirements, if one considers only the Hebbian learning system used in PCA and the global convergence properties which are demonstrated well in the literature [12]. The PCA linear transform is

$$\mathbf{y}(n) = \mathbf{W}\,\mathbf{x}(n), \quad \mathbf{y} \in R^M, \quad \mathbf{x} \in R^N, \quad \mathbf{W} \in R^{M \times N} \quad (19)$$

where $\mathbf{W}$ is the eigenvector submatrix of the form $\mathbf{U} = (\mathbf{u}_1, \mathbf{u}_2, ..., \mathbf{u}_M)^T$; that is, the rows of the $\mathbf{W}$ matrix are the first M principal eigenvectors corresponding to the largest eigenvalues of the autocorrelation matrix of the x signal. For the simplicity of presentation, we shall assume that the input signal is wide-sense stationary and has zero average.

From Equation (19), it results that a PCA network is a simple linear layer of additive processing elements (Figure 6) with the weight matrix $\mathbf{W}$, based on

Equation (19). After training, its rows $\mathbf{w}_j$ approximate the M principal eigenvectors of the autocorrelation matrix. Consequently, if the signal x has zero average, the variance probes obtained at the outputs y_j are estimates of the principal eigenvalues. The variance probes are estimated, under the assumption that the input signal is stationary, by the y_j signal energy.

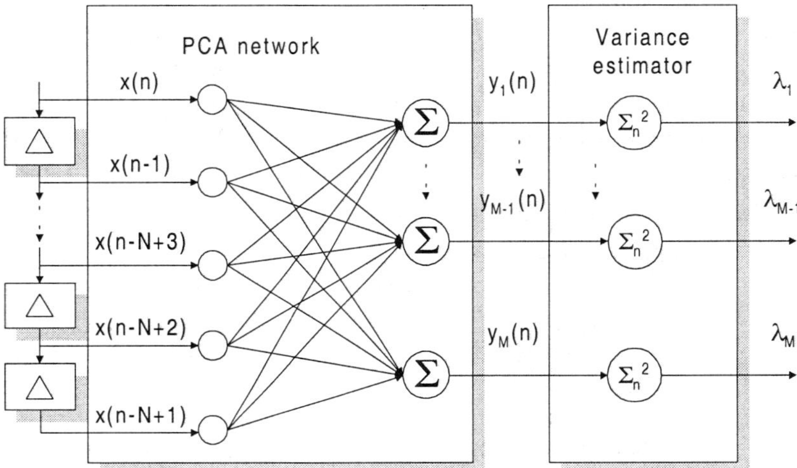

Figure 6. The PCA network and the eigenvalues estimation.

We consider an equal width R for each average window associated with the variance estimator.

3.4. PCA network adaptation procedure

There are many numerical methods, given by the so-called eigenvalues problem in algebra and numerical analysis [10], that may be used to derive the PCA network adaptation procedure. We emphasize that the PCA adaptation mechanism may be considered, like the unsupervised adaptation procedures, to be rooted in the natural neuronal learning mechanism. The neurobiological learning rule described in 1949 by Hebb states that the efficiency of the connection between two neural cells is directly dependent on the activity levels of both connected cells. Thus, only the axon impulses that traverse the connecting synapse and produce a significant activity level at the receiving cell will determine a growth in synapse efficiency. The Hebb principle was the first to explicitly introduce the notion of synaptic efficiency. The synapse strength is usually modeled in artificial neural systems by a real number that multiplies the output signal of the transmitter PE. In signal processing theory terms, the connection strength must be directly dependent on the correlation between the output signals of the connected PEs. Usually, if the connections are multiplicative, this is expressed in terms of input-output correlation of the receiver PE. For the connection weight w_{ij} at the input j of an additive processing element i, one can write the Hebb rule in the form

$$w_{ij}(n+1) = w_{ij}(n) + \eta\; y_i(n)x_j(n) \tag{20}$$

Equation (20) is the core of the more complex PCA adaptation algorithms. Supplemental constraints must be added to ensure the other important requirements on the PCA adaptation, namely, the decreasing order arrangement and the ortho-normalization of the eigenvectors in the **W** weight matrix defined in Equation (19).

In [13] the following learning rule is proposed:

$$w_{ij}(n+1) = w_{ij}(n) + \eta(n)y_i(n)\left[x_j(n) - \sum_{h=1}^{M} w_{hj}(n)y_h(n) \right] \tag{21}$$

$$i = 1,...,M \quad j = 1,...,N$$

where w_{ij} is the connection weight from the input j to the i-th processing element from the PCA layer. In Equation (21), a supplemental attenuation term is introduced. This regularization term represents the additive effect of other processing elements' output correlation measures with respect to the actual processing element output. Equation (21) defines the *symmetric subspace* learning rule, obtained from the gradient descent minimization of the quadratic cost function.

$$E = \frac{1}{2}\|\mathbf{e}\|^2 = \frac{1}{2}\|\mathbf{x} - \mathbf{x}_e\|^2 = \frac{1}{2}\|\mathbf{x} - \mathbf{W}^T\mathbf{y}\|^2$$
$$= \frac{1}{2}\left(\mathbf{x} - \mathbf{W}^T\mathbf{y}\right)^T\left(\mathbf{x} - \mathbf{W}^T\mathbf{y}\right) \tag{22}$$

where $\mathbf{e}$ identifies the effective error vector and $\mathbf{x}_e$ is the result of the inverse transform of the output $\mathbf{y}$ obtained with the actual weight matrix. The effective error considered in Equation (22) expresses the fact that the inverse of the eigenvector matrix may always be obtained from its transpose. Differentiating Equation (22) with respect to the weight matrix **W**, one obtains the error (Jacobian) matrix $\mathbf{J}_w(E)$, which directly gives the update rule of the form

$$\Delta \mathbf{W}(n) = \mathbf{W}(n+1) - \mathbf{W}(n) = -\eta(n)\,\mathbf{J}_W\,(E,n) =$$

$$= \eta(n)\,\mathbf{y}(n)\,\mathbf{e}^T(n) = \eta(n)\cdot\left[\mathbf{y}(n)\,\mathbf{e}^T(n) + \mathbf{W}(n)\,\mathbf{e}(n)\,\mathbf{x}^T(n)\right] \qquad (23)$$

The second term in the right hand of Equation (23) is usually very small, and it may be neglected. The update equation becomes

$$\Delta \mathbf{W}(n) = \eta(n)\cdot\left[\mathbf{y}(n)\,\mathbf{e}^T(n) + \mathbf{W}(n)\,\mathbf{e}(n)\,\mathbf{x}^T(n)\right]$$

$$= \eta(n)\,\mathbf{y}(n)\cdot\left[\mathbf{x}^T(n) - \mathbf{y}^T(n)\,\mathbf{W}(n)\right] \qquad (24)$$

$$= \eta(n)\cdot\left[\mathbf{W}(n)\,\mathbf{x}(n)\,\mathbf{x}^T(n)\left(\mathbf{I}_{n,n} - \mathbf{W}^T(n)\,\mathbf{W}(n)\right)\right]$$

This is an equivalent form of the updating rule Equation (21). In Equation (24), notice in the first term, the (autocorrelation) Hebbian term, and in the second term, the nonlinear degradation factor which ensures the normalization of the resulting eigenvectors.

The iteration procedure Equation (21) finds the global minimum of the cost function E; moreover, the resulting weight matrix consists of linear combinations of the input autocorrelation matrix eigenvectors [14]. This is, however, a drawback of the method because these linear combinations are not unique. That is, they are dependent on the specific input signal. A way to alleviate this problem was found by Oja, who used different weighting coefficients for the feedback contribution of each output y_h [15]. This weighting technique gives the *weighted subspace* learning rule and is expressed by the equation

$$w_{ij}(n+1) = w_{ij}(n) + \eta(n)y_i(n)\left[x_j(n) - \gamma_i \sum_{h=1}^{M} w_{hj}(n)y_h(n)\right] \qquad (25)$$

$$i = 1,\ldots,M \quad j = 1,\ldots,N \quad 0 < \gamma_1 < \gamma_2 < \ldots < \gamma_m$$

where the weighting coefficients γ_i induce the order of the extracted eigenvectors.

In fact, there is a simpler solution to this adaptation problem, namely, the use of particular combinations of the weighting coefficients for each PCA layer output. Sanger has shown [16] that for the same linear PCA structure, a sufficient condition for the convergence of the vector $\mathbf{w}_i$ to the associated eigenvector $\mathbf{u}_i$ is the use of unity feedback links only from the superior neighbor outputs. This means that the weight update equation is

$$w_{ij}(n+1) = w_{ij}(n) + \eta(n)y_i(n)\left[x_j(n) - \sum_{h=1}^{i} w_{hj}(n)y_h(n)\right] \tag{26}$$

$$i = 1,\ldots,M \quad j = 1,\ldots,N$$

Note that the summation index h in Equation (26) ranges in this case from 1 to i. This learning rule was named *the generalized Hebbian learning* rule. It was proved [17] that learning based on this rule converges from all initial conditions for reasonably small learning rates.

The stopping criterion in the case of the PCA network unsupervised adaptation procedures may be a general criterion. For instance, one may use limit ε for the average weight changes ($\|\Delta\mathbf{W}\| < \varepsilon$) as a stop condition. However, the accuracy of the final adaptation result must be checked using the specific properties of the eigenvector matrix. The orthogonality test on the resulting vectors is often used. The norms of the eigenvectors also provide useful information about the convergence of the PCA learning algorithm.

3.5. Nonlinear PCA networks

The PCA features extraction capabilities are intrinsically limited to the linear eigenvector transformation. There are several powerful PCA network extensions that use nonlinear elements to allow the extraction of high-order statistical moments [18]. The nonlinear characteristics may be introduced either at the connections level or at the processing elements level. The same learning rules are used, but the convergence is not guaranteed this time. This is not a serious limitation because the learning heuristics developed for usual artificial neural networks, like multilayer perceptrons or higher-order networks, also apply to the nonlinear PCA dynamics. Thus, in almost all contexts, small learning rates produce accurate and reproducible results in the PCA training process.

When the PCA uses nonlinear processing elements, the input-output mapping may be analyzed with the Taylor series expansion of each processing element output function. The Taylor expansion approximates the output function f by a polynomial. This approximation significantly facilitates the analysis of the PCA response. The higher order statistical moments are monomials in the same arguments. This allows the study of the cumulative moments composition of the PCA response using the desired accuracy. The Taylor series development around the origin $\mathbf{w}^T_i\mathbf{x} = 0$ of the scalar function $f(\mathbf{w}^T_i\mathbf{x})$ may be written as

$$y_i(\mathbf{x}) = f(\mathbf{w}_i^T \mathbf{x}) \cong \sum_{j=0}^{S} \frac{\left(\mathbf{w}_i^T \mathbf{x}\right)^j}{j!} f^{(j)}(0) = f(0) +$$

$$+ \frac{\mathbf{w}_i^T \mathbf{x}}{1!} f'(0) + \frac{\left(\mathbf{w}_i^T \mathbf{x}\right)^2}{2!} f''(0) + \dots + \frac{\left(\mathbf{w}_i^T \mathbf{x}\right)^S}{s!} f^{(s)}(0)$$

$$(27)$$

The local expansion Equation (27) is valid only in the neighborhood of the origin. Its local accuracy is given by the approximation order S. The nonlinear function f must be differentiable with respect to its scalar argument, at least for the approximation order S, i.e., the derivatives $f^{(j)}$ must exist for all values $j = 1,\dots,S$. The analysis usually retains only the quadratic and sometimes the cubic terms. For example, the quadratic approximation of Equation (27) leads to a second-degree polynomial output of the form

$$y_i(\mathbf{x}) = f(\mathbf{w}_i^T \mathbf{x}) \cong f(0) + \mathbf{w}_i^T \mathbf{x}\, f'(0) + \frac{1}{2}\left(\mathbf{w}_i^T \mathbf{x}\right)^2 f''(0) \qquad (28)$$

The relation equation (28) must be expanded as a polynomial of second degree in the $\mathbf{x}$ vector's components. Then, knowing the exact form of the function f, it is possible to evaluate its derivatives at the origin and to compute all the polynomial coefficients. Further analysis may be carried out with the classic statistical theory tools as we will detail in the following sections.

The other way to generate a nonlinear PCA input-output mapping is the use of nonlinear interconnections. For example, a linear processing element may have the input output mapping of the form

$$y_i(\mathbf{x}) = \sum_{k=1}^{N}\left(w_{ik} + \sum_{j=1}^{N} w_{ikj} x_j \right) x_k = \sum_{k=1}^{N} w_{ik} x_j + \sum_{j=1}^{N}\sum_{k=1}^{N} w_{ikj} x_j x_k \qquad (29)$$

where y_i denotes the scalar PE output, which depends on the inputs x_j using the connections set w_{ik}, but also on the intercorrelation sources given by the multiplicative inputs $x_k x_j$ using the multiplicative connection set w_{ikj}. Equation (29) describes a *second-order* processing element similar to the element obtained in Equation (28). We use the notations

$$y_i(\mathbf{x}) = \mathbf{w}_i^T \mathbf{z}$$

$$\mathbf{z} = \left(x_1, x_2, \ldots, x_N, x_1^2, x_1 x_2, \ldots, x_1 x_N, x_2^2, x_2 x_3, \ldots, x_{N-1} x_N, x_N^2\right)^T \tag{30}$$

$$\mathbf{w}_i = \left(w_{i1}, w_{i2}, \ldots, w_{iN}, w_{i11}, w_{i12}, \ldots, w_{i1N}, w_{i22}, w_{i23}, \ldots, w_{i,N-1,N}, w_{iNN}\right)^T$$

The intercorrelation matrix for the new variable vector $\mathbf{z}$ may be written in terms of the $\mathbf{x}$ vector elements and thus several matrix subblocks will contain the third- and fourth-order statistical moments [19]. Equation (30) may be obtained from a two-stage process: a linear process using a unit y fed with a $(N+1)(N+2)/2$-dimensional vector formed in a preprocessing stage which quadratically combines the $\mathbf{x}$ and $\mathbf{w}_i$ elements. After training with a PCA extraction algorithm, $\mathbf{w}_i$ will approximate one of the eigenvectors of the correlation matrix $\mathbf{A}(\mathbf{z})$ of the form

$$\mathbf{A} = \begin{pmatrix} \mathbf{A}_1 & \mathbf{A}_2 \\ \mathbf{A}_3 & \mathbf{A}_4 \end{pmatrix}$$

$$\mathbf{A}_1 = \begin{pmatrix} \langle x_1^2 \rangle & \langle x_1 x_2 \rangle & \cdots & \langle x_1 x_N \rangle \\ \langle x_2 x_1 \rangle & \langle x_2^2 \rangle & & \langle x_2 x_N \rangle \\ \vdots & & & \vdots \\ \langle x_N x_1 \rangle & \langle x_N x_2 \rangle & \cdots & \langle x_N^2 \rangle \end{pmatrix}$$

$$\mathbf{A}_2 = \begin{pmatrix} \langle x_1^3 \rangle & \langle x_1^2 x_2 \rangle & \cdots & \langle x_1 x_N^2 \rangle \\ \langle x_2 x_1^2 \rangle & \langle x_1 x_2^3 \rangle & & \langle x_2 x_N^2 \rangle \\ \vdots & & & \vdots \\ \langle x_N x_1^2 \rangle & \langle x_1 x_2 x_N \rangle & \cdots & \langle x_N^3 \rangle \end{pmatrix} \tag{31}$$

$$\mathbf{A}_4 = \begin{pmatrix} \langle x_1^4 \rangle & \langle x_1^3 x_2 \rangle & \cdots & \langle x_1^2 x_N^2 \rangle \\ \langle x_2 x_1^3 \rangle & \langle x_2^2 x_1^2 \rangle & & \langle x_1 x_2 x_N^2 \rangle \\ \vdots & & & \vdots \\ \langle x_N^2 x_1^2 \rangle & \langle x_N^2 x_2 x_1 \rangle & \cdots & \langle x_N^4 \rangle \end{pmatrix}$$

where <.,.> denotes the (statistical) mean. The $\mathbf{A}_1$ matrix is the first-order correlation matrix, $\mathbf{A}_2 = \mathbf{A}_3{}^T$ are the second-order moment matrices, and $\mathbf{A}_4$ is the fourth-order moment matrix.

The same applies in the first case. The nonlinear processing elements become polynomial, and the higher-order intercorrelation matrix may be built in a similar manner. If one allows higher-order terms in Equations (28) and (29), higher-order statistics correlation matrices will be obtained.

4. Radial basis function (RBF) networks

The RBF networks have a feedforward structure consisting of two layers of qualitatively different types of processing elements. The input layer provides a *selective response* to an input data vector depending on a *distance* between the input vector and each processing elements' weight vectors [20]. The output layer has additive processing elements, which linearly combine the resulting responses (Figure 7).

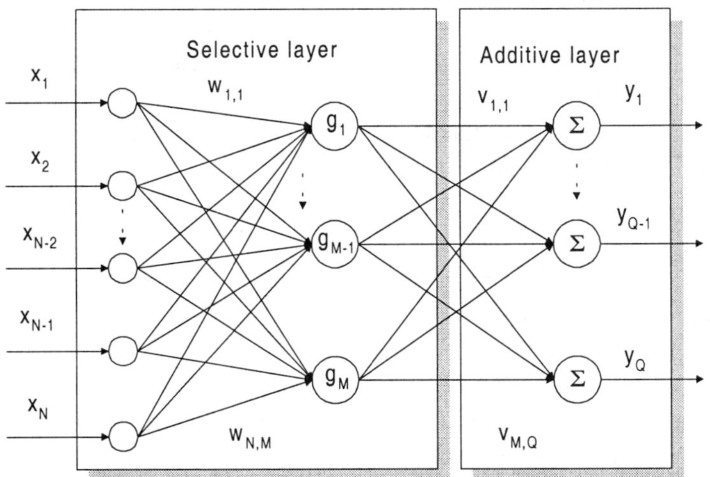

Figure 7. Radial basis function network.

The direct data flow through the RBF network is expressed by the equations

$$y_k(\mathbf{x}) = \sum_{j=1}^{M} v_{j,k}\, g_j(\mathbf{x}, \mathbf{w}_j) \quad \mathbf{w}_j = [w_{1,j}, \ldots, w_{N,j}]^T$$

$$g_j(\mathbf{x}, \mathbf{w}_j) = g_j\left(\left\| \mathbf{x} - \mathbf{w}_j \right\|\right) \quad k = 1, \ldots, Q \tag{32}$$

The output y_k is the weighted sum of the selective responses g_j of the hidden layer processing element outputs. The responses are computed based on a distance (similarity) measure $\|.\|$ between the N-dimensional input vector $\mathbf{x}$ and the weight vector $\mathbf{w}_j$. Note that this type of response represents the main difference between the RBF network and the multilayer perceptron (MLP) network. The MLP uses only the weighted additive activation mechanism (scalar product of the input and the weight vectors) for all processing elements. The usual distance measure is the Euclidean norm. This norm gives the radial symmetry property of the hidden layer processing element response with respect to the translation of the input N-dimensional input space origin onto the "center" $\mathbf{w}_j$.

The selective response to an input vector $\mathbf{x}$ means that the scalar function g must vanish rapidly when its argument moves away from zero. Usually g is "bell shaped," i.e., is a positive definite and symmetric function with a single maximum at zero. These types of radially symmetric basis functions are also encountered in modeling biological neuronal systems when a locally tuned response is required for a specific input excitation. A commonly used radial basis function is the Gaussian

$$g_j(\mathbf{x}, \mathbf{w}_j, \sigma_j) = \exp\left(-\frac{\left\| \mathbf{x} - \mathbf{w}_j \right\|}{2\sigma_j} \right) \tag{33}$$

The parameters of the Gaussian are the center position $\mathbf{w}_j$ and the response spread σ_j, also named the width of the receptive field. These parameters are adapted to feed the output layer with a selective response which expresses the maximum information extracted from the input data set.

The roots of the radial basis functions methods lie in both the interpolation and approximation theories. The hidden layer response is a nonlinear mapping between the N-dimensional input space and an M-dimensional features space providing simultaneously smooth interpolation and optimal approximation.

We introduce in the first subsection some basic notions from approximation theory which are directly related to the radial basis functions. The second subsection details the adaptation procedures designed for RBF networks training.

4.1. Approximation error and supervised RBF learning

Finding a continuous function **h** that approximates, in the least-mean-square (LMS) sense, the underlying mapping of a data set represents the main subject of the approximation theory. This function may be a linear combination of radial basis functions (see the Appendix), as is the output of the RBF neural network. From the optimal approximation point of view, the problem consists in finding a smooth mapping **h** able to represent the real complexity of the data set. The number of basis functions will express this complexity, regardless of the number of data points.

In the approximation case, the centers of the basis functions are obtained using an adaptation algorithm. The parameters of each basis function (like the receptive field width for the Gaussian) play an important role in the approximation procedure. The approximation function **h** is given by the equation

$$h_k(\xi) = \sum_{j=1}^{M} v_{j,k}\, g_j(\xi, \mathbf{w}_j) \quad \mathbf{w}_j = [w_{1,j}, \ldots, w_{N,j}]^T$$

$$g_j(\xi, \mathbf{w}_j) = g_j\left(\left\| \xi - \mathbf{w}_j \right\|\right) \quad k = 1, \ldots, Q \tag{34}$$

which has a direct equivalence in the forward data flow through the RBF network.

The LMS approximation error between the RBF network output and a desired function **y**(n) may be defined as

$$E = \frac{1}{2}\sum_{n=1}^{P}\sum_{k=1}^{Q}\left(h_k(\mathbf{x}(n)) - y_k(n) \right)^2$$

$$= \frac{1}{2}\sum_{n=1}^{P}\sum_{k=1}^{Q}\left(\sum_{j=1}^{M} v_{j,k} g_j(\mathbf{x}(n)) - y_k(n) \right)^2 \tag{35}$$

The minimum of the cost functional E may be found in two fundamentally different ways: with a fully supervised method and with a supervised-unsupervised method. The first method considers the nonlinear input-output function of the RBF network and finds the derivatives of the error with respect to the adaptive parameters (the output layer weight matrix **v** and the hidden layer RBF parameters). These partial derivatives are then used for back-propagating the error E through the network.

The partial derivatives of the approximation error E with respect to a generic RBF network parameters q are computed as

$$\nabla_q E = \frac{\partial E}{\partial q} = \sum_{n=1}^{P}\sum_{k=1}^{Q}\left[\left(h_k(\mathbf{x}(n)) - y_k(n)\right)\cdot\frac{\partial h_k(\mathbf{x}(n))}{\partial q}\right]$$

$$(36)$$

$$= \sum_{n=1}^{P}\sum_{k=1}^{Q}\left[\left(h_k(\mathbf{x}(n)) - y_k(n)\right)\cdot\frac{\partial}{\partial q}\sum_{j=1}^{M}\left(v_{j,k}\,g_j(\mathbf{x}(n)) - y_k(n)\right)\right]$$

The general updating equation following the gradient-descent technique may be written as

$$\Delta q(m+U) = -\eta\,\nabla_q E + \alpha\,\Delta q(m) \tag{37}$$

The symbol η denotes the update rate (learning rate). The right-hand term $\alpha\Delta q(m)$ in the above equation is usually added to provide smoother variations of the adapted parameter. The updating time step U is usually equal to the cardinality P of the input data set (full batch mode training), but any other value may be used, depending upon the specific learning strategy.

The error gradient components for the weights $v_{r,s}$ of the linear output layer are

$$\nabla_{v_{r,s}} E = \sum_{n=1}^{P}\left(h_s(\mathbf{x}(n)) - y_s(n)\right)g_r(\mathbf{x}(n)) \tag{38}$$

The partial derivatives of the radial basis function g_j with respect to the $w_{i,j}$ center parameter are

$$\frac{\partial g_j(\mathbf{x}(n))}{\partial w_{j,i}} = g'_j(\mathbf{x}(n))\cdot\frac{\partial}{\partial w_{j,i}}\left[\sum_{k=1}^{M}\left(x_k(n) - w_{j,k}\right)^2\right]$$

$$(39)$$

$$= 2g'_j(\mathbf{x}(n))\left(x_i(n) - w_{j,i}\right)x_i(n)$$

where $g_j'(n)$ denotes the *value* of the radial basis function first derivative (with respect to its scalar argument), computed with the actual input and center vectors.

The gradient components of the E function with respect to the center vectors of the hidden layer processing elements may be written as

$$\nabla_{w_{r,s}} E = \sum_{n=1}^{P} \sum_{k=1}^{Q} \left[\left(h_k(\mathbf{x}(n)) - y_k(n) \right) \cdot \sum_{j=1}^{M} v_{j,k} \frac{\partial}{\partial w_{r,s}} g_j(\mathbf{x}(n)) \right]$$

$$= \sum_{n=1}^{P} \sum_{k=1}^{Q} \left[\left(h_k(\mathbf{x}(n)) - y_k(n) \right) \cdot v_{r,k} \frac{\partial}{\partial w_{r,s}} g_r(\mathbf{x}(n)) \right] \qquad (40)$$

$$= 2 \cdot \sum_{n=1}^{P} \left[g'_r(\mathbf{x}(n)) \left(x_s(n) - w_{r,s} \right) \cdot \sum_{k=1}^{Q} \left(h_k(\mathbf{x}(n)) - y_k(n) \right) \cdot v_{r,k} \right]$$

The spread parameter gradient components depend on the particular form of the basis function and may be derived similarly.

Apart from the specific expressions of the gradient, this method is a direct application of the well-known error backpropagation algorithm used for MLP training. The main disadvantage of this method is the number of iterations needed to obtain a small enough error. However, the resulting RBF network has the same generalization ability as the MLP network.

The second method consists of two different steps. In the first step, the hidden layer processing elements (the radial basis function centers) are adapted using an unsupervised technique. This step depends only on the input data set; the adaptation procedure iteratively moves the RBF centers in the input space to obtain the maximum response for all input vectors from a detected data "cluster."

The unsupervised techniques generally detect the *prototypes* of an unlabelled input data set. The prototypes are representations of the probability density of the input data [21]. After the unsupervised training stage, the centers of the hidden layer RBF functions are the centers of detected data clusters. The processing element responses express the distance between the cluster center and the actual input vector.

The second training step assumes that the RBF parameters are fixed and the output layer weights are adapted to minimize the error E. The error E is a quadratic function with respect to the output layer weights $v_{j,k}$. This property allows the application of the direct method in finding the solution of the associated system of the normal equations. By differentiating the error E with respect to the unknown parameters $v_{j,k}$ and setting the derivatives to zero, one obtains

$$\frac{1}{2}\sum_{n=1}^{P}\frac{\partial}{\partial v_{j,k}}\sum_{k=1}^{Q}\left(\sum_{j=1}^{M}v_{j,k}g_j(\mathbf{x}(n))-y_k(n)\right)^2=0$$

$$\sum_{n=1}^{P}\sum_{k=1}^{Q}\left[\left(\sum_{j=1}^{M}v_{j,k}g_j(\mathbf{x}(n))-y_k(n)\right)\frac{\partial}{\partial v_{j,k}}\left(\sum_{j=1}^{M}v_{j,k}g_j(\mathbf{x}(n))-y_k(n)\right)\right]=0 \qquad (41)$$

$$\sum_{n=1}^{P}\sum_{k=1}^{Q}\left[\left(\sum_{j=1}^{M}v_{j,k}g_j(\mathbf{x}(n))-y_k(n)\right)g_i(\mathbf{x}(n))\right]=0, \qquad i=1,\dots,M$$

Equation (41) may be expressed in matrix form as

$$\left(\mathbf{G}^T\mathbf{G}\right)\mathbf{V}^T=\mathbf{G}^T\mathbf{Y} \qquad (42)$$

$\mathbf{G}\in\mathbf{R}^P\times\mathbf{R}^Q$ is the matrix of the hidden nodes' outputs for all the input vectors, $\mathbf{x}(n)$, $\mathbf{V}\in\mathbf{R}^Q\times\mathbf{R}^M$ denotes the output layer weights matrix, and $\mathbf{Y}\in\mathbf{R}^P\times\mathbf{R}^Q$ is the desired response vectors matrix. The matrix Equation (42) gives the exact closed form solution of the optimization problem above. Assuming that the inverse of the matrix $\mathbf{G}^T\mathbf{G}$ exists, one may compute the pseudo-inverse of the $\mathbf{G}$ matrix as

$$\mathbf{G}^+=\left(\mathbf{G}^T\mathbf{G}\right)^{-1}\mathbf{G}^T, \quad \mathbf{G}^+\in R^Q\times R^P \qquad (43)$$

Using the matrix $\mathbf{G}^{+,}$ the solution $\mathbf{V}^*$ can be expressed as

$$\mathbf{V}^*=\mathbf{G}^+\mathbf{Y} \qquad (44)$$

Thus, the solution $\mathbf{V}^*$ is obtained using only matrix inversion procedures and does not assume any iteration algorithm. This leads to fast adaptation, which is more appropriate for on-line applications.

The two-step training procedure has several important advantages. First, the unsupervised adaptation step may be performed separately, using another training data set. This is usually the case for rich unlabelled input data sets, when the unsupervised procedure finds the best RBF centers' values that fit the implicit data cluster prototypes. The second step may use a reduced labeled data set that is representative for the desired output mapping. In addition, the output layer adaptation may be performed several times, using the same RBF centers, obtained for a general input data set. This offers a greater accuracy of the RBF network response in a nonstationary input context. The main disadvantage of the noniterative training procedure employed for the output layer weights is the lower generalization abilities of the resulting RBF network. This is not true for iterative gradient algorithms, which may benefit from the various cross-validation techniques used to derive a stopping criterion for the adaptation and which ensure a maximum degree of generalization with respect to a representative testing data set.

4.2. Regularization with RBF networks

Controlling the smoothing degree for a mapping function is a problem of first interest in modeling theory. In the case of neural networks, the modeling context is parametric. This means that the model is obtained using a parametric mapping function. Its parameters are adapted to fit a set of input-output data pairs using an error function, e.g., the error function E from the previous sub-section.

The number of adaptive parameters expresses the model complexity. From the data fitting point of view, the best model ensures the minimum of the error $E,$ and, at the limit, may be considered as an equivalent formulation of the exact interpolation problem. Nevertheless, the modeling techniques try to express the systematic aspects (features) that are implicitly expressed in the data set. This will ensure the adequacy of the model to possible unknown inputs after the design stage and thus the generalization ability of the model. There is always a trade-off between the fitting quality with respect to a given finite data set and the generalization abilities of the model. One way to combine both of these modeling aspects is to add to the error function E a supplemental term which controls the regularity of the model function. The most used regularity feature is the mapping smoothness which depends on the derivatives of the model function.

Tikhonov was the first to study the concept of regularization [22]. Technically, taking into account a smoothing requirement for the model function is equivalent to adding a supplemental term to the modeling error functional. The sum of errors leads to an optimization problem with weak constraints when the supplemental error term depends on the derivatives of the model function. The modeling error functional E_M may be written as the sum of the fitting error term E and of the regularization term E_R.

$$E_M = E + \gamma E_R \quad 0 \leq \gamma \leq 1 \tag{45}$$

where γ is called the regularization factor.

When the desired model complexity is expressed using the smoothness degree of the model function $h\colon \mathbf{R}^N \to \mathbf{R}$ (we consider here, for clarity, a real-valued function), the regularization term E_R may be written as [20]

$$E_R = \| Dh \| = \int |Dh|^2\, d\mathbf{x} \tag{46}$$

D is a differential operator applied on the h function. When D is translation and rotation invariant, the general solution of the minimization problem involving the cost functional E_M is obtained as [21]

$$h(\mathbf{x}) = \sum_{n=1}^{P} v_j\, g(\mathbf{x}, \mathbf{x}(n)) = \sum_{n=1}^{P} v_n\, g(\|\mathbf{x} - \mathbf{x}(n)\|) \tag{47}$$

$g(.)$ is a radial-basis type Green function for the operator D, which satisfies [23].

$$D^* Dg(\mathbf{u}, \mathbf{v}) = \delta(\mathbf{u} - \mathbf{v}) \tag{48}$$

D^* denotes the adjoint of the differential operator D. The local solution around a given input data vector $\mathbf{x}(n)$ satisfies

$$h(\mathbf{x}(n)) - y^n + \gamma\, v_n = 0 \tag{49}$$

Using Equation (47) in Equation (49) for each input data vector $\mathbf{x}(n)$, one obtains the linear system of equations.

$$(\mathbf{G} + \gamma\, \mathbf{I})\mathbf{v} = \mathbf{y}$$
$$\mathbf{G} = \{g_{pq}\} \quad g_{pq} = \mathbf{G}(\|\mathbf{x}(p) - \mathbf{x}(q)\|) \tag{50}$$
$$\mathbf{v} \in R^P, \mathbf{y} \in R^P \quad p, q = 1, \ldots, P$$

Here, $\mathbf{I}$ denotes the P-order unit matrix. The operator D may have the form

$$\int |Dh|^2\, d\mathbf{x} = \sum_{r=0}^{\infty} \frac{\sigma^{2r}}{r!\,2^r} \int |\nabla^r h(\mathbf{x})|^2\, d\mathbf{x} \tag{51}$$
$$\nabla^{2r} = (\nabla^2)^r \quad \nabla^{2r+1} = \nabla(\nabla^{2r})$$

where ∇ is the gradient operator and ∇^2 is the Laplacian operator. In this case, the Green functions g are Gaussian functions (as in Equation (33)) with the same width parameter σ [21].

It is interesting to note that a zero value of the regularization factor γ in Equation (50) will lead to the exact interpolation solution (see the Appendix). When the regularization factor increases, the solution is a smoother data model. Simpler regularization terms may be used based on the elements of the Hessian matrix of the input-output modeling function. The regularization technique may be similarly applied to the approximation problem, using the same arguments as in the previous section.

Moreover, extending this technique to a general context, the *a priori* information related to the model may be expressed as a regularization term in the cost functional. As we shall see in the next sections, the combination of the fitting error term and a *features* error term significantly improves the model from the general semantic point of view.

4.3. Unsupervised basis function parameter optimization

As mentioned earlier, there are two distinct methods for the RBF network training: the iterative gradient descent method and the two-stage (unsupervised-supervised) method. For the second method, the output layer weight matrix is computed directly using matrix inversion, but any other method for solving linear overdetermined systems of equations may be used. We focus in this section on the frequently used unsupervised techniques, which lead to the RBF input space decomposition.

Several schemes have been suggested to find the receptive field centers and widths using only the input data set properties. The main principle applied in this context is to follow the input data set probability distribution. The RBF centers are distributed randomly over the input data space and a clustering algorithm is used to iteratively adjust the centers to represent only a small region of the input space which corresponds to a data cluster. The k-means clustering algorithm is often used. This algorithm may be regarded as a special case of the more general competitive adaptation scheme [24]. A cost functional to be minimized in the RBF network centers adaptation may be defined as

$$E = \frac{1}{2}\sum_{n=1}^{P}\sum_{k=1}^{M} \mathbf{M}_{n,k} \left\| \mathbf{x}(n) - \mathbf{w}_k \right\|^2 \tag{52}$$

Here, $\mathbf{M}_{n,k}$ is a dynamically evolving scalar function that determines whether or not the processing element k responds (wins the competition) when the $\mathbf{x}(n)$ input is presented to the network. When the Euclidean norm is used in

Equation (52), the gradient of the error E with respect to the $\mathbf{w}_k$ vector has the form

$$\nabla_{\mathbf{w}_k} E = -\sum_{n=1}^{P} M_{n,k} \left(\mathbf{x}(n) - \mathbf{w}_k \right)$$

$$\Delta \mathbf{w}_k = -\eta \, \nabla_{\mathbf{w}_k} E = \eta \sum_{n=1}^{P} M_{n,k} \left(\mathbf{x}(n) - \mathbf{w}_k \right)$$

(53)

This is equivalent to the batch-mode version (over the whole training data set) of the competitive learning rule [24]

$$\Delta \mathbf{w}_k = \begin{cases} \eta \left(\mathbf{x}(n) - \mathbf{w}_k \right) & \text{if unit } i \text{ is a winner for input } n \\ 0 & \text{otherwise} \end{cases}$$

(54)

The k-mean clustering algorithm starts with an initial random selection of the RBF centers as vectors from the input data set. These values give the initial labeling for the M clusters, one for each RBF center. The remaining training vectors are labeled as being elements of the closest cluster in terms of Euclidean distance. In the second step, the RBF centers are computed using all the data vectors from the formed clusters. A new labeling operation will be performed and new center positions will be further determined.

This two-step process is invoked until a stable configuration of the centers is reached. The method needs storage for the data vector labels for the entire training set. This is avoided if an incremental method is applied. In this case, for each input data vector, the closest cluster center is computed. Then, the detected center vector is adjusted following the new membership information acquired (the input vector position) using Equation (54). The learning rate η is chosen to be small enough to avoid large center oscillation when each new input vector adds its position information to the cluster characterization.

Other, more refined clustering techniques, such as Learning Vector Quantization [25], may be used. All methods are based on the similarity measures between the training data vectors. It is noteworthy to observe that the competitive learning mechanism is possible in the RBF case only when the hidden units' response is local. This allows the application of the competitive updating rule Equation (54) following the direct comparison of the Euclidean norms because, implicitly, the output unit response vanishes for larger norm values.

Another parameter, directly related to the quality of the input-output mapping performed by the RBF networks, is the spread of the receptive field. Generally, the spread is a common parameter (in the semantic sense) for all radial-basis function types. The spread parameter controls the distance-based response of the RBF unit. Thus, it is directly related to the selectivity degree of the unit. There are no general methods to adapt the spread parameters of the radial basis functions. A simple solution is to leave the spreads equal for all processing elements and, depending on the particular function used, to allow a 50% average overlapping degree between the function centers. More refined schemes have been suggested in the literature. An estimate of the Gaussian spreads, proposed in [26], is the mean of the distances between all the centers of the processing elements in the hidden layer. A local spread selection criterion may be dependent on the distances to the nearest neighbor centers, as has been suggested in [24].

As pointed out at the beginning of this section, the two-stage training technique is able to cope with different data sets for the same modeling problem. That is, one may use a large unlabeled data set for the center position adjustment and a small, labeled (or with a corresponding target data vector associated) representative data set for the output layer adaptation. This technique does not give satisfactory results when the input data set has significant variance and small correlation to the target values. In this case, the number of hidden units that result is large, following the unsupervised training step. Moreover, the linear output layer will fail to extract the target model, due to its low (linear) modeling capabilities, when the hidden layer decomposition is not very accurate.

When the hidden-to-desired output linear correlation is not strong enough, a better choice is a nonlinear output layer. This will enhance the modeling capability of the network, but will also change the training rule. The classic gradient descent techniques must be applied to cope with the nonlinear character of the network mapping.

5. Adaptive hybrid systems

Many papers in the literature refer to neural approaches which integrate the features extractor and the data preprocessor (filter) into a single neural system. The integration effort is focused on attenuating the composite hybrid system characteristics using new global learning schemes. This is the way to design specific neural stand-alone processors [18], like principal component analysis networks [16, 27, 28], blind signal identification networks [29, 30], or wavelet networks [31].

Many researchers have reported the limits and drawbacks of the existing paradigms for adaptive signal filtering. Several ways to overcome the lack of connection between the embedded semantics (features) of the signals and traditional signal processing methods have been proposed. An important part of the recent signal processing literature focuses on finding different useful signal representations. Recent developments in this respect propose time-frequency representations used in wavelet adaptive filters [32], general representation models like cone classes described in [33], or higher order cumulants such as representation features in [34, 35].

In this context, the neural hybrid solution, which attempts to embed various features extractors in complex processing systems, may take advantage of both types of development [36]. Moreover, using the features space processing approach, these apparently heterogeneous processing methods may benefit from superior integration, which provides a better overall system quality.

Two specific features space filtering systems are presented in the following sections. The first system uses an adaptive finite impulse response (FIR) filter and an RBF features extractor. The Gaussian basis decomposition space is used to adapt the filter coefficients, following an imposed pattern in the features space [37, 38].

The second hybrid system combines a multilayer perceptron filter and a PCA features extractor. The adaptation process is driven by an error function in the decomposition space of the principal components.

5.1. FIR filter – RBF features extractor hybrid system

The discrete time FIR filter equation may be written as

$$y_{OD}(n) = \sum_{i=1}^{N_{ID}} w_{i,FIR} x_{ID}(n-i+1) \tag{55}$$

where $w_{i,FIR}$ are the N_{ID} components of the filter vector of coefficients and x_{ID} is the input data vector in the N_{ID}-dimensional input space [39]. The output data space signal y_{OD} feeds a radial basis function features extractor (Figure 8), employed by a Gaussian basis function neural network. The filter and the features extractor are coupled using a delay line with N_{OD} unity taps. The RBF network input vector at each instant n is denoted by

$$\mathbf{y}_{OD}(n) = \left[y_{OD}(n-N_{OD}+1),\ldots,y_{OD}(n)\right]^{T} \tag{56}$$

The RBF network parameters form the output features space, that is, the Gaussian centers of the hidden processing elements and the weight vector of the output layer processing elements are the extracted features. For a RBF network with N_{OD} inputs, H hidden processing elements, and a single output processing element h_{OD}, the extracted features vector has the form

$$\mathbf{y}_{OF} = \left[\mathbf{w}_1^T, \mathbf{w}_2^T, \dots \mathbf{w}_H^T \mathbf{v}^T\right]^T$$

$$\mathbf{w}_h = \left[w_{h1}, w_{h2}, \dots, w_{hN_{OD}}\right]^T \quad h = 1, \dots, H \tag{57}$$

$$\mathbf{v} = \left[v_1, \dots, v_H\right]^T$$

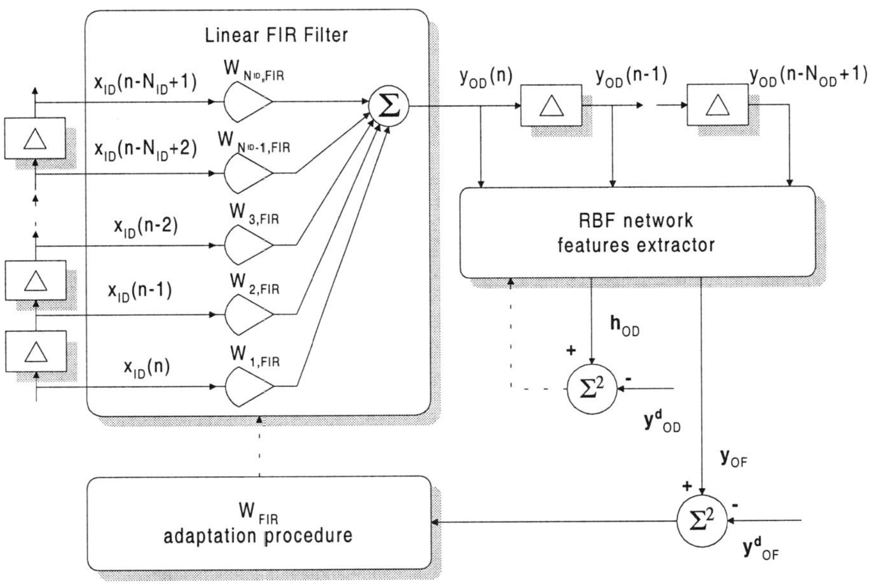

Figure 8. Linear FIR filter – RBF features extractor hybrid system.

The parameters of the RBF hidden processing elements and the filter coefficients are adapted to minimize the distance in the features space E_{OF} between a reference features vector $\mathbf{y}_{OF}^d$ and the actual features vector $\mathbf{y}_{OF}$ obtained from a noisy data set.

$$E_{OF} = \left\| \mathbf{y}_{OF}^d - \mathbf{y}_{OF} \right\|^2 \tag{58}$$

The norm used in Equation (58) is defined as the weighted L_2 distance between the actual features vector and the reference features vector.

$$E_{OF} = \gamma_w \sum_{i=1}^{N_{OD}} \sum_{j=1}^{H} \left(w_{i,j} - w_{i,j}{}^d\right)^2 + \gamma_v \sum_{i=1}^{H} \left(v_i - v_i{}^d\right)^2 \tag{59}$$

The weighting factors γ_w and γ_v are positive constants that control the contribution of each class of adaptive parameters to the feature space error.

However, the weighting factors γ_w and γ_v in Equation (59) are difficult to estimate in a very crisp manner. Moreover, different users could indicate various values. Furthermore, the subjective effect of quality is not necessarily a quadratic function of the distance in the features space. Consequently, in such situations, fuzzy membership functions could be defined such as in [8, 40].

$$\mu[E_{OF}] = \mu_w \left[\sum_{i=1}^{N_{OD}} \sum_{j=1}^{H} \left(w_{i,j} - w_{i,j}^{\,d} \right)^2 \right] + \mu_v \left[\sum_{i=1}^{H} \left(v_i - v_i^{\,d} \right)^2 \right] \tag{60}$$

where the $\mu[.]$ is a fuzzy membership function. The reference RBF decomposition $\mathbf{y}^d{}_{OF}$ is obtained using a clean signal in a separate training session of the RBF network.

The features space filtering method can be formally regarded in this case as a generalization (in the nonlinear sense) of the linear parametric filtering when the features vectors contain the adaptive parameters of the system. This approach is useful when the radial-basis function decomposition of the data set is motivated by physical evidence.

The relation between the input signal space and the output space is nonlinear and noninvertible, due to the RBF network decomposition. The direct propagation through the system is expressed as

$$
\begin{aligned}
y_{OD}(n) &= \sum_{i=1}^{H} v_i g_i \left(\mathbf{y}_{OD}(n) \mathbf{w}_i^{\,T}, \sigma_i \right) = \sum_{i=1}^{H} v_i \exp\left(-\frac{\left\| \mathbf{y}_{OD}(n) - \mathbf{w}_i^{\,T} \right\|}{2\sigma_i} \right) \\
&= \sum_{i=1}^{H} v_i \exp\left(-\frac{1}{2\sigma_i} \sum_{j=1}^{N_{OD}} \left(y_{OD}(n-j+1) - w_{i,j} \right)^2 \right) \\
&= \sum_{i=1}^{H} v_i \exp\left(-\frac{1}{2\sigma_i} \sum_{j=1}^{N_{OD}} \left(\sum_{k=1}^{N_{ID}} w_{k,FIR} x_{ID}(n-j-k+2) - w_{i,j} \right)^2 \right)
\end{aligned}
\tag{61}
$$

The relation between the feature space *OF* and the input signal space *ID* during learning depends *on overall history* of the adaptation procedure of the RBF network parameters. A general explicit form of this dependence does not exist. The filter coefficients depend on the RBF decomposition parameters. These parameters obey a nonlinear and discrete-time varying equation as explained in Section 2.4. The error function E_{OF} depends on the RBF network parameters and on the reference features vector $\mathbf{y}^d{}_{OF}$.

In the first stage, the filter is adapted with the same clean signal used during the extraction of the reference parameter vector $\mathbf{y}^d{}_{OF}$. This filter is fed with a noisy signal and its outputs are used for the first RBF network training. Thus, the RBF network realization and, consequently, the features space vector $\mathbf{y}_{OF}$ is obtained using a data space error of the form

$$E_{OD} = \frac{1}{2}\left(y_{OD}{}^d - h_{OD}\right)^2 \tag{62}$$

An unsupervised training procedure exclusively using the $\mathbf{y}_{OD}(n)$ input vector is also possible for the centers of the Gaussian functions. The receptive field widths σ_j are fixed to the values obtained for the reference RBF decomposition. The RBF decomposition $\mathbf{y}_{OF}$ is compared with the reference decomposition and the features space error is computed.

A perturbation of the filter coefficient $w_{k,FIR}$ produces a change in the output signal y_{OD}. A new RBF network is trained with this signal using the E_{OD} error from Equation (8), with the same clean signal as target. The features space error E_{OF} is computed using Equation (4). If this error is greater than the error previously obtained, the perturbation and the last RBF decomposition are discarded. Otherwise, the changes are preserved. Another iteration will be started, with a new perturbation of the filter coefficients.

The following steps summarize the system training procedure:

1. *Obtain a reference filter FIR* and a reference decomposition RBF* using the clean signal $y^d{}_{OD}$.*

2. *Obtain the filter FIR(0) and the associated Gaussian decomposition RBF(0) using a noisy input signal. FIR(0) is obtained from FIR* with a small parameter perturbation. The RBF(0) is obtained using the FIR(0) output signal y_{OD} and the clean desired signal $y^d{}_{OD}$, using a random initial state.*

3. *Repeat until the system error is smaller than a given value or the system is settled in a stable state (error changes are smaller than a given value for a prespecified number of steps).*

   3.1. *Obtain the filter FIR(i) from the filter FIR(i-1), with a small parameter perturbation.*

   3.2. *Obtain the Gaussian decomposition RBF(i), using the FIR(i) filter output signal y_{OD} the clean desired signal $y^d{}_{OD}$ and the RBF(i-1) centers as initial values for RBF(i).*

   3.3. *Compute the error $E_{OF}(i)$ using RBF(i) and RBF* output signals.*

3.4. If $E_{OF}(i) > E_{OF}(i-1)$

Replace FIR(i) with FIR(i-1), RBF(i) with RBF(i-1) and $E_{OF}(i)$ with $E_{OF}(i-1)$ (reject the whole i-th iteration).

If $E_{OF}(i) < E_{OF}(i-1)$

Go to 3.5.

3.5. $i = i+1$.

When the error E_{OF} decreases, one obtains a better Gaussian decomposition for the linear filter output signal, and the perturbed filter parameters are retained. When the E_{OF} increases, one restarts the algorithm with the previous filter coefficients and with the previous RBF decomposition. It is interesting to note that the memory of the learning system refers only to the features-space error in this algorithm. That is, the retained initial states for the system components depend only on the features-space error.

In the above adaptation algorithm, the error used for the perturbation learning procedure may be considered as a binary function. This function is derived from the features-space error function, E_{OF}, and decides if the perturbation is accepted / rejected at the system level.

5.2. MLP filter – PCA features extractor hybrid system

In this subsection, a multilayer perceptron (MLP) neural network is used for the adaptive filter. The features extractor is based on the information obtained from the second order statistics of the signal. The statistics are extracted with a PCA network, as detailed in Section 3. The training procedure uses an error signal computed as the difference between the desired and actual signals in the principal decomposition space.

We propose an MLP neural network, designed as an adaptive filter. Nonlinear processing elements are used, which have sigmoid-like input-output functions of the form

$$x_j^L = f(a_j^L) = \frac{1}{1+\exp(-a_j^L)} \tag{63}$$

The activation a_j^L of the j-th processing element of the layer L follows the additive equation.

$$a_j^L = \sum_{i=1}^{n_{L-1}} w_{ij} x_{ij}^L + b_j^L \tag{64}$$

where $w_{ji}{}^{L}$ parameters form the weights inset to the j-th processing element of layer L, and b_j^L is the bias term. The index L denotes a specific layer of the network, and $L = 0$ is assigned to the input of the MLP. In vector notation, the direct data flow through the MLP may be written, layer by layer, as

$$\mathbf{x}_j^L = \mathbf{f}(\mathbf{W}_j^L \mathbf{x}^{L-1}) \tag{65}$$

$\mathbf{f}$ is a vector of scalar operators, i.e., its scalar function components operate only on the corresponding elements from the vector argument.

We use a refined form of the MLP, namely, the asymmetric pyramidal ($n_L < n_{L-1}$) topology. Each processing element of the layer L is connected only to its right-handed counterparts in the layer above (Figure 9). This asymmetric connection scheme is particularly adequate for filtering operations [41]. The MLP network implicitly performs a weighting operation on each input sample. In this particular case, this is driven not only by the symmetric back-propagation of the error function gradient, but also by the topological constraint. The triangular constraint allows a progressively reduced number of connections for the oldest delayed input signal samples. Consequently, this produces an attenuation of their contributions to the output signal.

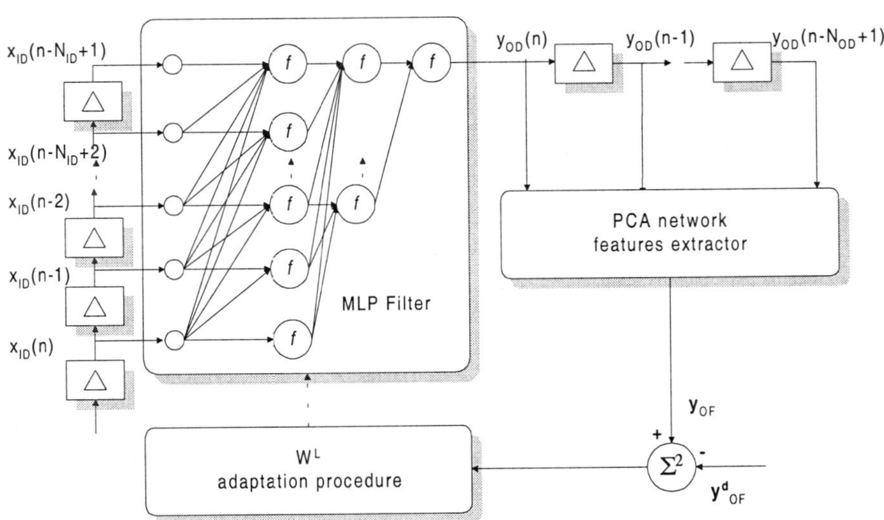

Figure 9. MLP filter – PCA features extractor hybrid system topology.

As a feature extractor, we use a hierarchical PCA network. The MLP feeds the PCA layer using a tap delay line. The input vector to the PCA at each instant n is denoted by

$$\mathbf{y}_{OD}(n) = \left[y_{OD}(n - N_{OD} + 1), ..., y_{OD}(n) \right]^T \quad \mathbf{y}_{OD}(n) \in R^{N_{OD}} \tag{66}$$

The PCA realizes the principal subspace transform

$$\mathbf{y}_{OF}(n) = \mathbf{W}_{PCA}\, \mathbf{y}_{OD}(n), \quad \mathbf{y}_{OF} \in R^{N_{OF}} \quad \mathbf{W}_{PCA} \in R^{N_{OD} \times N_{OF}} \tag{67}$$

where $N_{OF} < N_{OD}$ in the usual data compression case.

The feedforward data flow through the system may be written as

$$y_{i,OF}(n) = \mathbf{w}_{i,PCA}^T \mathbf{y}_{OD}(n) \quad \mathbf{w}_{i,PCA} \in R^{N_{OD}} \quad i = 1, ..., N_{OF}$$
$$y_{i,OF}(n) = \mathbf{w}_{i,PCA}^T \mathbf{f}^L \left[\mathbf{W}_{MLP}^L \left[\mathbf{f}^{L-1} ... \mathbf{f}^1 \left[\mathbf{W}_{MLP}^1 \mathbf{x}_{ID}(n - N_{OD} + 1) \right] \right] \right] \tag{68}$$

The number of nested square brackets in Equation (68) is equal to the number of layers in the MLP network.

The features space error function uses the L_2-norm to measure the distance between the desired reference signal in the principal space $\mathbf{y}^d_{OF}(n)$ and the actual output vector $\mathbf{y}_{OF}(n)$ of the feature extractor.

$$E_{OF} = \sum_{i=1}^{N_{OF}} \gamma_i \sum_{n=1}^{R} \left(y_{i,OF}^d(n) - y_{i,OF}(n) \right)^2 \tag{69}$$

The E_{OF} is the mean square error over a time interval R between the desired and actual signals at the output of the PCA layer. Each term in the outer sum of Equation (69) is multiplied by a positive coefficient γ_i. These coefficients control the contribution of each principal component to the features space error. Depending on the characteristics of the signal to be filtered, the weights γ_i are chosen to express a specific supplemental constraint in the features space.

It is interesting to point out that the information extracted from the signal $\mathbf{y}_{OD}$ at the output of the MLP is passed through the decorrelation PCA layer. This layer has a linear transfer function. The error function E_{OF} derivatives with respect to the MLP network weights exist and may be used in the system training procedure.

The relevance of the mapping $\mathbf{y}_{OF} = \mathbf{y}_{OF}(\mathbf{x}_{ID})$ is dependent on both the MLP network and the PCA layer adaptation procedures. The latter uses the unsupervised Generalized Hebbian algorithm (GHA), detailed in Section 3. This algorithm converges to globally stable solutions in a relatively small number of iterations. In contrast, the MLP training procedure is more difficult and requires a considerable number of iterations.

Because of these different learning dynamics, we separate the training procedure of the system into two stages: an open-loop direct pretraining stage and a closed-loop, indirect adaptation stage. In the case of the MLP network, the open-loop pretraining is performed as a standard backpropagation procedure, based on a representative selection of input signals and desired output signals. We use the instantaneous mean squared error between the reference and actual output signal of the MLP, measured in the data space.

$$E_{OD} = \left(y_{OD}^{d}(n) - y_{OD}(n) \right)^{2} \tag{70}$$

The signal $y^{d}{}_{OD}$ is a reference signal in the data space. The weight update equation, in vector form, is

$$\Delta \mathbf{w}_{j}^{L^{T}}(n+1) = -\eta\, g_{j}^{L}(n)\mathbf{x}^{L-1^{T}} + \alpha\, \Delta \mathbf{w}_{j}^{L-1^{T}}(n) \tag{71}$$

where g_{j}^{L} is the backpropagated gradient of the error function to the j-th processing element of the layer L, η is the learning rate parameter, and α the momentum coefficient. The transposed unfolding of backpropagation paths is constrained in the asymmetric MLP topology as it is shown in the scalar form of Equation (70).

$$\Delta w_{ij}^{L}(n+1) = -\eta\, g_{j}^{L}(n)\, x_{i}^{L-1} + \alpha\, \Delta w_{ij}^{L-1}(n),\ i \le j + n_{L-1} - n_{L} \tag{72}$$

by the limited variation of the subscript index i. Once the pretrained MLP network performs the reference input-output mapping in the signal space with a given accuracy, the MLP outputs are used to pretrain the PCA layer with GHA (Section 3.3).

After the pretraining stage, when all the adaptive system components are settled in a favorable state, the loop is closed and the system is fed with the noisy signal. This will change the decomposition signals at the output of the PCA. The features space error E_{OF} is used to drive the indirect adaptation of the MLP. It is possible to use two techniques for FSF training: a perturbation technique as in the FIR-BBF system case, and a gradient backpropagation algorithm. The former technique uses the direct propagation paths of the system, with a small computational load. The latter technique exploits the inverse propagation path of the system as a whole.

The perturbation technique consists of changing by a small amount a weight parameter of the MLP. Each perturbation is directly propagated through the system and modifies the cost function E_{OF}. If the change produces an increase of the error, the change is discarded and another weight is perturbed. The weight selection procedure follows a uniform probability density.

The gradient backpropagation through the system follows the same steps as the standard BP algorithm. Starting at the output of the variance estimator, the gradient of the error function with respect to the weights of the MLP is computed. This computation involves the time unfolding of the MLP subsystem [42], [43] due to the tap delay-line between the MLP and PCA layer. We may consider that this type of temporal coupling between the system components needs a *trajectory learning* procedure, that is, the gradient is back-propagated simultaneously through the PCA network *for each delayed component of the MLP network output* up to the delay-line dimension N_{OD}. The instantaneous gradient for each MLP weight parameter, at each time step, is cumulated and the weights update is made after a discrete time interval T.

6. ECG filtering in features space

In this section, two electrocardiographic signal filtering examples are presented. The first uses the MLP filter – PCA features extractor system and the second the FIR filter – RBF features extractor system detailed in the previous section.

The electrocardiographic (ECG) signal characteristics are generally difficult to model, and elaborate pattern detection schemes must be used to accurately recover it from noise [44-46]. The main difficulty for a classic neural network based filtering system is the use of incremental learning techniques. These learning methods are generally stochastic, and consequently, are well suited for stationary signals with a *uniform* probability density function. The neural network is able to form accurate representations of the temporal correlation between the signal samples and to reject the uncorrelated noise-like components in these cases.

The ECG signal features are not expressed in the statistical contents of the probability density function. For example, the extreme value of the QRS wave (Figure 10a) may be readily considered as a statistical outlier (Figure 10b). This is also due to its slight temporal displacement in the cardiac cycle [47] and to its high frequency constituents, which extend to 40 Hz. The P and T waves generally have frequencies under 10 Hz (Figure 10c).

Special signal processing methods must be considered to alleviate this drawback, mainly robust filtering methods [48], multiband techniques, such as wavelet decomposition [44] or filter-bank approaches [45].

We explore the ECG filtering capabilities of the features space processing systems described in the previous section. Using different features space representations, this complex filtering problem may be solved accurately. Moreover, it is possible to outline the characteristics of the signal, which are useful in the subsequent processing stages.

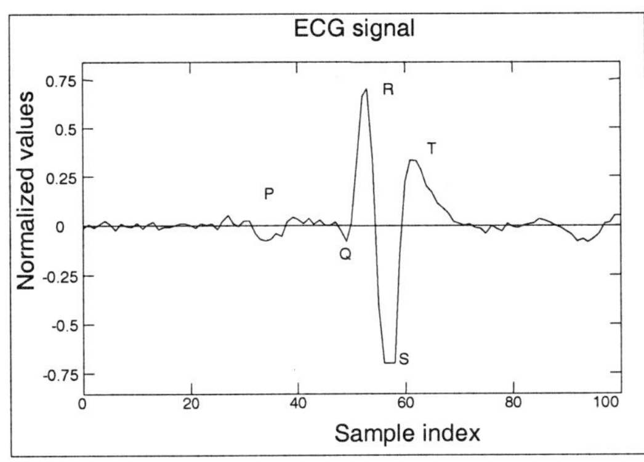

(a) Sample ECG signal

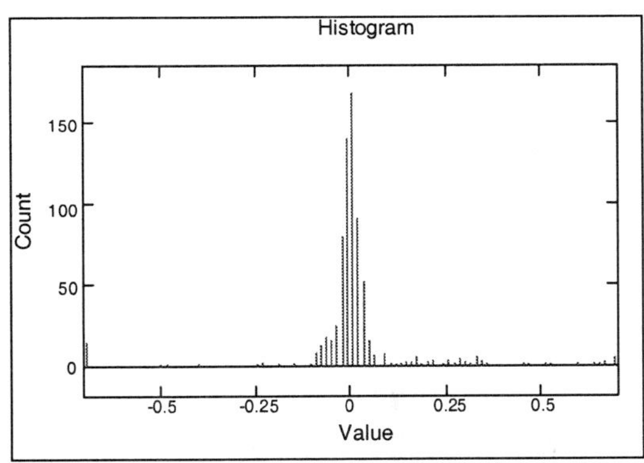

(b) Typical ECG signal histogram

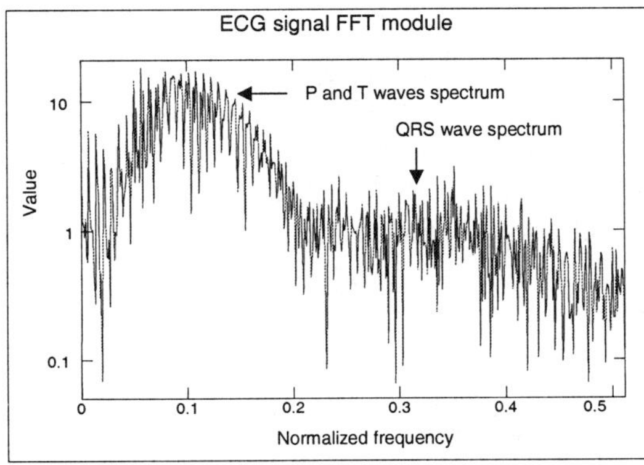

(c) Typical ECG Fourier spectrum (modulus)

Figure 10. Typical ECG signal characteristics.

6.1. ECG filtering with PCA features extractor

For the MLP-PCA filtering system, the features space is the PCA decomposition space. In this space it is possible to obtain various features of the filtered signal, based on the eigenvalues and the eigenvectors of the autocorrelation matrix of the filtered signal. The eigenvalues are obtained as the second statistical moment (the variance) of the decomposition signals (the signals have zero mean).

$$E_{OF} = \sum_{i=1}^{N_{OF}} \gamma_i (\lambda_i^d - \lambda_i^i)^2, \quad \lambda_i^{(d)} = \sum_{n=1}^{R} \left(y_{i,OF}^{(d)}(n) \right)^2 \tag{73}$$

This approach was explored in [41, 36]. The temporal window width R gives the accuracy of the variance estimations. The eigenvalues λ_i are global measures for the reference and actual output signals. The adaptation algorithm tries to minimize the differences between these measures.

In this chapter, another approach is proposed, namely, the direct comparison of the desired and the actual decomposition signals.

$$E_{OF} = \sum_{i=1}^{N_{OF}} \gamma_i \sum_{n=1}^{R} \left(y_{i,OF}^d(n) - y_{i,OF}(n) \right)^2 \tag{74}$$

Here, the temporal window width R is given by the adaptation strategy and may be reduced to unity for instantaneous gradient learning.

The simulations use a MLP-PCA system realized with a 100:75:1 MLP network and a 10:2 PCA features extractor. The temporal window width is $R = 1$. Following the procedure described in the previous section, we pretrain the MLP with an ECG reference signal (Figure 11). The output signal of the MLP network is used to train the PCA layer until convergence is achieved. The principal eigenvector norm evolution during adaptation is plotted in Figure 12.

The reference decomposition signals obtained after PCA adaptation $y_{i,OF}^d(n)$ are stored and used in the second training stage as the target for the error (74). Two ECG signals corrupted with additive Gaussian noise are used (Figure 13 and Figure 14). The noise signal has zero mean, with the variance $\sigma_{na}^2 = 0.001$ and $\sigma_{nb}^2 = 0.02$. The reference signal has the variance $\sigma_s^2 = 0.02$. Consequently, the signal-to-noise ratio (computed as SNR = 10 log $(\sigma_s^2 / \sigma_n^2)$) is SNR$_1$ = 13 dB and SNR$_2$ = 0 dB for the signals plotted in Figure 13 and Figure 14, respectively.

The system is trained using the gradient adaptation procedure described in Section 5. The error evolutions during learning are plotted in Figure 15 and

Figure 16 and the features-space filtered signals after adaptation of the MLP-PCA system are plotted in Figure 17 and in Figure 18.

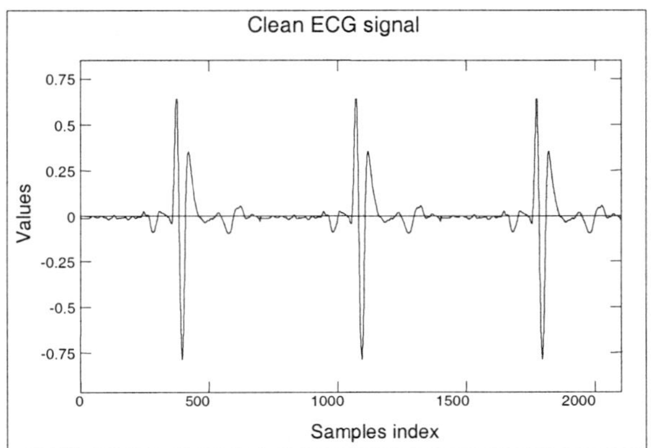

Figure 11. Clean ECG signal.

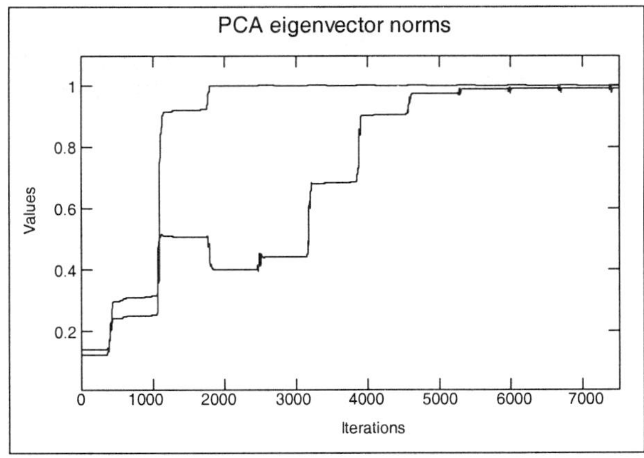

Figure 12. Eigenvector norms during PCA adaptation.

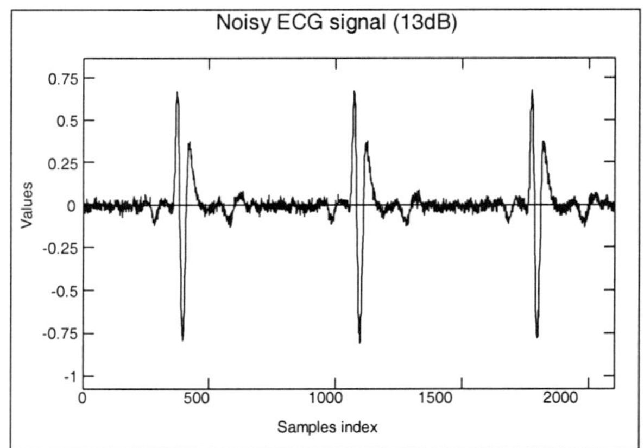

Figure 13. Noisy ECG signal ($SNR_{in} = 13$ dB).

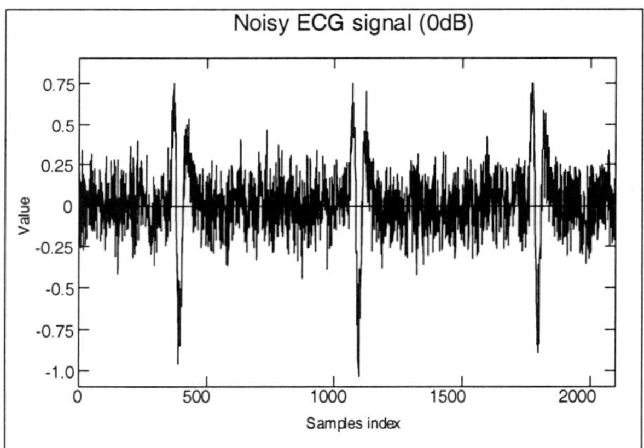

Figure 14. Noisy ECG signal ($SNR_{in} = 0$ dB).

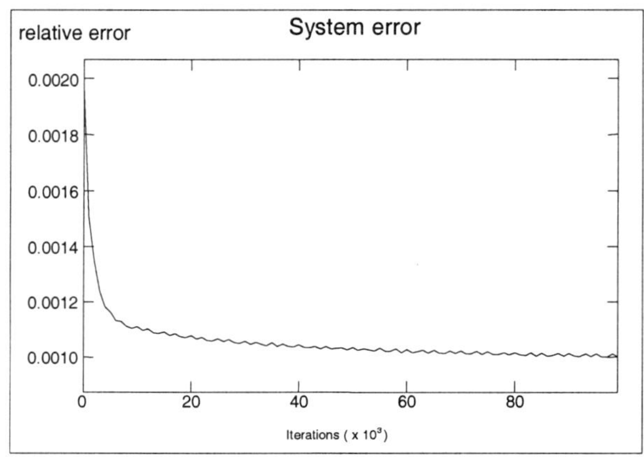

Figure 15. MLP-PCA system error evolution ($SNR_{in} = 13$ dB).

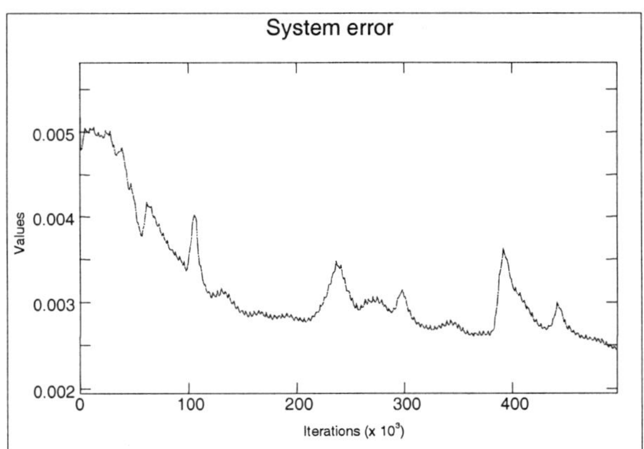

Figure 16. MLP-PCA system error evolution ($SNR_{in} = 0$ dB).

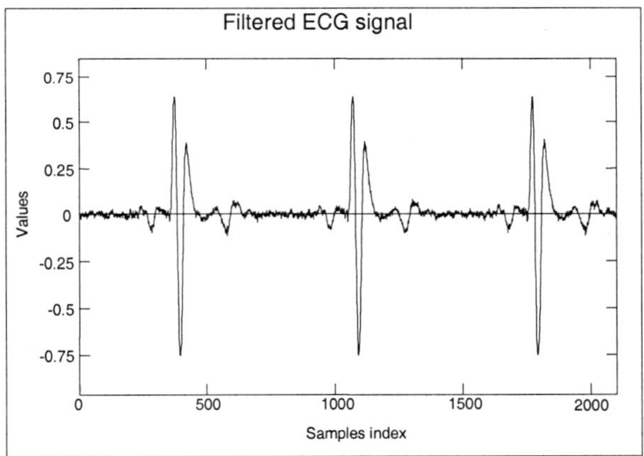

Figure 17. Filtered ECG signal ($SNR_{in} = 13$ dB).

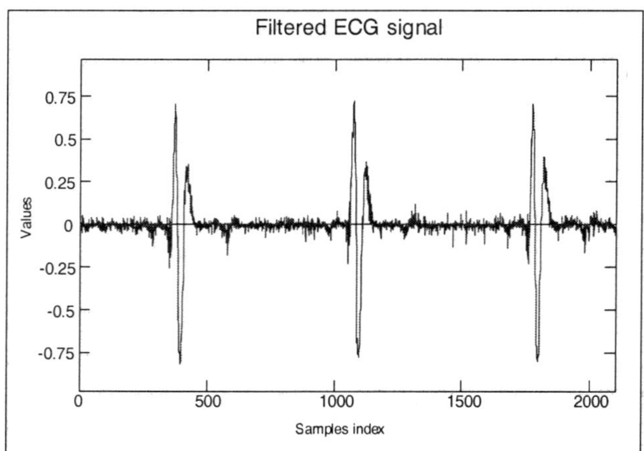

Figure 18. Filtered ECG signal ($SNR_{in} = 0dB$).

These experiments show that even when the features space system components are loosely coupled using a delay line, the learning is convergent and the filter has a good performance. The noise rejection ratios (computed as $NRR = 10 \log (\sigma^2_{n,output} / \sigma^2_{n, input})$) obtained with the trained systems are $NNR_1 = -8$ dB and $NRR_2 = -13.5$ dB.

6.2. ECG filtering with RBF features extractor

The same ECG signals feed the linear FIR filter – RBF features extractor system described in the previous section. The system is composed of a 40:1 adaptive linear filter and a 20:30:1 RBF network. In the first training stage, the system reference components are obtained using the clean signal (Figure 11). An approximation performance measure, expressed in terms of absolute percent error lower than 1%, is obtained for both the linear FIR filter and the RBF reference network. We use in this simulation a subvector of the features vector containing the center weight vectors $\mathbf{w}_i$ and the output network layer weight vector $\mathbf{v}_0$.

$$\mathbf{y}_{OF} = \left[\mathbf{w}_1^T, \mathbf{w}_2^T, ... \mathbf{w}_H^T \mathbf{v}^T\right]^T$$

$$\mathbf{w}_h = \left[w_{h1}, w_{h2}, ..., w_{hN_{OD}}\right]^T \quad h = 1, ..., H \tag{75}$$

$$\mathbf{v} = \left[v_1, ..., v_H\right]^T$$

For the system training, we use the noisy signals from Figure 13 and Figure 14. Each learning system iteration i is composed of the perturbation of a randomly chosen FIR filter parameter, followed by a complete training session of the RBF network using the output signal of the filter and the desired reference signal in

Figure 11. The perturbation value is $\eta_{FIR} = 0.001$. The RBF network is trained on-line with the centers' learning rate $\eta_w = 0.1$ and the output layer weights' learning rate $\eta_v = 0.01$. The training cycle has $300 \cdot 10^3$ steps. The system error is formed with the difference between the reference and the actual RBF decompositions.

$$E_{OF} = \left\| \mathbf{y}_{OF}{}^d - \mathbf{y}_{OF} \right\|^2 \tag{76}$$

A typical system error evolution is plotted in Figure 19 for the input signal of Figure 13 and the final FIR filter output is plotted in Figure 21. Similarly, the input signal in Figure 14 produces the error evolution from Figure 20 and the output signal from Figure 22.

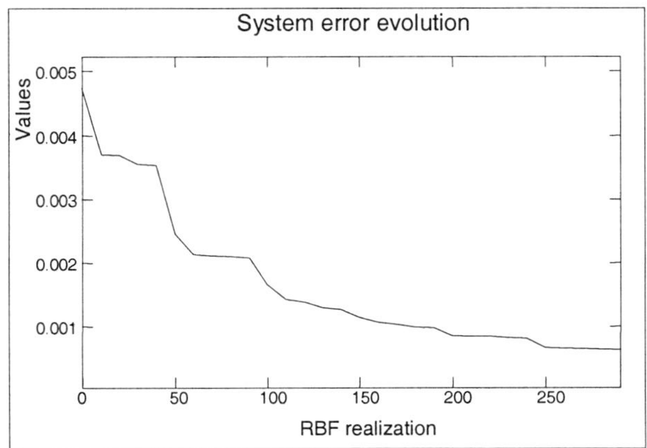

Figure 19. FIR filter-RBF network system error evolution $(SNR_{in} = 13 \text{ dB})$.

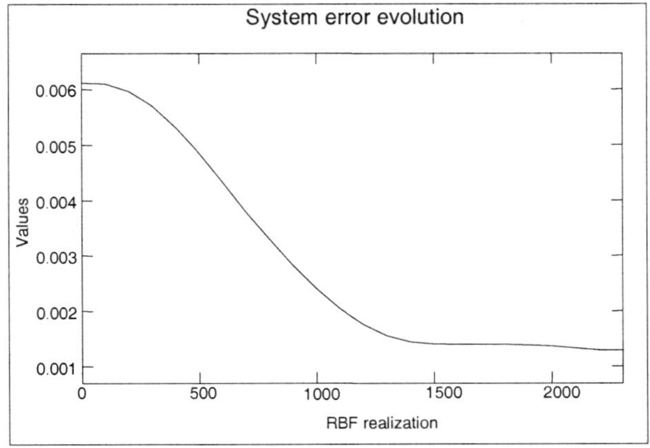

Figure 20. FIR filter-RBF network system error evolution $(SNR_{in} = 0 \text{ dB})$.

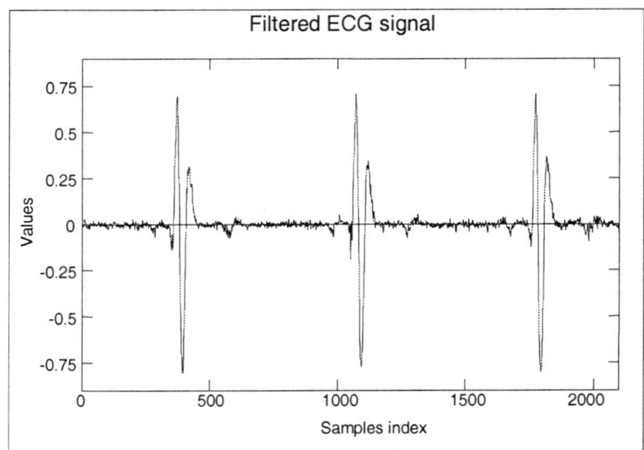

Figure 21. FIR filter output after a FIR filter – RBF network system training session (SNR_{in} = 13 dB).

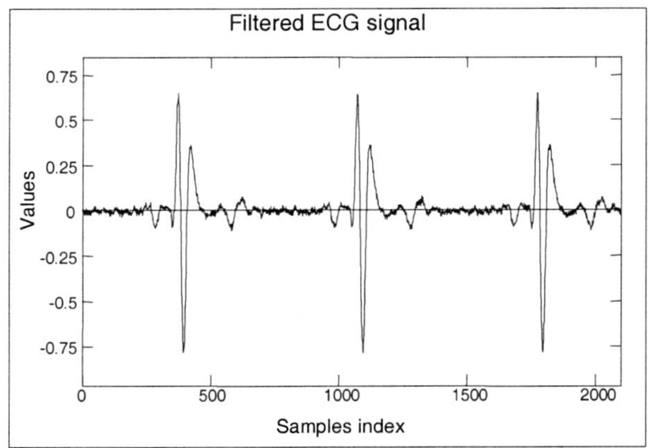

Figure 22. FIR filter output after a FIR filter – RBF network system training session (SNR_{in} = 0 dB).

The obtained NRR ratios are close to those obtained for the MLP-PCA system (approximately –8 dB for the input signal from Figure 13 and –14 dB for the input signal from Figure 14). It is worth noting that the learning systems add important constraints to the filter realizations. These constraints are imposed in different features spaces, by means of principal component or by Gaussian function decompositions, which are the targets of the learning system.

6.3. Discussion

These experiments show that the filtering systems above are able to reject noise from the ECG signal without distorting the signal characteristics. Moreover, when compared to a linear FIR filter performance, the features space filtering is significantly better for lower signal-to-noise ratios.

For a 40:1 linear FIR filter, trained with the plain LMS algorithm, the obtained noise rejection ratio is approximately the same, regardless of the signal-to-noise ratio of the input signal. The output signals, after the filter adaptation with the input signals from Figure 13 and Figure 14, and with the desired target signal from Figure 11 are plotted in Figure 19 and Figure 20, respectively.

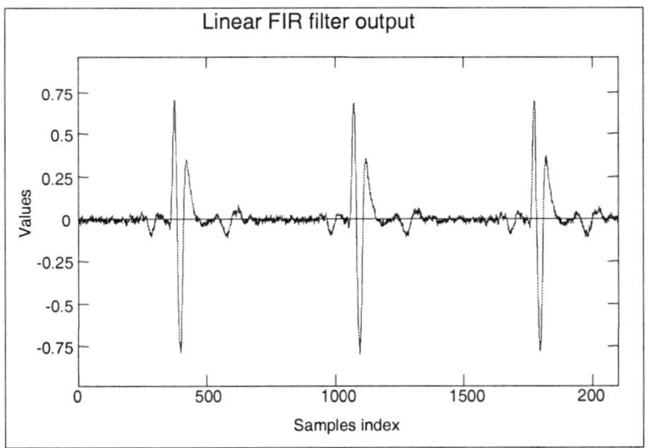

Figure 23. FIR filter output after an LMS training session in data space ($SNR_{in} = 13$ dB).

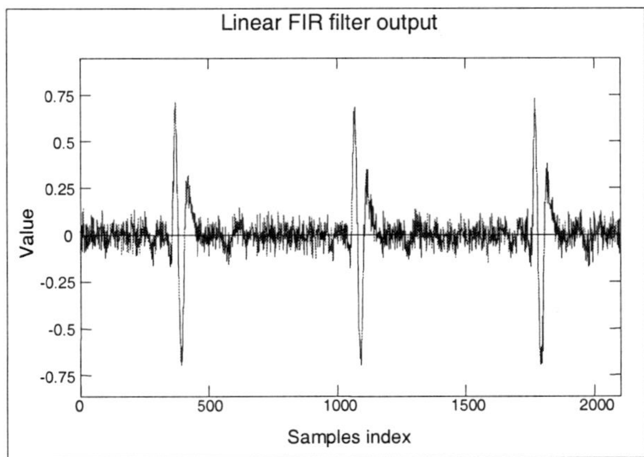

Figure 24. FIR filter output after an LMS training session in data space ($SNR_{in} = 0$ dB).

The above systems are better for lower signal-to-noise ratios, due to the intrinsic increased processing capability and to the features space learning constraints.

7. Concluding remarks

Two hybrid architectures, based on neural networks, were used to illustrate the features space filtering method: the FIR filter – RBF network features extractor system and the MLP filter – PCA features extractor system. The former uses patterns obtained with RBF neural network decomposition parameters to adapt the coefficients of a linear FIR filter. The latter uses the principal components of the autocorrelation matrix of the input data to adapt a multilayer asymmetric perceptron.

The filtering performance in the sample space is comparable to that obtained with classic methods, but the "perceiveness" of the result is enhanced, and the subsequent processing stages in features space are more accurate. This means that in applications where the filtered signals are to be further recognized by humans or machines, the use of a specific pattern-extraction procedure enhances the recognition results. Moreover, the FSF systems principle clearly outperforms the classic two-stage adaptive systems in complex, dedicated tasks when a filtering criterion in the samples space can hide the features of interest, i.e., the signal specificity.

The presented system architectures are quite general and may produce several effective implementations. The neural hybrid approach described has the advantage of exploiting the intrinsic nonlinear features of the input data set and enables a large class of application-specific pattern extraction procedures.

The targeted applications area of the features-space systems is real time control systems [36, 49], where increased capabilities of temporal processing, especially for discrete time event systems, and sequences recognition may be well employed. The features-space systems are especially useful in complex systems control when the underlying dynamic model is hard to obtain analytically.

Appendix. Interpolation and approximation with radial basis functions

In the following we consider a set of P data pairs $\{\mathbf{x}(n), \mathbf{y}(n)\}$, $\mathbf{x}(n) \in \mathbf{R}^N$, $y(n) \in \mathbf{R}^M$, $n = 1,...,P$. The exact interpolation problem consists in finding a continuous differentiable function $\mathbf{h}(\mathbf{x}(n))$ such that

$$\mathbf{h}(\mathbf{x}(n)) = \mathbf{y}(n) \overset{\Delta}{=} y^n \quad n = 1,\ldots,P$$
$$\mathbf{h} = [h_1,\ldots,h_M]^T, \quad y^n = [y^n_1,\ldots,y^n_M]^T \tag{77}$$

The Powell approach to the multidimensional exact interpolation [50] uses a set of radial basis functions, *one for each data point*, which depends on the Euclidean distance between a generic input vector $\xi \in \mathbf{R}^N$ and the associated data vector $\mathbf{x}(n)$. These basis functions are defined as

$$\mathbf{g}^n : R^N \to R^M, \, \mathbf{g}^n\big(\|\xi - \mathbf{x}(n)\|\big) = [\mathbf{g}^n_1, \mathbf{g}^n_2,\ldots,\mathbf{g}^n_M]^T \, n = 1,\ldots,P \tag{78}$$

A general interpolation function may be defined as a linear combination of these basis functions.

$$h_k(\xi) = \sum_{n=1}^{P} v_{n,k} g^n_k\big(\|\xi - \mathbf{x}(n)\|\big) = \mathbf{G}_k \mathbf{v}_k \quad k = 1,\ldots,M \tag{79}$$

The vector $\mathbf{v}_k \in \mathbf{R}^P$ denotes all the linear combination coefficients and $\mathbf{G}_k \in \mathbf{R}^P \times \mathbf{R}^P$ are square matrices with the elements $g^{n,m}_k = g^n_k (\|\mathbf{x}(n) - \mathbf{x}(m)\|)$, m, $n = 1,\ldots,P$.

A more restrictive interpolation function, which better matches the RBF network architecture, will use the same basis functions in the linear combinations corresponding to each output k. That is, for the k-th output, only the weighting coefficients will change.

$$h_k(\xi) = \sum_{n=1}^{P} v_{n,k} g^n\big(\|\xi - \mathbf{x}(n)\|\big) = \mathbf{G}\mathbf{v}_k \quad k = 1,\ldots,M$$
$$g_1^{\,n} = g_2^{\,n} = \ldots = g_M^{\,n} \overset{\Delta}{=} g^n \tag{80}$$

The interpolation condition Equation (77) may be written with the notations from Equation (80) as

$$\mathbf{G}\mathbf{v}_k = \mathbf{y}_k \quad k = 1,\ldots,M \quad \mathbf{y}_k = [y^1_k,\ldots,y^P_k]^T \tag{81}$$

If the inverse of the matrix $\mathbf{G}$ exists, the above system may be solved for the $\mathbf{v}_k$ unknowns. The solution has the form

$$\mathbf{v}_k = \mathbf{G}^{-1}\mathbf{y}_k \quad k = 1,...,M \tag{82}$$

The matrix $\mathbf{G}^{-1}$ exists for a large class of functions $\mathbf{g}^n$ when all pairs of data points $\{\mathbf{x}^n, \mathbf{y}^n\}$ are distinct [51]. The interpolation function $\mathbf{h}$ is relatively insensitive to the exact form of the basis functions [50].

In the neural network context, localized functions (like Gaussian functions) are used, but any other distance-dependent function may be employed. The choice of the basis function type depends on the semantic contents assigned to the function image space. The significance of the function values must always express the *selectivity* property of the response. For example, for a localized response of Gaussian type, a significant difference between the input vector and the center vector corresponds to a zero response. When a nonlocalized function is used, e.g., the hyperbolic tangent, the difference between these vectors is mapped to the unity value and the perfect matching between these vectors is mapped to the zero value.

In many practical contexts, the above exact interpolation scheme is not very efficient, for two main reasons. First, the (possible) noisy input and/or output data sets will produce high oscillatory interpolation mappings. Second, the number of basis functions needed to build the interpolation function is equal to the cardinality of the interpolation data set.

A continuous function $\mathbf{h}$ that approximates in the least mean square (LMS) sense the underlying mapping of the data set has a larger applicability. This function may use a reduced number of radial basis functions. From the optimal approximation point of view, the problem consists of finding a smooth mapping $\mathbf{h}$ able to represent the real complexity of the data set. The number of basis functions will express this complexity, regardless of the number of data points.

It has been shown in [52] that the RBF networks have the *universal approximation* property for a large class of radial basis functions, providing that a sufficiently large number of hidden layer processing elements exist. Girossi and Poggio showed that the RBF network also has the *best approximation* property [53], i.e., there exists a single combination of basis functions parameters that ensures the minimum of the approximating error for any given function to be approximated.

Acknowledgments

The authors are indebted to Prof. L.K. Jain and to Mr. Adam Schenker for several comments on preliminary versions of this chapter. The first author also acknowledges the support of the Institute for Information Science of the Romanian Academy and the support of a research grant in 1996 from FNS.

References

[1] Bezdek, J.C., What is computational intelligence? *Computational Intelligence: Imitating Life*, J.M. Zurada, R.J. Marks, C.J. Robinson, Eds., Piscataway, NJ, IEEE Press, pp. 1-11, 1994.

[2] Jacobs, R.A., Jordan, M.I., Nowlan, S.J., and Hinton, G.E., Adaptive mixtures of local experts, *Neural Computation*, Vol. 3, pp. 78-97, 1991.

[3] Cho, S-B. and Kim, J.H., Multiple network fusion using fuzzy logic, *IEEE Transactions on Neural Networks*, Vol. 6, No. 2, pp. 497-501, 1995.

[4] Rodriguez, C., Rementeira, S., Martin, J.I., Lafuente, A., Muguerza, J., and Perez, J., A modular neural network approach to fault diagnosis, *IEEE Transactions on Neural Networks*, Vol. 7, No. 2, pp. 326-340, 1996.

[5] Matsuyama, Y., Harmonic competition: a self-organizing multiple criteria optimization, *IEEE Transactions on Neural Networks*, Vol. 7, No. 3, pp. 652-669, 1996.

[6] Rosenblatt, F., The perceptron: a probabilistic model for information storage and organization in the brain, *Psychological Review*, Vol. 65, No. 6, pp. 386-408, 1958.

[7] Pineda, F.J., Dynamics and architecture for neural computation, *Journal of Complexity*, Vol. 4, pp. 216-275, 1988.

[8] Teodorescu, H.N., Yamakawa, T., Uchino, T., Miki, T., Inagawa, N., Sofron, E. and Suceveanu, S., Pattern oriented neuro-fuzzy filtering, *Proc. of the 3rd Int. Conf. on Fuzzy Logic, Neural Nets and Soft Computing*, Iizuka, Japan, pp. 657-660, 1994.

[9] Bellanger, M.G., Adaptive Digital Filters and Signal Analysis, *Marcel Dekker, Inc.*, New York, 1987.

[10] Wilkinson, J.H., *The Algebraic Eigenvalue Problem*, Oxford University Press, 1985.

[11] Max, J. and Lacoume, J-L., *Methodes et techniques de traitement du signal et applications aux mesures physiques,* Fifth edition, Masson & Cie, Paris, 1996.

[12] Plumbey, M.D., Lyapunov functions for convergence of principal component algorithms, *Neural Networks*, Vol. 8., No. 1, pp. 11-23, 1995.

[13] Oja, E. and Karhunen, J., On stochastic approximations of the eigenvectors and eigenvalues of the expectation of a random matrix, *Journal of Mathematical Analysis and Applications*, Vol. 104, 1985.

[14] Krogh, A. and Hetz, J., Hebbian learning of principal components, *Parallel Processing in Neural Systems and Computers,* R. Eckmiller, G. Hartmann and G. Hauske, (Eds.), North-Holland, Amsterdam, 1990.

[15] Oja, E., Principal components, minor components and linear neural networks, *Neural Networks*, Vol. 5, pp. 927-935, 1992.

[16] Sanger, T.D., Optimal unsupervised learning in a single-layer linear feedforward neural network, *Neural Networks*, Vol. 2, 1989.

[17] Yan, W-O., Helmke, U., and Moore, J.B., Global analysis of Oja's flow for neural networks, *IEEE Transactions on Neural Networks*, Vol. 5., 1994.

[18] Cichocki, A. and Unbehauer, R., *Neural Networks for Optimization and Signal Processing*, John Wiley & Sons, Chichester, 1994.

[19] Haykin, S., *Neural Networks: A Comprehensive Foundation*, IEEE Press, 1994.

[20] Poggio, T. and Girossi, F., Networks for approximation and learning, *Proceedings of the IEEE*, Vol. 78, No. 9, pp. 1481-1497, 1990.

[21] Bishop, C.M., *Neural Networks for Pattern Recognition,* Clarendon Press, Oxford, 1995.

[22] Tikhonov, A.V. and Arsenin, V.Y., *Solutions of Ill-Posed Problems*, W.H. Winston, Washington, D.C., 1977.

[23] Courant, R. and Hilbert, D., Methods of mathematical physics, Vol. 1, chapters IV and V, *Interscience Publishers Inc.*, New York, Eighth reprint, 1970.

[24] Hassoun, M., *Fundamentals of Artificial Neural Networks*, MIT Press, Cambridge, 1995.

[25] Kohonen, T., *Self-Organization and Associative Memories,* Springer-Verlag, Berlin, second edition, 1988.

[26] Moody, J. and Darken, C., Fast Learning in networks with locally tuned processing units, *Neural Computation*, Vol. 1, No. 2, pp. 281-294, 1989.

[27] Silva, F.M. and Almeida, L.B. A distributed decorrelation algorithm, *Neural Networks: Advances and Applications*, E. Gelenbe (Editor), Elsevier Science Publishers B.V., pp. 145-163, 1991.

[28] Karhunen, J. and Joutsensalo, J., Generalizations of principal component analysis, optimization problems and neural networks, *Neural Networks*, Vol. 8, No. 4, pp. 549-562, 1995.

[29] Jutten, C. and Herault, J., Blind separation of sources, part I: an adaptive algorithm based on neuromimetic architecture, *Signal Processing*, Vol. 24, No. 1, pp. 1-10, 1991.

[30] Karhunen, E., Oja, E., Wang, L., Vigario, R., and Joutsensalo, J., A class of neural networks for independent component analysis, *IEEE Transactions on Neural Networks*, Vol. 8, No. 3, pp. 486-504, 1997.

[31] Zang, Q. and Benveniste, A., Wavelet networks, *IEEE Transactions on Neural Networks*, Vol. 3, No. 6, pp. 889-898, 1992.

[32] Erdol, N. and Basbug, F., Wavelet transform based adaptive filters: analysis and new results, *IEEE Transactions on Signal Processing*, Vol. 44, No. 9, pp. 2163-2171, 1996.

[33] Ramprashad, S., Parks, T.W., and Shenoy, R., Signal modeling and detection using cone classes, *IEEE Transactions on Signal Processing*, Vol. 44, No. 2, pp. 329-338, 1996.

[34] Rajan, J.J. and Rayner, P.J.W., Generalized features extraction for time-varying autoregressive models, *IEEE Transactions on Signal Processing*, Vol. 44, No. 10, pp. 2498-2508, 1996.

[35] Sadler, B.M., Detection in cumulated impulsive noise using fourth- and second-order cumulants, *IEEE Transactions on Signal Processing*, Vol. 44, No. 11, pp. 2793-2800, 1996.

[36] Teodorescu, H.N. and Bonciu, C., Features space neural filters and controllers, *Intelligent Adaptive Control. Industrial Applications*, L.C. Jain and C.W. de Silva, Eds., CRC Press, 1998.

[37] Bonciu, C. and Teodorescu, H.N., Features space filtering with RBF networks, *EUFIT'97*, Aachen, Germany.

[38] Teodorescu, H.N. and Bonciu, C., Learning algorithm for RBF networks as features extractors, *First Int. Conf. on Conventional & Knowledge-Based Intelligent Electronic Systems KES'97*, Adelaide, Australia, 1997.

[39] Widrow, B. and Stearns, A., *Adaptive Signal Processing*, Prentice Hall, 1985.

[40] Teodorescu, H.N., Kandel, A., Anghelescu, M., and Bonciu, C., Feature-oriented filtering hybrid systems, *Int. Journal of Knowledge-Based Intelligent Engineering Systems*, Vol. 2, No. 2, pp. 72-79, 1998.

[41] Teodorescu, H.N. and Bonciu, C., Feedforward neural filter with learning in features space, *Proc. First Int. Symp. on Neuro-Fuzzy Systems AT'96*, Laussane, Switzerland, 1996.

[42] Waibel, A., Hanazawa, T., Hinton, G.E., Shikano, K., and Lang, K.J., *Phoneme Recognition Using Time Delay Neural Networks*, Technical Report TR-1-0006, Japan, Advanced Telecommunications Research Institute, 1987.

[43] Lang, K.J. and Hinton, G.E., *The Development of the TDNN Architecture for Speech Recognition*, Technical Report CMU-CS-88-152, Carnegie-Mellon University, 1988

[44] Suzuki, Y., Self-organizing QRS-wave recognition in ECG using neural networks, *IEEE Transactions on Neural Networks*, Vol. 6, No. 6, pp. 1469-1477, 1995.

[45] Alfonso, V.X., Tompkins, W.J., Nguyen, T.Q., Michler, K., and Luo, S., Comparing stress ECG enhancement algorithms, *IEEE Engineering in Medicine and Biology*, Vol. 15, No. 3, pp. 37-44, 1996.

[46] Sahambi, J.S., Tandon, S.N., and Bhat, R.K.P., Using wavelet transforms for ECG characterization, *IEEE Engineering in Medicine and Biology*, Vol. 16, No. 1, pp. 77-83, 1997.

[47] Barro, S., Fernandez-Delgado, M., Villa-Spbrino, J.A., Regueiro, C.V., and Sanchez, E. Classifying multi-channel ECG patterns with an adaptive neural network, *IEEE Engineering in Medicine and Biology*, Vol. 17, No. 1, pp. 45-55, 1998.

[48] Connor, J.T., Martin, R.D., and Atlas, L.E., Recurrent neural networks and robust time series prediction, *IEEE Transactions on Neural Networks,* Vol. 5. No. 2, pp. 240-253, 1994.

[49] Bonciu, C. and Teodorescu, H.N., Features space neural systems for identification and control, *World Multiconference on Systemics, Cybernetics and Informatics WMSCI'98,* Vol. 1, Orlando, Florida, 1998.

[50] Powell, M.J.D., Radial Basis Functions for Multivariable Interpolation: A Review, *Algorithms for Approximations,* J.C. Mason, M.G. Cox, (Eds.), Clarendon Press, Oxford, UK, 1987.

[51] Miccelli, C.A., Interpolation of scattered data: distance matrices and conditionally positive definite functions, *Constructive Approximations,* Vol. 2, No. 1, pp. 11-22, 1986.

[52] Park, J. and Sandberg, I.W., Approximation and radial basis functions, *Neural Computation,* Vol. 5, No. 2, pp. 305-316, 1993.

[53] Girossi, F. and Poggio, T., Networks and the best approximation property, *Biological Cybernetics,* Vol. 63, pp. 169-176, 1990.

Part 3.

Applications in Psychology, Nutrition, and Professional Evaluation

Chapter 9

An emotion-processing system based on fuzzy inference and subjective observations

Naruki Shirahama, Torao Yanaru, and Masahiro Nagamatsu

The two theories concerning mixed emotions adopted in this chapter are briefly explained. Also discussed are the image codes linked to the mixed emotional words, and the way to realize a mechanism using fuzzy inference in which the internal emotion of a simulated person reacts as a sequence of inputted terms that evokes some emotional change. Next, the relevant part of the theory for a subjective observation model to the application of an emotion-processing system is briefly explained. The construction methodology of the system, which has two functions, is described. One function is that the evoked emotion is transitive depending on the observation, and the other is that the aggregated emotion by several subjective observations settles to the objective emotion. Then, some interesting results obtained by the simulated emotion-processing system are shown, namely, what kind of emotions are evoked, and how the emotional transition is done by subjective observations when a poem is used for the input signal. Furthermore, we obtain and analyze several emotional clustering diagrams processed by pair vectors such as [optimism, curiosity], which is an interesting result from a psychological viewpoint.

1. Introduction

In general, fuzzy inference technology is effective when it is applied to objects whose strict analysis and formulization are almost impossible by classic methods. Thus, by constructing a mathematical model, several emotional reactions are studied from two engineering viewpoints, i.e., for general emotional reactions, fuzzy inference technology is applied, and for the transitional emotions evoked from a person's temporal condition, the theory of subjective observation model [1-5] is applied.

In Section 4 a mathematical description based on vectorial representations is introduced to describe emotions. The reader can skip this section without loss of understanding of the main ideas in this chapter.

2. Mechanism for emotional variation by input words

2.1. Image codes of words

The emotions considered here are based on the theories of Plutchik and Young [6, 7, 8], (see Appendix). The four attributes are introduced corresponding to the four pairs of pure emotional words, considering the Postulate 5 introduced by Plutchik (see Appendix A): [joy-sadness], [anger-fear], [expectation-surprise], and [hate-acceptance]. These attributes are expressed later by [JOY], [ANG], [EXP], and [ACC], respectively, for simplicity. The mixed emotions can be defined on the four attributes and expressed by the four-dimensional vectors. Weights on the attributes of each emotion are done within the range [-1, +1] by referring to the Plutchik standard. He interviewed thirty students, and presented thirty-four synonyms for primary mixed emotions and their intensities in eleven stages (see Appendix A, Table 9). He also proposed the secondary mixed emotions generated from these primary thirty-four mixed emotions with some relationship. We chose the additional thirty-four synonyms from his proposed synonyms set for secondary thirty-four mixed emotions, dropping some synonyms which almost have the same feeling as those chosen. That is, sixty-eight mixed emotional words are treated here. The image codes of the words are based on a value in the range [-1, +1]. As an example, the value in Table 9 for [happiness] is 7.1, which yields 7.1/11 = 0.65. We thus assign a value of 0.65 to the attribute for [JOY]. We also considered that it is natural that the mixed emotion "happiness" will include some weights on the attributes, not only "pure emotions" as [JOY], but also [EXP] and [ACC]. Based on the consideration, we assigned the values 0.50 for [EXP] and 0.30 for [ACC].

Table 1. An image codes table of sixty-eight mixed emotional words

No.	JOY	ANG	EXP	ACC	No.	JOY	ANG	EXP	ACC
1 ecstasy	0.91	0.00	0.30	0.30	35 disgrace	0.00	-0.55	0.00	-0.55
2 joy	0.74	0.00	0.50	0.30	36 discreet	0.00	-0.42	0.00	-0.42
3 happiness	0.65	0.00	0.50	0.30	37 grief	-0.80	0.00	-0.50	-0.40
4 pleasant	0.52	0.00	0.30	0.30	38 sadness	-0.68	0.00	-0.40	-0.40
5 quiet	0.40	0.00	0.10	0.30	39 discouragement	-0.57	0.00	0.00	-0.30
6 calm	0.30	0.00	0.10	0.30	40 gloominess	-0.50	0.00	0.00	-0.30
7 pride	0.55	0.55	0.00	0.30	41 meditation	-0.40	0.00	0.00	-0.20
8 optimism	0.48	0.00	0.48	0.30	42 despair	-0.75	-0.75	0.00	-0.40
9 hope	0.67	0.00	0.67	0.30	43 disappointment	-0.60	0.00	-0.60	-0.30
10 unhealthy	0.45	0.00	0.30	-0.45	44 sentimentality	-0.45	0.00	0.00	0.45
11 rage	0.00	0.90	-0.50	0.00	45 shudder	-0.10	-0.92	-0.30	-0.30
12 anger	0.00	0.76	-0.50	0.00	46 confusion	-0.10	-0.89	-0.30	-0.30
13 perplexity	-0.45	0.45	-0.45	0.00	47 fear	-0.10	-0.72	-0.30	-0.30
14 attack	0.00	0.80	0.80	0.00	48 anxious	-0.10	-0.58	-0.20	-0.20
15 obstinate	0.00	0.55	0.55	0.00	49 timid	-0.10	-0.37	0.00	-0.10
16 abhorrence	0.00	0.78	-0.50	-0.78	50 awe	0.00	-0.55	-0.55	0.00
17 hostility	0.00	0.50	-0.46	-0.50	51 astonishment	0.00	-0.85	-0.85	0.00
18 contempt	0.00	0.43	-0.45	-0.43	52 obedience	0.00	-0.65	0.00	0.65
19 envy	-0.42	0.42	-0.44	0.00	53 modesty	0.00	-0.30	0.00	0.30
20 expectation	0.20	0.00	0.66	0.30	54 guilt	0.45	-0.45	0.00	0.00
21 anticipation	0.10	0.00	0.61	0.35	55 amaze	0.00	0.00	-0.85	0.00
22 careful	-0.10	0.00	0.53	0.30	56 astonish	0.00	0.00	-0.75	0.00
23 posture	0.00	-0.20	0.32	0.30	57 surprise	0.00	0.00	-0.67	0.00
24 irony	0.00	0.00	0.48	-0.48	58 curiosity	0.00	0.30	-0.50	0.50
25 pessimism	-0.59	0.00	0.59	0.00	59 delight	0.80	0.00	-0.80	0.00
26 uneasiness	0.00	-0.63	0.63	0.00	60 violence	0.00	0.73	-0.73	0.00
27 anxiety	0.00	-0.50	0.50	0.00	61 wrath	0.00	0.67	-0.67	0.00
28 detest	0.00	0.83	0.00	-0.83	62 admission	0.00	0.00	0.40	0.42
29 hatred	0.00	0.30	0.00	-0.69	63 acceptance	0.00	0.00	0.40	0.36
30 dislike	0.00	0.30	0.00	-0.50	64 union	0.00	0.00	0.40	0.32
31 boredom	0.00	0.30	0.00	-0.43	65 affection	0.70	0.00	0.40	0.70
32 trouble	0.00	0.00	0.00	-0.41	66 friendship	0.59	0.00	0.40	0.59
33 unhappiness	-0.60	0.00	0.00	-0.60	67 superiority	0.00	0.50	0.00	0.50
34 regret	-0.46	0.46	0.00	-0.46	68 fate	0.00	0.00	0.40	0.40

Table 1 is an image code table that depends strongly on personal subjectivity. However, we confirmed experimentally that individuals with generally normal emotions assign codes with similar trends, except when he/she possesses abnormal emotions. Although the values of image codes are subjective, and contain randomness and vagueness, our simulated results demonstrate that common objective words are obtained in the model output which were discussed in [3]. Thus, we introduce a system that is capable of dynamically modifying an image code according to the subjective observation.

2.2. Fuzzy inference for pure emotions

The internal emotional state of a person is expressed by aggregation of the four pure emotional situations. The transition of the internal emotional state is supposed to be caused by the inputted terms and performed by a fuzzy inference mechanism. It is also supposed that, for each pure emotion as an attribute, fuzzy inference is generally applied in such a way that the emotional state of a pure emotion is strengthened in proportion to the coded intensity of the inputted term. Thus, we adopt a simple system consisting of nine fuzzy inference rules, shown in Figure 1.

The four defuzzified values (coefficients on four-dimensional vectors) can be regarded as an expression of the new emotional state of the simulated person evoked by the inputted terms.

3. Expression of emotional transition based on subjective observations

3.1. Expression of emotions by vectors and conditional Euclidean space

Image codes of mixed emotions $\{x_k\}$ ($k = 1, 2, \ldots, 68$) can be expressed by vectors consisting of coefficients on the four attributes (pure emotions) to a normalized rectangular basal coordinate (NRBC) system which is denoted by $\{e_i\}$ for $i = 1,2,3,4$; inner product $\mathbf{e}_i \cdot \mathbf{e}_j = 0$ ($i \neq j$), $\mathbf{e}_i \cdot \mathbf{e}_j = 1$ ($i = j$). The origin of the reference system is dropped here for simplicity.

$$x_k = x_{k1}e_1 + x_{k2}e_2 + x_{k3}e_3 + x_{k4}e_4, \tag{1}$$

where

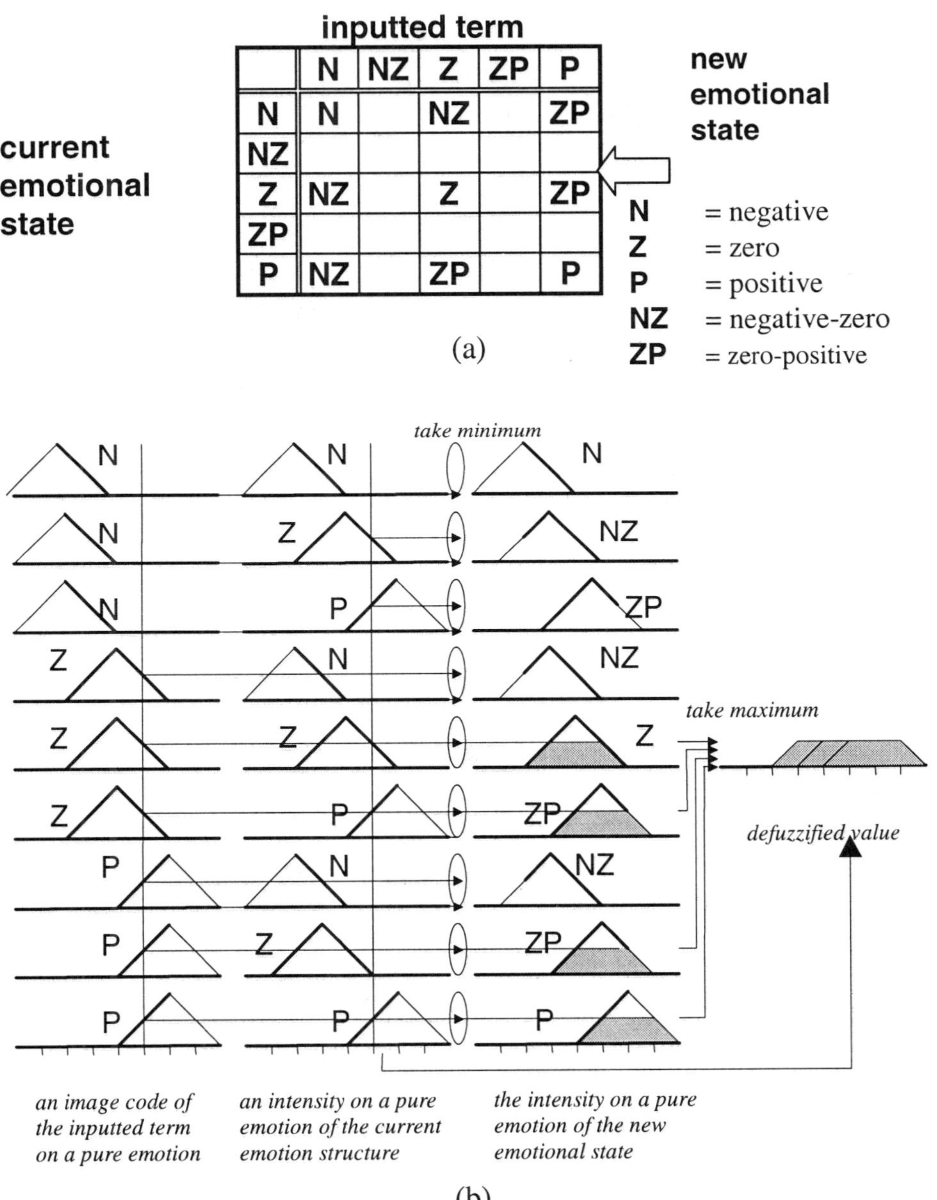

Figure 1. (a) The nine fuzzy rules for a pure emotion, (b) An example of a fuzzy inference process on a pure emotion and defuzzification.

$$(e_1, e_2, e_3, e_4) = ([\text{JOY}], [\text{ANG}], [\text{EXP}], [\text{ACC}]). \tag{2}$$

A term s_k (the suffix k means the term in order k in a sequence of terms, like a sentence, in general) can also be expressed by the image code combining the mixed emotional words,

$$s_k = s_{k1}e_1 + s_{k2}e_2 + s_{k3}e_3 + s_{k4}e_4, \tag{3}$$

s_{ki} $(i = 1,2,3,4) \in \mathbf{R}$ (real number).

Consider a processor, $\mathbf{P}_1 = (p_{11}, p_{12}, p_{13}, p_{14})$, whose function is to transform the inputted signal, $\{s_k\}$, consisting of a sequence of image code vectors into the output signal $\{s_{kout}\}$. We can express each member of the output signal as follows:

$$s_{kout} = \sum_{i=1}^{4} p_{1i}(s_{ki}) \cdot e_i = \sum_{i=1}^{4} y_{ki} e_i. \tag{4}$$

On the other hand, if we want to express the output signal of Equation (4) as appropriate mixed emotional words corresponding to the transformed image code, it is natural to introduce a norm, $\left\| s_{kout} - x_k \right\|$ (distance between two vectors). Moreover, it is natural to order the words based on the norm; i.e., for an assigned constant δ, we list the words as to satisfy the following equation:

$$\left\| s_{kout} - x_k \right\| = \sqrt{\sum_{i=1}^{4} (y_{k1} - y_{ki})^2} < \delta. \tag{5}$$

It is easily understood that, in general, the larger the value δ, the higher the number of terms listed. Sometimes, a case occurs where no terms are selected, which is analogous to a person's condition in daily life, e.g., such as expressing internal emotion only with tears, unable to find an appropriate term. We call this selection the soft matching method.

For clearer understanding, an image of the flow and the process of transformation mentioned above is illustrated in Figure 2 (a), (b), but they are drawn in three-dimensional normalized rectangular basal coordinate, (e_1, e_2, e_3)

in place of the strict drawings in four-dimensional NRBC because drawing them on the plane is essentially impossible.

A physical image of the model for the emotion-processing system is shown in Figure 2 (a), which consists of the following five parts:

1. The NRBC that consists of $\{e_i'\}$ corresponding to the attributes $\{e_i\}$ as a combination, and of the origin O_{E1},
2. The layer for the set of mixed emotional words as a set of genetic elements, $\{x_k\}$,
3. The higher layer for the newly produced elements by linear combination of the genetic mixed emotional words, $\{y_k\}$,
4. The processor for transformation, E_1, from symbols to the image code vectors, e.g., $s_k \in S_1 \rightarrow s_k \in \mathbf{S}_1$,
5. The fuzzy inference processor, $\mathbf{P}_1 = \{p_{1i}\}$ $(i = 1,2,3,4)$.

Note that suffix 1 of the symbols, S_1, $\mathbf{S}_1$, $\mathbf{P}_1$, E_1, and Ω_1 in Figure 2 means implicitly further existence of a number of local subsystems like this model (a local subsystem).

The model for an emotion-processing system can be described by mathematical notations as follows.

All of the elements, including the newly produced elements, can be equivalently drawn on a conditional Euclidean space (or Euclidean subspace), $(X_1, V_1^4 \mid E_1)$ [see Figure 2 (b)]. Here, the condition E_1 is denoted by $(\Omega_1, \{x_k\})$ which is a tuple of NRBC frame and the genetic elements as an infrastructure; X_1 is a set of the starting points of the vectors; V_1^4 is a set of four-dimensional vectors related with inner product operation to each other (usually called by "inner product vector space") i.e., $\Omega_1 = (O_{E1} : e_1, e_2, e_3, e_4)$; O_{E1} is the origin (location) of the system.

Human beings are, in general, almost unable to understand in a direct way the absolute meanings of the objects or the relationships among the objects in more than three-dimensional space. Usually, we recognize and understand the meanings concerning the objects by dropping the order of dimensions and aggregating the observed information from several angles.

Considering this human property, a specialized two-dimensional Euclidean space for observation is developed here. The model stands on the philosophical point that all the recognition and understanding can be done only on the observation space, by mapping the objects defined on the high-dimensional space onto the observation space.

If we consider again the concern related to Equation (5), taking into account the principles mentioned above, the direct inverse transformation of the output signals into emotional words on the defined original space may look like nonsense. However, the function for the mapping still remains meaningful for a special usage of diagnostics, for example.

Thus, the condition for the observation space E_O can be denoted by

$$E_O = (\Omega_O, \varepsilon) \quad (\varepsilon \text{ means empty})$$

and the coordinates frame, Ω_O, is written as

$$\Omega_O = \{O_O : \boldsymbol{o}_1, \boldsymbol{o}_2\}. \tag{6}$$

Consequently, applying affine mapping theory [9] to the mapping in this model, not only all of the vectors for mixed emotions as the genetic members and for produced elements in higher order, but also transition of the vectors caused by a sequence of the inputted signals and of output signals can be observed on the two-dimensional space (plane) from several angles. Thus, the emotional words depending on observation can be selected by the soft matching method (see Figure 2 (c)).

3.2. Affine mapping and pair vectors for subjective observation

We first review the concepts in the general theory of affine mapping [9], under the assumption of the existence of a number of subspaces (local subsystem, LS).

Consider the mapping of the i-th LS, $(X_i, V_i^n | E_i)$ onto the observation space, $(X_O, V_O^n | E_O)$, and suppose that the coordinate frames are denoted by Ω_1 and Ω_O respectively, i.e.,

$$\Omega_1 = (O_{E1} : \boldsymbol{e}_1, \boldsymbol{e}_2, \cdots, \boldsymbol{e}_n), \ O_{E1} \in X_1$$

$$\Omega_O = (O_O : \boldsymbol{o}_1, \boldsymbol{o}_2), \ O_O \in X_O$$

where $(\boldsymbol{e}_1, \boldsymbol{e}_2, \ldots, \boldsymbol{e}_n)$ is a basal coordinate system of E_i, and $(\boldsymbol{o}_1, \boldsymbol{o}_2)$ is a particular coordinate for mapping. O_{E1} and O_O are the origins of the frames, respectively.

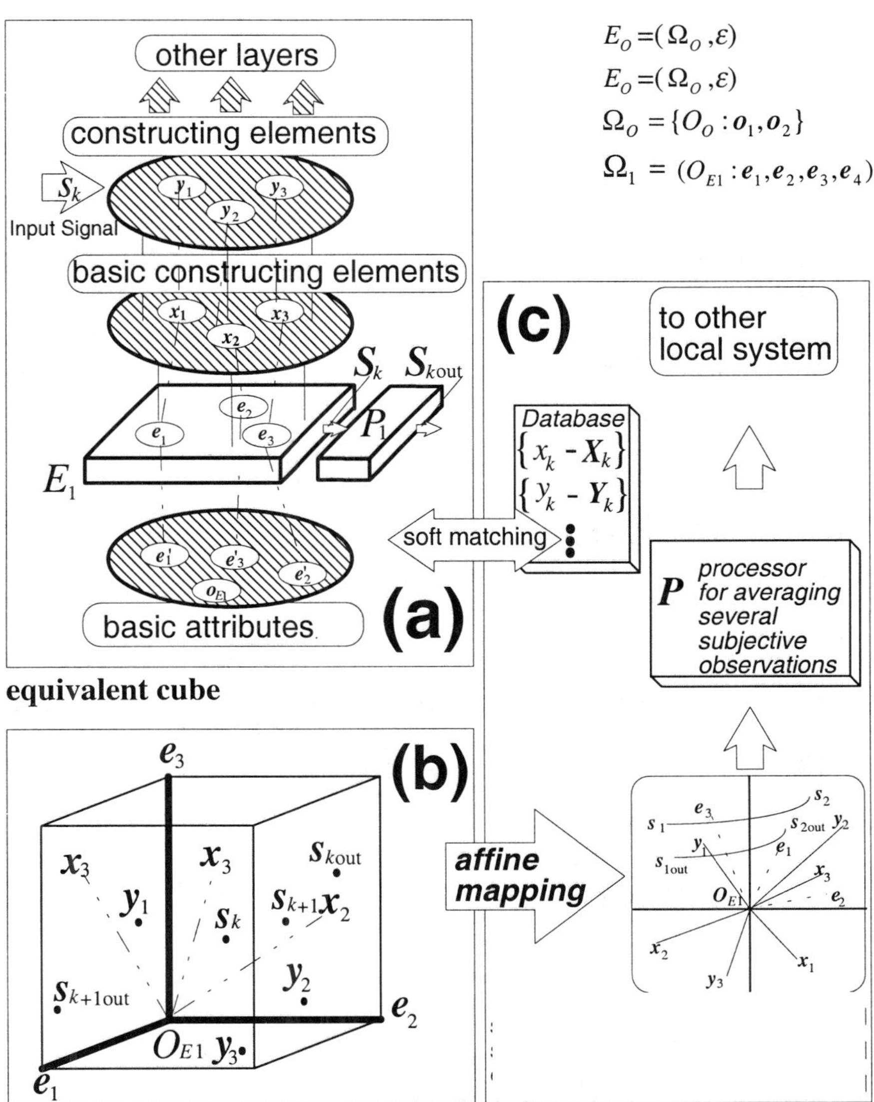

Figure 2. Diagram of a subjective observation model.

Thus, in general, an affine mapping (γ, ϕ) is expressed as follows:

1. For the origins, mapping is performed by a function γ as follows:

$$f_O = \overrightarrow{O_O \gamma(O_{Ei})} = \alpha_{i1} o_1 + \alpha_{i2} o_2, \tag{7}$$

where α_{i1} and α_{i2} are coefficients depending on the function γ in the application in hand. Note that $\alpha_{11} = \alpha_{12} = 0$ in this model for the most simple case, but, for the advanced model thinking of two emotional subspaces with cross communication, the mapping function with nonzero coefficients will be introduced.

2. For basal coordinates, mapping is performed by the function ϕ in the following way:

$$\begin{pmatrix} \phi(e_1) \\ \phi(e_2) \\ \vdots \\ \phi(e_n) \end{pmatrix} = \begin{pmatrix} \varepsilon_1 \delta_1 \\ \varepsilon_2 \delta_2 \\ \vdots \\ \varepsilon_n \delta_n \end{pmatrix} \cdot (o_1, \quad o_2) \tag{8}$$

3. For any other vector, $A \in V_i^n$, constructing the LS linear transformation by the function ϕ is done in the following way:

$$A = a_1 e_1 + a_2 e_2 + \cdots + a_n e_n \tag{9}$$

$$\phi(A) = a_1 \phi(e_1) + a_2 \phi(e_2) + \cdots + a_n \phi(e_n), \tag{10}$$

$$= \left(\sum_{i=1}^{n} a_i \,_i \right) \cdot o_1 + \left(\sum_{i=1}^{n} a_i \delta_i \right) \cdot o_2 \tag{11}$$

Suppose that the two vectors, (ζ, η) are arbitrarily selected from the LS, i.e.,

$$\phi_{\zeta-\eta}(e_i) = (\zeta \cdot e_i) \cdot o_1 + (\eta \cdot e_i) \cdot o_2 \quad \text{(for } i = 1, 2, \ldots, n) \tag{12}$$

where

$$\zeta = \zeta_1 e_1 + \zeta_2 e_2 + \cdots + \zeta_n e_n, \quad \eta = \eta_1 e_1 + \eta_2 e_2 + \cdots + \eta_n e_n \tag{13}$$

Equation (12) can be written as

$$\begin{pmatrix} \phi_{\zeta-\eta}(e_1) \\ \phi_{\zeta-\eta}(e_1) \\ \vdots \\ \phi_{\zeta-\eta}(e_n) \end{pmatrix} = \begin{pmatrix} \zeta_1 \eta_1 \\ \zeta_1 \eta_1 \\ \\ \zeta_n \eta_n \end{pmatrix} \cdot (o_1, \quad o_2), \tag{14}$$

because the inner product, $\zeta \cdot \eta$, becomes the only coefficient ζ_i by rectangularity, i.e.,

$$\zeta \cdot e_i = \zeta_i \text{ (for } i=1, 2,\ldots, n). \tag{15}$$

It should be noted that Equation (14) becomes the same as Equation (8). Consequently, we can make the replacements: function $\phi_{\zeta-\eta} \to \phi$ and coefficients, $\zeta_i \to \varepsilon_i$, $\eta_i \to \delta_i$, (for $i = 1, 2,\ldots, n$). Furthermore, concerning an arbitrary vector $A \in V_i^n$, we can define the following function:

$$\phi_{\zeta-\eta}(A) = (\zeta \cdot A) \cdot o_1 + (\eta \cdot A) \cdot o_2 \tag{16}$$

which is made coincident with Equation (11) in the corresponding way. Thus, we can conclude that any pair of the vectors constructing the LS can be selected and treated as the mapping vectors for subjective observation, and thus, all of the vectors can be mapped on the space, Ω_O, depending on the subjective observation by the pair vectors (ζ, η).

The way of thinking and the resultant properties are significant, not only for the theoretical expansion, but also for various applications.

3.3. How to estimate the coefficients of a true vector in a certain LS by several subjective observations

Let A be a vector:

$$A = a_1 e_1 + a_2 e_2 + \cdots + a_n e_n, \tag{17}$$

then

$$R(A, e_i) = A \cdot e_i = a_i. \tag{18}$$

Therefore, the coefficient a_i of the coordinate e_i can be computed by the inner product. In the same way, we can define the relationship between the mapped vectors by an inner product operation, under the condition that the mapped origin is made coincident with the origin of the observation space, as follows:

$$R_O(\phi(A), \phi(e_i)) = \phi(A) \cdot \phi(e_i). \tag{19}$$

Substituting a pair of the vectors (ζ, η) for the mapping function ϕ and using Equations (12) and (16), Equation (19) can be written as

$$\phi(A) \cdot \phi(e_i) = \{(\zeta \cdot A)o_1 + (\eta \cdot A)o_2\} \cdot \{(\zeta \cdot e_i)o_1 + (\eta \cdot e_i)o_2\} \tag{20}$$

$$= (\zeta \cdot A)\zeta_i + (\eta \cdot A)\eta_i, \tag{21}$$

$$= \left(\sum_{j=1}^{n} \zeta_j a_j\right) \cdot \zeta_i + \left(\sum_{j=1}^{n} \eta_j a_j\right) \cdot \eta_i. \tag{22}$$

On the other hand, as mentioned above, in order to realize the objective observation of the coefficients by aggregating the information based on several subjective observations, i.e., selecting several pairs of vectors (ζ, η), the following Equation (26) must hold.

First, we regard the value in Equation (22) as a pseudo coefficient by a subjective observation, and denote it by

$$a_i' = \left(\sum_{j=1}^{n} \zeta_j a_j\right) \cdot \zeta_i + \left(\sum_{j=1}^{n} \eta_j a_j\right) \cdot \eta_i, \text{ (for } i = 1, 2, \ldots, n) \tag{23}$$

The pseudo vector A' can be expressed by

$$A' = a_1' e_1 + a_2' e_2 + \cdots + a_n' e_n. \tag{24}$$

Then,

$$E(\tilde{a}_i') = E\left(\left(\sum_{j=1}^{n} \tilde{\zeta}_j a_j\right) \cdot \tilde{\zeta}_i + \left(\sum_{j=1}^{n} \tilde{\zeta}_j a_j\right) \cdot \tilde{\zeta}_i\right) \tag{25}$$

$$E(\tilde{a}_i') = a_i \tag{26}$$

where $E(\cdot)$ means expectation of $(\cdot)$. $\tilde{a}_i'$, $\tilde{\zeta}_j$, $\tilde{\zeta}_i$, $\tilde{\eta}_j$, and $\tilde{\eta}_i$ are all random variables corresponding to a_i', ζ_j, ζ_i, η_j, and η_i, respectively. The reason is that the meaning of several observations is equivalently regarded as the procedure to replace a_i' (consequently A') with random variables $\tilde{a}_i'$ (consequently $\tilde{A}'$). This is equivalent to replacing the coefficients, ζ_j, ζ_i, η_j, η_i with the random variables, $\tilde{\zeta}_j$, $\tilde{\zeta}_i$, $\tilde{\eta}_j$, $\tilde{\eta}_i$, respectively.

$$\sum_{j=1}^{n} a_j E(\tilde{\zeta}_i \tilde{\zeta}_j) + \sum_{j=1}^{n} a_j E(\tilde{\eta}_i \tilde{\eta}_j) = a_i \tag{27}$$

taking a_i outside,

$$\sum_{\substack{j=1 \\ j \neq i}}^{n} a_j \left[E(\tilde{\zeta}_i \tilde{\zeta}_j) + E(\tilde{\eta}_i \tilde{\eta}_j)\right] + a_i E\left(\tilde{\zeta}_i^2 + \tilde{\eta}_i^2 - 1\right) = 0. \tag{28}$$

Consequently, in order for Equation (28) to always hold for any of the vectors A, i.e., for any values $\{a_i\}$ ($i = 1, 2, \ldots, n$), all coefficients concerning $\{a_i\}$ must become zero, i.e.,

$$E(\tilde{\zeta}_i \tilde{\zeta}_j) + E(\tilde{\eta}_i \tilde{\eta}_j) = 0 \tag{29}$$

and

$$E(\tilde{\zeta}_i^2 + \tilde{\eta}_i^2 - 1) = 0. \tag{30}$$

Thus, Equations (29) and (30) are regarded as the necessary condition for Equation (26). Let us consider the condition that the mapped NRBCs ($\phi(e_i)$, $i = 1, 2, \ldots, n$) distribute around a unit circle without grouping. The following equations define the above condition:

$$E(\tilde{\zeta}_i) = E(\tilde{\eta}_i) = 0 \tag{31}$$

$$E(\tilde{\zeta}_i^2 + \tilde{\eta}_i^2) = 1 \tag{32}$$

$$E(\tilde{\zeta}_i\tilde{\zeta}_j) = E(\tilde{\eta}_i\tilde{\eta}_j) = 0 \;\; (i \neq j) \tag{33}$$

It will become clear by the following explanation that the definition is natural. Furthermore, Equation (33) means the condition that each random variable $\tilde{\zeta}_i$ (or $\tilde{\eta}_i$) distributes in weak independence of the other variables $\tilde{\zeta}_j, j \neq i$ (or $\tilde{\eta}_j, (j \neq i)$) [10].

Thus, Equations (31) to (33) are regarded as the sufficient condition to hold Equation (26). In other words, the strategy to see the true coefficients of the original vector is to make several mappings so that the mapped coordinates distribute around a unit circle without grouping.

3.4. Theory for time-dependent subjective observations

"The mixed emotions of a person are transitive
(or evoked) depending on the duration and the
repetition of his personal experience with a certain object"
(Matuyama et al., 1974).

In order to incorporate this psychological phenomenon into our model, the obtained pseudo vector A' from the real vector A in Equation (24) by a subjective observation is used again as the pair of vectors for subjective observation instead of ζ, replacing ζ with η. That is, the obtained pseudo coefficients after t-times repetition, which are denoted by $\zeta_i(t)$ ($i = 1, 2,...,n$), can be written by the following recursive equations:

$$
\begin{aligned}
a_i'(t) &= \zeta_i'(t) \\
&= \left(\sum_{i=1}^{n}\zeta_j'(t-1)a_j\right)\zeta_i'(t-1) + \left(\sum_{i=1}^{n}\eta_j'(t-1)a_j\right)\eta_i'(t-1),
\end{aligned}
\tag{34}
$$

$$\eta_i'(t) = \zeta_i'(t-1) \tag{35}$$

$$\zeta_i'(0) = \zeta_i, \;\; \eta_i'(0) = \eta_i \tag{36}$$

$$A'(t) = a_1'(t)e_1 + a_2'(t)e_2 \cdots + a_n'(t)e_n \tag{37}$$

$$\zeta(t) = \zeta_1'(t)\mathbf{e}_1 + \zeta_2'(t)\mathbf{e}_2 + \cdots + \zeta_n'(t)\mathbf{e}_n \tag{38}$$

$$\eta'(t) = \eta_1'(t)\mathbf{e}_1 + \eta_2'(t)\mathbf{e}_2 + \cdots + \eta_n'(t)\mathbf{e}_n \tag{39}$$

It should be noted that Equations (34) and (35) construct a system for nonlinear (two dimensions, in this case) recursive equations, which is regarded as a discrete type system of nonlinear derivative equations. Consequently, the behavior of $(\zeta'(t), \eta'(t))$ will be complicated, depending on the initial pair of vectors for subjective observation ($\zeta'(0) = \zeta$, $\eta'(0) = \eta$)).

4. Computer simulations and results

4.1. Experiments for objectivity on the selected mixed emotional words

Let us consider the following five Japanese poems [11] as examples:

<table>
<tr><td>

トランプをならべる夜
ひとりでトランプ
ならべる夜は
やるせない日に　きまってる

</td><td>

Shuffling cards in the night.
It's dreary to shuffle cards alone
in the night.

</td></tr>
<tr><td>

炬燵が家にある
炬燵がある
炬燵が家にある
こう思うとキモチがよいのです

</td><td>

There is a fireplace in my house.
There is a fireplace in my house.
That makes me feel good.

</td></tr>
<tr><td>

おふくろにおこられない日は
おふくろに
おこられない日は
ものたりない　ものたりない

</td><td>

On the day my mother doesn't scold me.
On the day my mother doesn't scold me,
I feel something is missing,
something is missing.

</td></tr>
<tr><td>

雪がふる
雪がふる　雪がふる
てのひらに　それを受け
すぐにとけるのを　悲しむ

</td><td>

It is snowing.
It is snowing, snowing.
I laid the falling snow on the palm of my
hand. I feel sad the snow has melted quickly.

</td></tr>
</table>

一番苦手なのは

一番苦手なのは
おふくろの涙です
何にもいわずに
こっちを見ている涙です

My weakest point.
My weakest point is a tear of my mother,
the tear staring at me in silence.

Translated into English, the meaning may contain some differences in nuances between the original meaning in Japanese and the translated one. In this sense, it may be necessary to have the natives themselves make the image code dictionary. However, the nuance is less important than the research for finding a capability to construct a person-oriented system able to deal with such a poem.

First we make a sequence of image codes of the keywords constructing each of these poems based on the indirect way as shown in Table 2, under supposition that the constructing words (terms) have already been extracted by some lexical analysis. That is, the mixed emotional words related with the constructing words were chosen by students in our laboratory by way of a questionnaire. In the questionnaire, mixed emotional words are associated with fewer than three words to each student. Then, the image code of the constructing words was made by computing the linearly combined values of the selected words.

Table 2. Associated mixed emotional words from the key words constructing the poem

(a) *Shuffling cards in the night.*

Constructed Words	Associated Mixed Emotional Words			Image Codes			
				JOY	ANG	EXP	ACC
alone	uneasiness	gloominess		-0.25	-0.31	0.31	-0.15
cards	joy	envy		0.16	0.21	0.03	0.15
shuffle	expectation			0.20	0.00	0.66	0.30
night	uneasiness	meditation		-0.20	-0.31	0.31	-0.10
dreary	discouragement	gloominess	disappointment	-0.56	0.00	-0.20	-0.30
obvious	anticipation	irony	pessimism	-0.16	0.00	0.56	-0.04

(b) *There is a fireplace in my house.*

Constructed Words	Associated Mixed Emotional Words			Image Codes			
				JOY	ANG	EXP	ACC
fireplace	happiness	pleasant		0.58	0.00	0.40	0.30
house	happiness	union	affection	0.45	0.00	0.43	0.44
feel	meditation			-0.40	0.00	0.00	-0.20
good	joy	pleasant		0.63	0.00	0.40	0.30

(c) *On the day my mother doesn't scold me.*

Constructed Words	Associated Mixed Emotional Words			Image Codes			
				JOY	ANG	EXP	ACC
mother	happiness	affection	fate	0.45	0.00	0.43	0.47
not scold	anxiety	timid		-0.05	-0.44	0.25	-0.05
missing	uneasiness	wrath		0.00	0.02	-0.02	0.00

(d) *It is snowing.*

Constructed Words	Associated Mixed Emotional Words			Image Codes			
				JOY	ANG	EXP	ACC
snow	calm	gloominess		-0.10	0.00	0.05	0.00
fall	posture	uneasiness		0.00	-0.41	0.47	0.15
palm	hope	careful		0.28	0.00	0.60	0.30
catch	acceptance	union		0.00	0.00	0.40	0.34
melt	anticipation	acceptance	union	0.03	0.00	0.47	0.34
sad	sadness	sentimentality		-0.56	0.00	-0.20	0.02

(e) *My weakest point.*

Constructed Words	Associated Mixed Emotional Words			Image Codes			
				JOY	ANG	EXP	ACC
weakest	careful	uneasiness	fear	-0.07	-0.45	0.29	0.00
mother	joy	affection	fate	0.48	0.00	0.43	0.47
tear	sadness			-0.68	0.00	-0.40	-0.40
silence	timid	acceptance		-0.05	-0.19	0.20	0.13

Table 3 shows the process of the emotions evoked by the poems in Table 2. These results are obtained by a fuzzy inference mechanism. In the rightmost column in Table 3, the evoked mixed emotional words are listed, which are selected by soft matching method, i.e., the words arranged in the order of smaller distance by Equation (5). The following properties became evident after examining the experimental results. Emotional words "meditation," "pessimism," and "gloominess" are evoked last in the poem *Shuffling cards in the night* (Poem 1), see Table 3 (a). This result reflects well the mood of loneliness in the poem. Emotional words "meditation," "gloominess" and "discouragement" are evoked last in the poem *My weakest point* (Poem 5) (see Table 3 (e)). Both Poem 1 and Poem 5 have a similar mood like loneliness, and two words "meditation" and "gloominess" are evoked as common emotional words of these poems. Emotional words "pleasant," "optimism," and "calm" are evoked last in the poem *There is a fireplace in my house* (Poem 2) (see Table 3 (b)). Actually, many students in our laboratory said, "I was impressed by the poem with some delightful emotions."

Interesting facts can be discovered in the evoked words of the poem *On the day my mother doesn't scold me* (Poem 3). With this poem, the emotional word "modesty" is strongly evoked. Emotional words "modesty," "timid," and "calm" are evoked last (see Table 3(c)). In the first half of the poem *It is snowing* (Poem 4), (the repetition of the phrase "*It is snowing*"), "posture" is evoked frequently; in the final part, the emotional word "sentimentality" is more frequently evoked than "posture." Of course, there are subtle differences in the results depending on the personal situation. Anyway, these results are in good agreement with the emotions of a vast majority of people.

The value of δ is remarkable. If $\delta < 0.35$, no emotional words are selected in Poems 1, 3, and 4, which is analogous to the human's situation of being unable to find any appropriate term. However, we need more to demonstrate that these kinds of evoked emotional words have a fair resemblance to human feeling when the poem is read.

Table 3. Process of evoked emotion by the inputted poem

(a) *Shuffling cards in the night.*

Words	Defuzzified Value				Evoked Mixed Emotional Words					
	JOY	ANG	EXP	ACC	Words			Distances		
alone	-0.13	-0.16	0.16	-0.08	timid	meditation	trouble	0.27	0.37	0.42
cards	0.01	0.02	0.11	0.03	calm	posture	union	0.39	0.40	0.41
shuffle	0.12	0.01	0.40	0.18	union	acceptance	fate	0.18	0.22	0.25
night	-0.04	-0.15	0.38	0.04	posture	union	careful	0.27	0.32	0.34
dreary	-0.31	-0.09	0.08	-0.13	meditation	gloominess	discouragement	0.16	0.28	0.34
obvious	-0.27	-0.05	0.33	-0.11	meditation	pessimism	gloominess	0.37	0.43	0.45

(b) *There is a fireplace in my house.*

Words	Defuzzified Value				Evoked Mixed Emotional Words					
	JOY	ANG	EXP	ACC	Words			Distances		
fireplace	0.29	0.00	0.20	0.16	calm	quiet	pleasant	0.18	0.21	0.29
fireplace	0.45	0.00	0.33	0.26	pleasant	optimism	quiet	0.08	0.16	0.24
house	0.46	0.00	0.41	0.38	optimism	pleasant	happiness	0.11	0.14	0.22
feel	0.02	0.00	0.20	0.07	union	posture	acceptance	0.31	0.32	0.35
good	0.33	0.00	0.33	0.21	pleasant	optimism	calm	0.22	0.23	0.25

(c) *On the day my mother doesn't scold me.*

Words	Defuzzified Value				Evoked Mixed Emotional Words					
	JOY	ANG	EXP	ACC	Words			Distances		
mother	0.23	0.00	0.22	0.23	calm	quiet	union	0.15	0.22	0.30
not scold	0.09	-0.22	0.27	0.09	posture	union	modesty	0.23	0.35	0.36
missing	0.05	-0.10	0.13	0.05	posture	modesty	calm	0.33	0.34	0.37
missing	0.03	-0.05	0.06	0.03	modesty	timid	calm	0.37	0.38	0.38

(d) *It is snowing.*

Words	Defuzzified Value				Evoked Mixed Emotional Words					
	JOY	ANG	EXP	ACC	Words			Distances		
snow	-0.06	0.00	0.03	0.00	timid	meditation	modesty	0.39	0.4	0.42
fall	-0.03	-0.21	0.26	0.08	posture	union	modesty	0.23	0.35	0.35
snow	-0.08	-0.11	0.17	0.05	posture	timid	modesty	0.32	0.34	0.37
fall	-0.05	-0.29	0.35	0.12	posture	anxiety	union	0.21	0.29	0.36
palm	0.12	-0.15	0.48	0.24	posture	union	anticipation	0.22	0.22	0.23
catch	0.07	-0.08	0.46	0.32	union	acceptance	fate	0.12	0.13	0.14
melt	0.07	-0.05	0.47	0.36	acceptance	fate	union	0.11	0.12	0.12
sad	-0.23	-0.03	0.11	0.20	sentimentality	posture	modesty	0.35	0.37	0.39

(e) *My weakest point.*

Words	Defuzzified Value				Evoked Mixed Emotional Words					
	JOY	ANG	EXP	ACC	Words			Distances		
weakest	-0.04	-0.23	0.15	0.00	timid	modesty	posture	0.24	0.35	0.35
mother	0.21	-0.12	0.32	0.23	posture	calm	union	0.24	0.27	0.27
tear	-0.20	-0.07	-0.03	-0.07	meditation	timid	gloominess	0.25	0.32	0.39
silence	-0.15	-0.15	0.09	0.03	timid	modesty	posture	0.27	0.35	0.38
tear	-0.42	-0.08	-0.14	-0.18	meditation	gloominess	discouragement	0.17	0.22	0.25

4.2. Experiments for emotional transition in time by several subjective observations

Figures 3 and 4 show the results for emotional transition in time by subjective observations based on the image codes in the case of the poem *It is snowing* in Table 3. Figure 3 parts (a)-(c) are the results for a simulated person whose current emotion (or maybe the person's nature) is supposed to be [optimism, curiosity] before reading the poem, whose image codes are used for the pair of vectors for subjective observation. The sequence of the figures shows that the emotion converges (settles) quickly into the objective one.

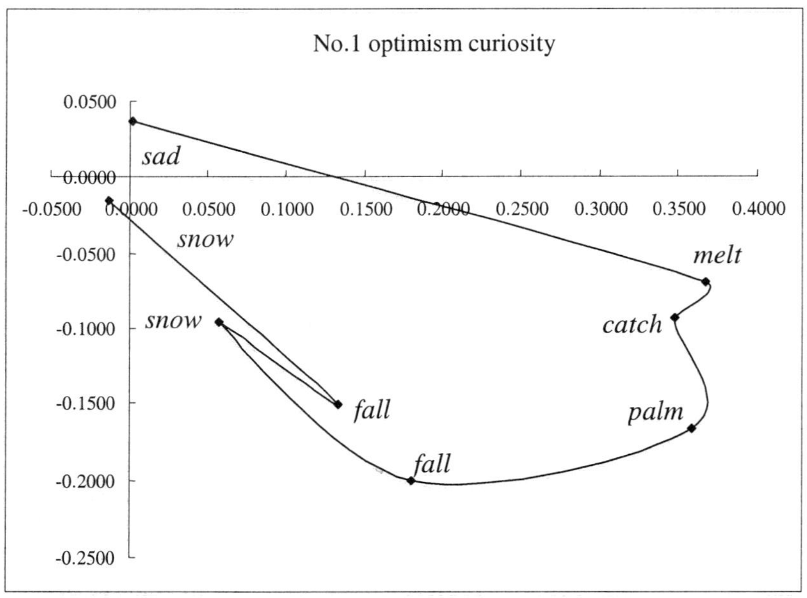

(a) Pair of vectors for subjective observation is [optimism, curiosity].

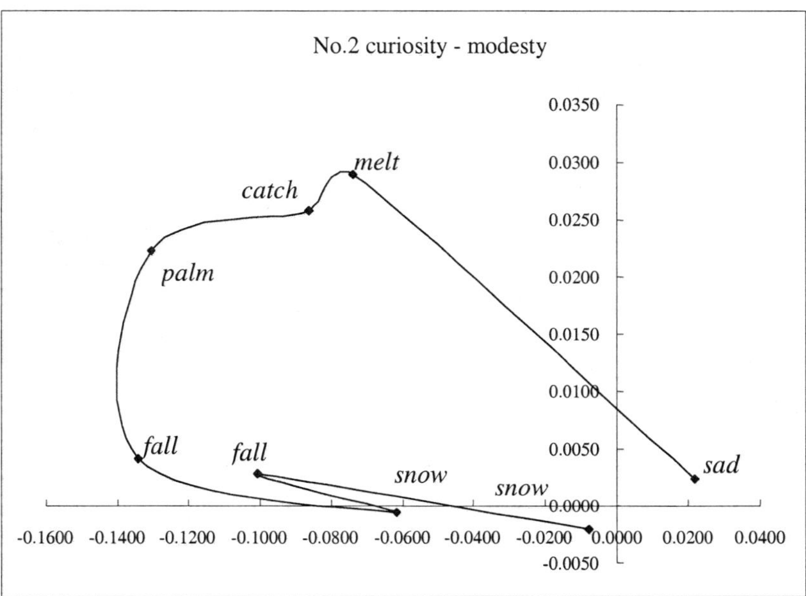

(b) Pair of vectors for subjective observation is [curiosity, modesty].

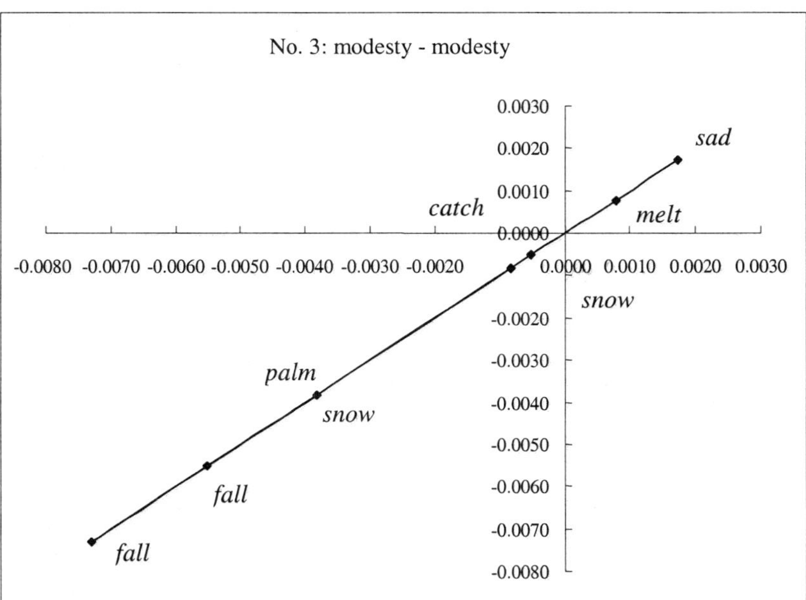

(c) Pair of vectors for subjective observation is [modesty, modesty].

Figure 3. An example of the emotional transition process when the initial pair of vectors for subjective observation is [optimism, curiosity].

On the other hand, the emotional transition process of the person who has fallen into an emotion like [abhorrence, violence] for some reason, just before reading this poem, converges into the objective emotion five times, as shown in Figure 4.

Besides these results, we could obtain several interesting results on behavior in the chaotic or oscillatory mode. These phenomena may be interesting, even from the psychological viewpoint, although they cannot be shown here for lack of space. A detailed explanation of the phenomenon is given in [4].

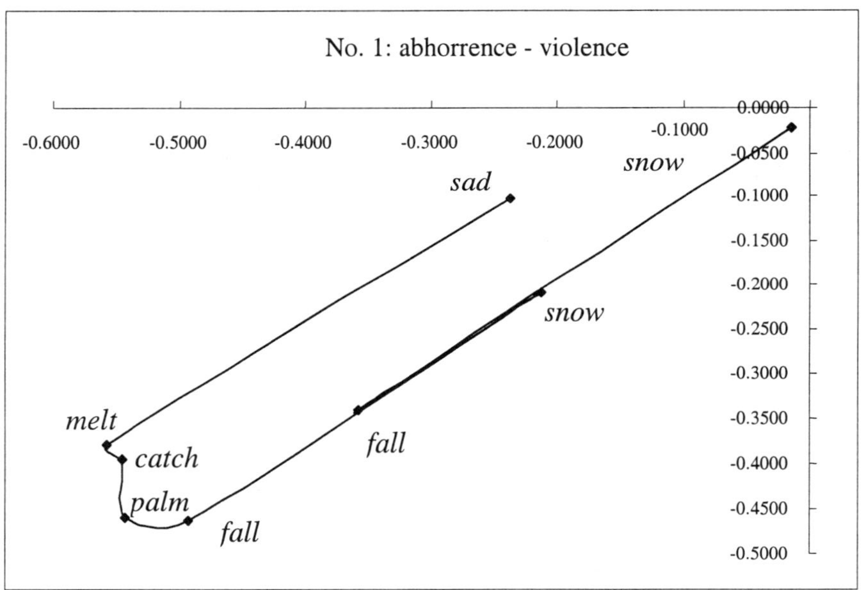

(a) Pair of vectors for subjective observation is [abhorrence, violence].

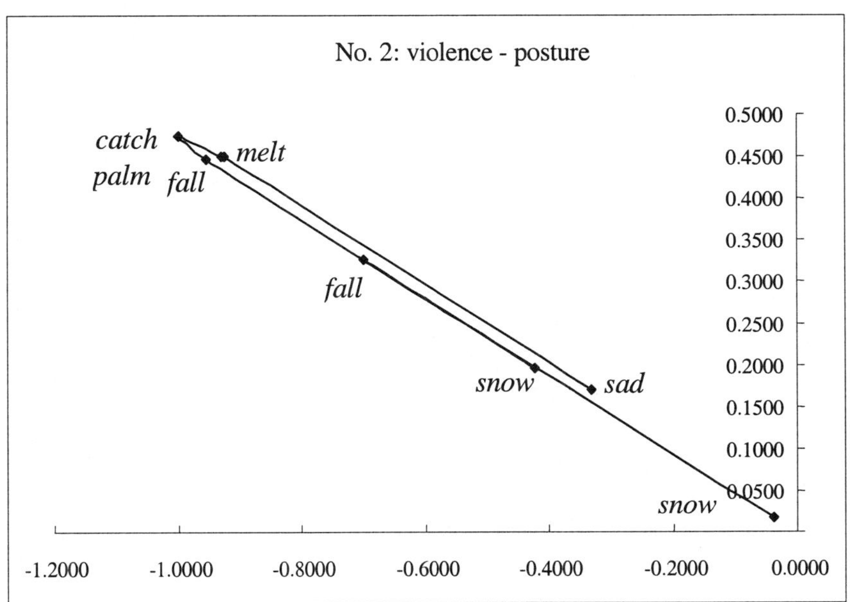

(b) Pair of vectors for subjective observation is [violence, posture].

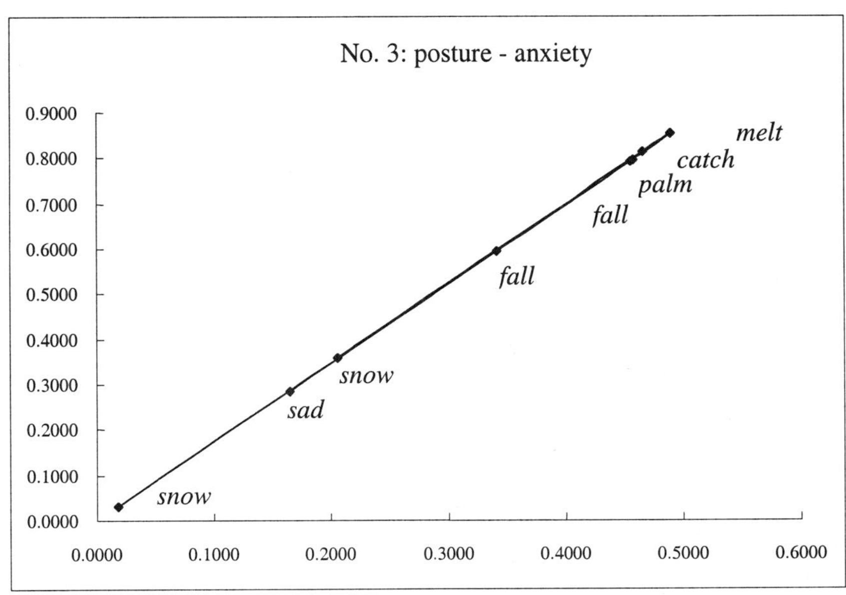

(c) Pair of vectors vector for subjective observation is [posture, anxiety].

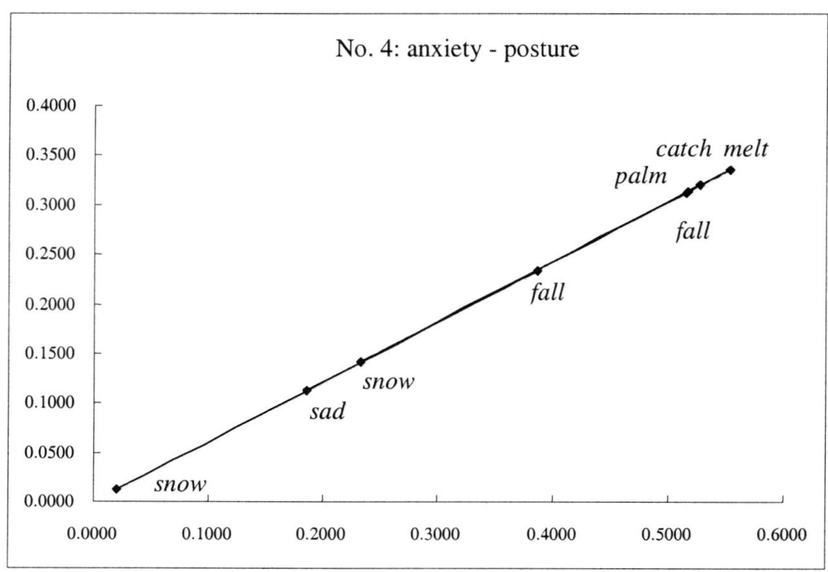

(d) Pair of vectors for subjective observation is [anxiety, posture].

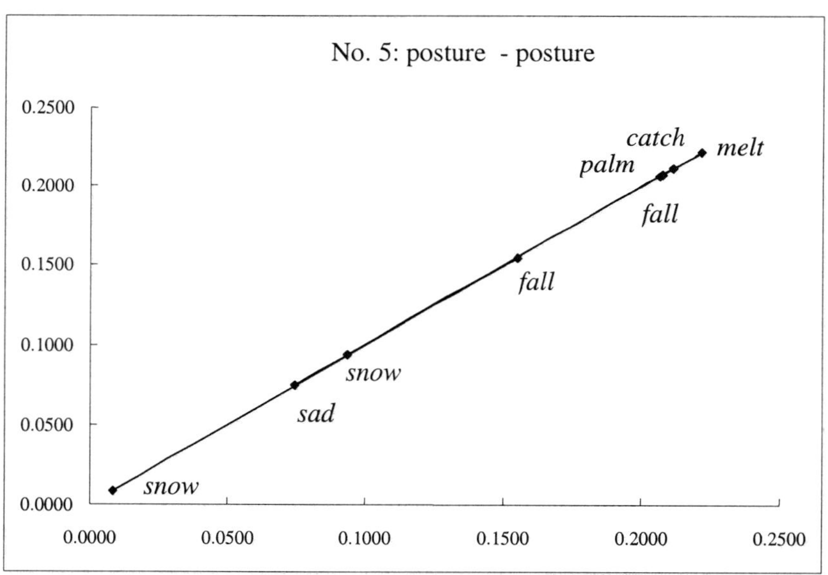

(e) Pair of vectors for subjective observation is [posture, posture].

Figure 4. An example of the emotional transition process when the initial pair of vectors for subjective observation is [abhorrence, violence].

Next we describe an experiment to clear the effect of a pair of vectors for a subjective observation. We set five pairs of vectors for subjective observation. These five pairs of vectors are selected considering the following five simulated persons:

1. An optimist having much curiosity: [optimism, curiosity].
2. A person in despair and rage: [despair, rage].
3. An ironical person in fear of something: [fear, irony].
4. A violent person having abhorrence to something: [abhorrence, violence].
5. An affectionate person in joy: [affection, joy].

In Table 4 the results for converged emotional words of the five poems are shown by subjective observation using five pairs of vectors.

Table 4. Converged emotional words of five poems by subjective observation

Pair of vectors		Poem 1	Poem 2	Poem 3	Poem 4	Poem 5
optimism	curiosity	trouble	calm	calm	modesty	trouble
despair	rage	timid	calm	timid	timid	timid
fear	irony	timid	calm	timid	calm	timid
abhorrence	violence	trouble	posture	posture	posture	trouble
affection	joy	grief	affection	calm	meditation	grief

The results of subjective observations are more dependent on the pair of vectors than the poems themselves. Specifically, all five poems are observed as only two emotional words, "posture" or "trouble" by the pair [abhorrence, violence]. On the other hand, results obtained by pair [affection, joy] are four emotional words, "grief," "affection," "calm," and "meditation," which reflect well the characteristics of each poem, respectively. It is necessary to investigate statistically whether or not real persons whose nature is similar to the simulated person's one is really impregnated with the resultant emotions listed in Table 4. However, these results are in approximate agreement with human's feelings. Table 5 (a), (b), (c), (d), and (e) show the results for processes of emotional transition in time. Table 5 (d) shows that the number of convergence times for the pair of vectors [abhorrence, violence] is larger than for other pairs of vectors.

Table 5. Results for emotional transition in time.

(a) [optimism, curiosity]

Poem	1	2	3	4
Poem 1	meditation	timid	timid	timid
Poem 2	calm	calm	calm	
Poem 3	calm	calm	calm	
Poem 4	modesty	modesty	modesty	
Poem 5	meditation	trouble	trouble	trouble

(b) [despair, rage]

Poem	1	2	3	4
Poem 1	timid	timid	timid	
Poem 2	quiet	calm	calm	calm
Poem 3	timid	timid	timid	
Poem 4	timid	timid	timid	
Poem 5	calm	calm	calm	

(c) [fear, irony]

Poem	1	2	3
Poem 1	timid	timid	timid
Poem 2	calm	calm	calm
Poem 3	timid	timid	timid
Poem 4	calm	calm	calm
Poem 5	timid	timid	timid

(d) [abhorrence, violence]

Poem	1	2	3	4	5
Poem 1	timid	timid	timid		
Poem 2	posture	anxiety	posture	posture	posture
Poem 3	posture	anxiety	posture	posture	posture
Poem 4	posture	anxiety	posture	posture	posture
Poem 5	trouble	trouble	trouble		

(e) [affection, joy]

Poem	1	2	3	4
Poem 1	sadness	grief	grief	grief
Poem 2	affection	affection	affection	
Poem 3	calm	calm	calm	
Poem 4	meditation	meditation	meditation	
Poem 5	sadness	grief	grief	grief

In order to clarify the general features of subjective observation as related to pairs of vectors, we perform the same experiment considering sixty-eight image codes in place of the five poems. Table 6 shows an example of emotional transitions of sixty-eight mixed emotions obtained by the pair of vectors ([affection, joy]).

The sixty-eight mixed emotional words can be classified into several groups. For example, mixed emotions, "abhorrence," "hostility," "contempt," and "envy" are converged to "grief," and "admission," "acceptance," and "union" are converged to "hope." These five tables can be represented by the pie-graphs in Figures 5 (a), (b), (c), (d), and (e), respectively. They are more intuitively understandable than the tables.

Table 6. An example of emotional transition of sixty-eight mixed emotional words

No.	Emotion	1	2	3	4	5	6	Result
1	**ecstasy**	affection	affection	affection				**affection**
2	**joy**	affection	affection	affection				**affection**
3	**happiness**	affection	affection	affection				**affection**
4	**pleasant**	affection	affection	affection				**affection**
5	**quiet**	friendship	affection	affection	affection			**affection**
16	**abhorrence**	grief	grief	grief				**grief**
17	**hostility**	sadness	grief	grief	grief			**grief**
18	**contempt**	sadness	grief	grief	grief			**grief**
19	**envy**	sadness	grief	grief	grief			**grief**
62	**admission**	pleasant	joy	joy	hope	hope	hope	**hope**
63	**acceptance**	pleasant	joy	joy	hope	hope	hope	**hope**
64	**union**	pleasant	joy	joy	hope	hope	hope	**hope**
65	**affection**	affection	affection	affection				**affection**
66	**friendship**	affection	affection	affection				**affection**
67	**superiority**	quiet	pleasant	quiet	calm	calm	calm	**calm**
68	**fate**	pleasant	joy	joy	hope	hope	hope	**hope**

When the observation is done by the pair of vectors [optimism, curiosity], we can see several converged emotions such as "calm," "trouble," "surprise," "irony," "curiosity," "grief," and "modesty," have the percentages 38%, 37%, 12%, 6%, 3%, 3%, and 1%, respectively, in Figure 6 (a). This means that the observed emotions, in this case, mostly converge to "calm" or "trouble." Also, in the case that the air of vectors is [despair, rage], the observed emotions are "timid," "calm," "rage," "pride," "despair," "boredom," "meditation," "uneasiness," and "violence" by 22%, 19%, 18%, 13%, 12%, 7%, 4%, 4%, and 1%, respectively, in Figure 6 (d). Similarly, we can find several interesting tendencies in these figures. The case of the observation [fear, irony] is similar to the case [despair, rage] with respect to the fact that they converge mostly (with some exceptions) to the same emotional words "timid" and "calm."

Emotional words "timid" and "calm" are observed mostly in Figures 5 (a), (b), and (c) below. This is because the image codes are mapped repeatedly and the resultant value of each attribute of the image codes is decreased, step by step.

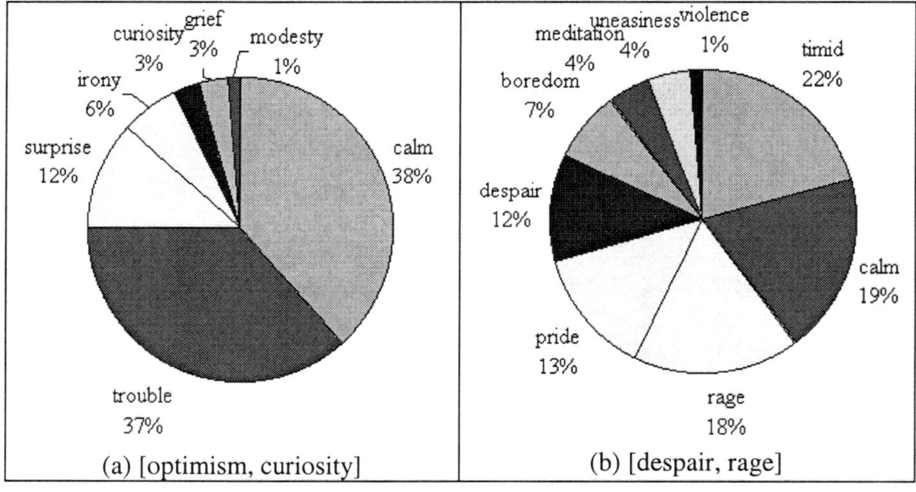

(a) [optimism, curiosity]   (b) [despair, rage]

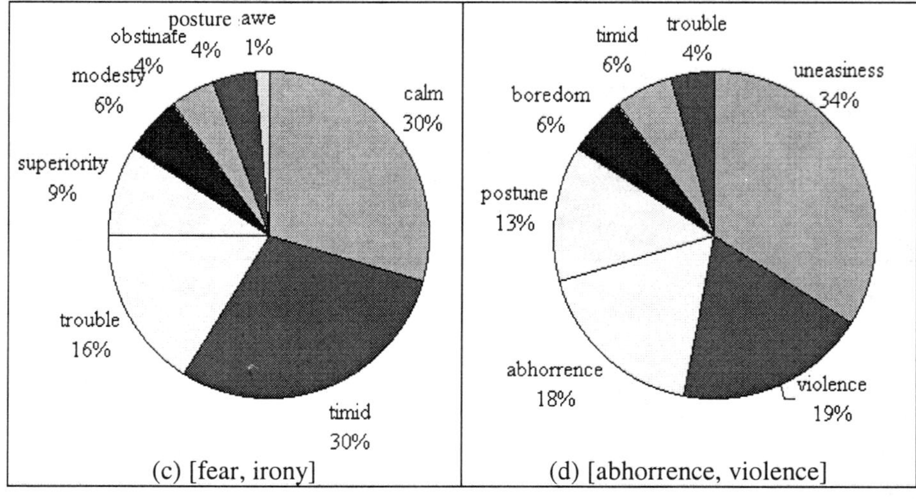

(c) [fear, irony]   (d) [abhorrence, violence]

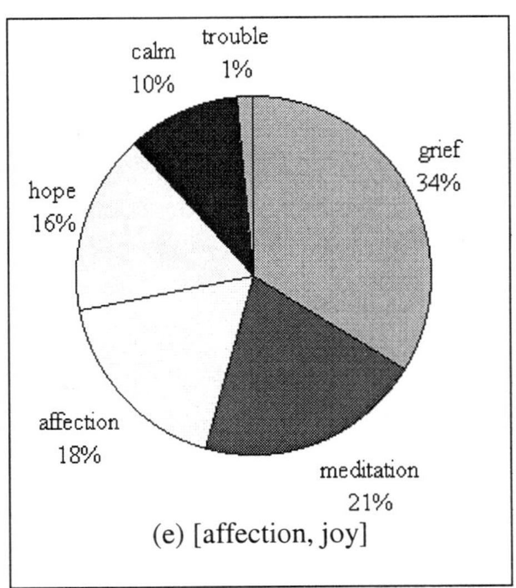

Figure 5. Circle graphs drawn by computing the percentage of the converged sixty-eight mixed emotional words.

On the other hand, there are some pairs of vectors such as [abhorrence, violence] or [affection, joy] that increase the value on each attribute for image codes by mapping repeatedly. The image codes observed vectors are strongly dependent on the pair of vectors. In the case of [abhorrence, violence], only the emotional words are observed, such as "uneasiness," "violence," "abhorrence," "posture," "boredom," "timid," and "trouble."

The following properties become evident after the experimental results. Converged emotional words are strongly dependent on a pair of vectors for subjective observation. A relationship between converged emotional words and a pair of vectors is similar to a human's. For example, Figure 5 (d) shows an interesting relationship where the subjective observation by [abhorrence, violence] strongly derives similar emotional words. A violent person having some abhorrence actually tends to consider all things around him as "uneasiness," "violence," "abhorrence," "posture," "boredom," "timid," and "trouble." For a further example, let us consider the result obtained by the pair of vectors [affection, joy] in Figure 5 (e). An affectionate and joyful person tends to consider the negative emotion (which are the emotions classified into "grief" and "meditation" in Table 8) as "grief" or "meditation" and considers the positive emotions (which are the emotions classified into "affection" in Table 8) as "affection."

It is important to be clear on what emotions are classified into the emotional group by a pair of vectors for subjective observation. Table 7 shows what and how many mixed emotions are classified into the emotional group by the pair of vectors [abhorrence, violence].

Table 7. Emotional words classified by the pair of vectors [abhorrence, violence]

uneasiness	violence	abhorrence	posture	boredom	timid	trouble
23	13	12	9	4	4	3
joy	pride	rage	ecstasy	attack	irony	unhealthy
happiness	dislike	anger	pleasant	trouble	discreet	obstinate
optimism	boredom	perplexity	quiet	discouragement	awe	meditation
hope	unhappiness	abhorrence	calm	gloominess	astonishment	
expectation	grief	hostility	sentimentality			
anticipation	sadness	contempt	fear			
careful	disappointment	envy	anxious			
posture	amaze	detest	timid			
pessimism	astonish	hatred	modesty			
uneasiness	surprise	regret				
anxiety	curiosity	violence				
disgrace	delight	wrath				
despair	superiority					
shudder						
confusion						
obedience						
guilt						
admission						
acceptance						
union						
affection						
friendship						
fate						

Take the emotional group "abhorrence," for example. The twelve mixed emotional words belonging to this group have common features. This feature is shown in Figure 6 by the line graph.

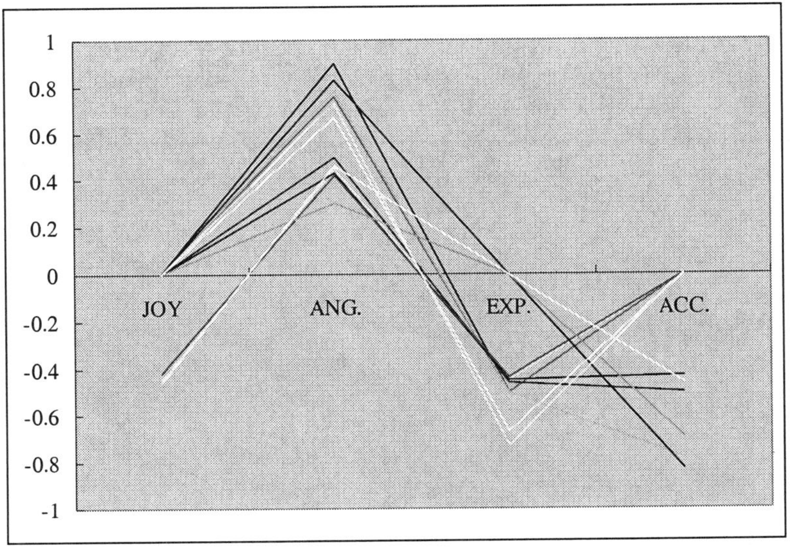

Emotion	JOY	ANG	EXP	ACC
rage	0.00	0.90	-0.50	0.00
anger	0.00	0.76	-0.50	0.00
perplexity	-0.45	0.45	-0.45	0.00
abhorrence	0.00	0.78	-0.50	-0.78
hostility	0.00	0.50	-0.46	-0.50
contempt	0.00	0.43	-0.45	-0.43
envy	-0.42	0.42	-0.44	0.00
detest	0.00	0.83	0.00	-0.83
hatred	0.00	0.30	0.00	-0.69
regret	-0.46	0.46	0.00	-0.46
violence	0.00	0.73	-0.73	0.00
wrath	0.00	0.67	-0.67	0.00

Figure 6. The line graph of twelve image codes belonging to group "abhorrence" in Table 7.

It is obvious that the values of attribute ANG are higher than the values of other attributes.

Here is another example. Table 8 shows what and how many mixed emotional words are classified into each emotional group by the pair of vectors [affection, joy].

Table 8. Emotional words classified by the pair of vectors [affection, joy]

grief	meditation	affection	hope	calm	trouble
23	14	12	11	7	1
perplexity	rage	ecstasy	calm	unhealthy	irony
abhorrence	anger	joy	attack	obstinate	
hostility	pessimism	happiness	careful	anxiety	
contempt	dislike	pleasant	posture	modesty	
envy	boredom	quiet	uneasiness	curiosity	
detest	trouble	pride	obedience	delight	
hatred	disgrace	optimism	guilt	superiority	
unhappiness	discreet	hope	admission		
regret	sentimentality	expectation	acceptance		
grief	anxious	anticipation	union		
sadness	timid	affection	fate		
discouragement	awe	friendship			
gloominess	surprise				
meditation	wrath				
despair					
disappointment					
shudder					
confusion					
fear					
astonishment					
amaze					
astonish					
violence					

Take the emotional group "affection," for example. The twelve mixed emotional words belonging to this group have a common feature. Figure 7 shows this feature in line graph.

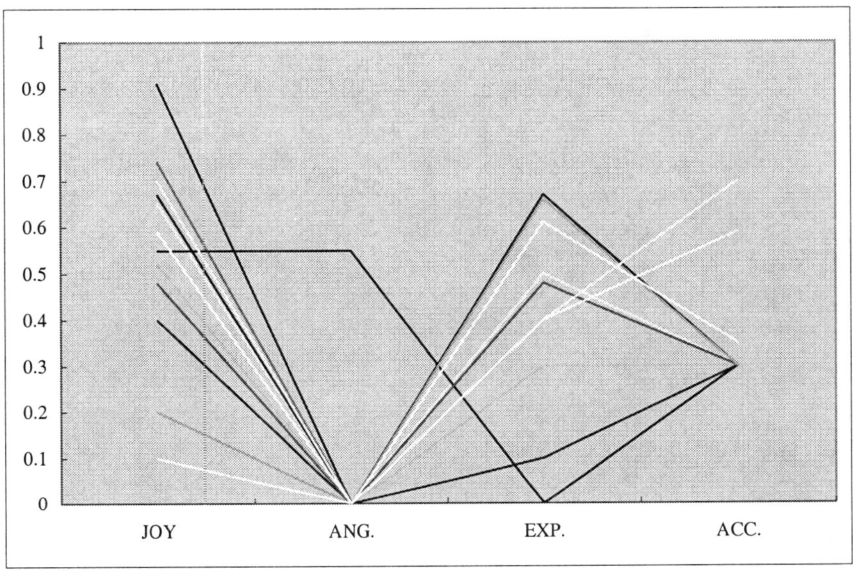

Emotion	JOY	ANG	EXP	ACC
ecstasy	0.91	0.00	0.30	0.30
joy	0.74	0.00	0.50	0.30
happiness	0.65	0.00	0.50	0.30
pleasant	0.52	0.00	0.30	0.30
quiet	0.40	0.00	0.10	0.30
pride	0.55	0.55	0.00	0.30
optimism	0.48	0.00	0.48	0.30
hope	0.67	0.00	0.67	0.30
expectation	0.20	0.00	0.66	0.30
anticipation	0.10	0.00	0.61	0.35
affection	0.70	0.00	0.40	0.70
friendship	0.59	0.00	0.40	0.59

Figure 7. The line graph of twelve image codes belonging to group "affection" in Table 8.

It is obvious that the values of attribute ANG are lower than the values of other attributes. Thus, it can be said in general that similar image codes are classified into an emotional group by a pair of vectors for subjective observation. Furthermore, classification of emotional words in this mapping way (subjective observation) is useful for producing something acceptable to human emotion.

4.3. Emotional clustering diagram

In order to make the mapping effect by pair vectors clearer, the explanation using the maps onto a two-dimensional plane is introduced here. First we select two vector pairs (ζ, η), each of which is constructed by two emotional words, such as [optimism, curiosity] and [violence, rage]. The vector pairs are used for mapping functions ϕ_{OPT_CUR} and ϕ_{VIO_RAG} Equation (16). We consider that the mapping function ϕ_{OPT_CUR} corresponds to the character of a person for whom the point of view is optimistic and curious. The mapping function ϕ_{OPT_CUR} maps the sixty-eight emotional image code vectors x_k ($k = 1,2,...,68$) in four-dimensional emotional space onto the two-dimensional observational space. The distribution of the mapped points $\phi_{OPT\_CUR}(x_k)$ ($k = 1,2,...,68$) is shown in Figure 7. Also shown in Figure 8 is that of $\phi_{VIO\_RAG}(x_k)$. The sixty-eight emotions are represented by numbers. The number "2" means "joy," the number "3" means "happiness," and so on (see Table 1).

Second we get the pseudo vectors x_k' Equation (24) for the subjective observation applying the mapping function ϕ_{OPT_CUR}. But x_k' is still merely a numerical vector. Then, we express x_k' by the corresponding appropriate emotional word x_k, applying the soft matching method. We obtained some attractive results from the mapping functions ϕ_{OPT_CUR} and ϕ_{VIO_RAG}. When we applied the mapping function ϕ_{OPT_CUR}, the emotional words "joy," "happiness," and "hope" are categorized and understood to be "hope"; on the other hand, when we applied the mapping function ϕ_{VIO_RAG}, these emotional words are observed to be "uneasiness." These kinds of phenomena reflect well on the human subjective emotion.

Finally, for any point in the observation space, it can be categorized to some emotional words as well as the mapped point $\phi(\mathbf{x}_k)$. Considering the point $P_m(p_{1m}, p_{2m})$ in the observation space and performing the inverse mapping operation, we can obtain the corresponding image code in four-dimensional space and find the emotional word closest to where it is located. In more mathematical detail, computing the equation

$$q_{im} = p_{1m}\zeta_i + p_{2m}\eta_i \qquad \text{(for } i = 1,2,3,4)$$

we can obtain the vector $Q_m(q_{1m}, q_{2m}, q_{3m}, q_{4m})$ and find the emotional words. In this way we can obtain the map of the categorized emotion and draw a clustering map of emotional space into regions of emotional classes.

The subjective emotional space spanned by the vector pair [optimism, curiosity] is classified into thirteen groups, as seen in Figure 8. The vector pair [violence, rage] classifies the emotional space into six groups in Figure 9. These six groups are "rage," "anger," "uneasiness," "anxiety," "timid," and "violence." This result analogizes that a violent and irritable person cannot interpret what objects are. These kinds of emotions are often observed in a person whose nature is emotionally unstable.

Furthermore, this result has a possibility of showing the mapping function-oriented clustering algorithm.

5. Conclusions

We applied the basic theory for a subjective observation model, including a fuzzy inference technique that we recently created, to an emotion-processing system.

In order to make the general feature of subjective observation clear with a pair of vectors, we performed several experiments. The following properties were evidenced by the experimental results regarding the emotional transition in time for several subjective observations.

Converged emotional words are strongly dependent on a pair of vectors for subjective observation. Moreover, the relationship between converged emotional words and a pair of vectors is similar to human's. For example, a violent person having some abhorrence cannot actually tend to consider all things around him as happy.

It can be said in general that similar image codes are classified into an emotional group by a pair of vectors for subjective observation. Furthermore, the classification of emotional words according to this mapping version (subjective observation) is useful for producing something similar to a classification performed by humans.

The diagram of mapped emotional two-dimensional plane has a possibility of showing the mapping function-oriented clustering algorithm. We defined the mapping function as an operator that interprets image codes expressed by emotional words and vectors. The mapping method is regarded as a useful mechanism to automate the rule generator regarding the emotional space. The results presented in this chapter may be useful in creating new types of processing systems that include emotional functions in the near future. However, several issues should be addressed by further research.

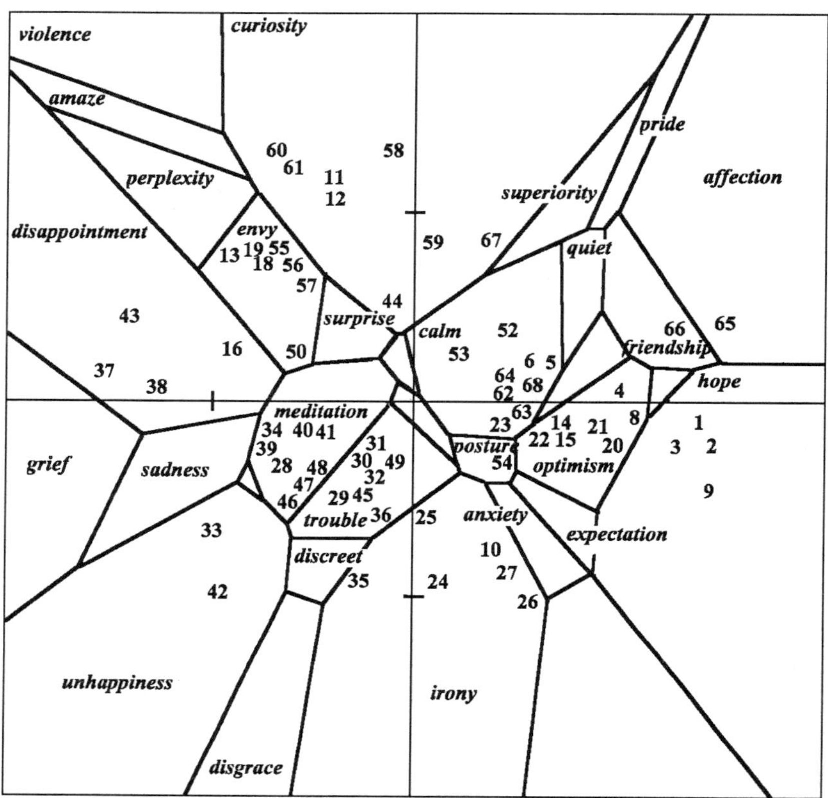

calm	quiet, calm, pride, posture, obedience, modesty, admission, acceptance, union, fate
optimism	pleasant, optimism, attack, obstinate, expectation, anticipation, careful
hope	ecstasy, joy, happiness, hope
envy	perplexity, contempt, envy, awe, amaze, astonish, surprise
posture	guilt
irony	unhealthy, irony, pessimism, uneasiness, anxiety, disgrace
trouble	hatred, dislike, boredom, trouble, discreet, shudder, timid
unhappiness	unhappiness, despair
meditation	detest, regret, discouragement, gloominess, meditation, confusion, fear, anxious
disappointment	abhorrence, hostility, grief, sadness, disappointment, astonishment
curiosity	rage, anger, sentimentality, curiosity, delight, violence, wrath, superiority
affection	affection
friendship	friendship

Figure 8. Result of mapping sixty-eight emotions by pair vectors [optimism, curiosity]. The axes correspond to the intensity of the two emotions.

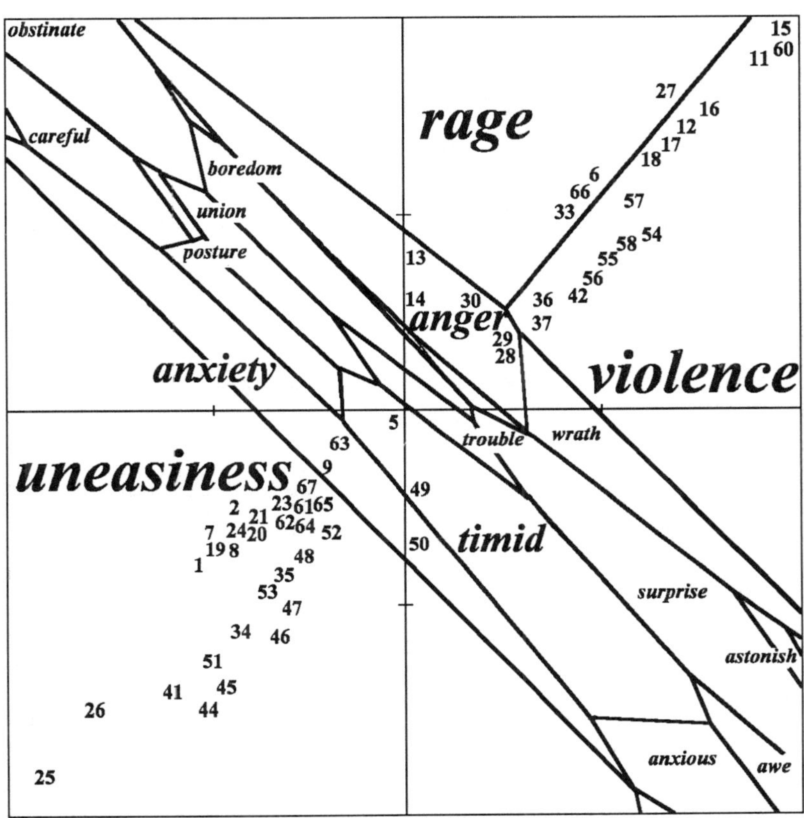

rage	pride, detest, regret, superiority
anger	attack, obstinate, hatred, dislike, boredom
uneasiness	joy, happiness, optimism, hope, expectation, anticipation, careful, posture, irony, pessimism, uneasiness, anxiety, disgrace, discreet, despair, shudder, confusion, fear, anxious, timid, obedience, modesty, guilt, admission, acceptance, affection, friendship, fate
anxiety	ecstasy, pleasant, unhealthy, astonishment, union
timid	quiet, calm, trouble, unhappiness, discouragement, gloominess, meditation, sentimentality, awe
violence	rage, anger, perplexity, abhorrence, hostility, contempt, envy, grief, sadness, disappointment, amaze, astonishment, surprise, curiosity, delight, violence, wrath

Figure 9. Result of mapping sixty-eight emotions by pair vectors [violence, rage]. The axes correspond to the intensity of the two emotions.

Appendix A.

Outline of Plutchik's theory (adapted after [7]) and basic behavior dimensions

Some human behaviors cause happiness; others result in pain. Plutchik ordered such adaptational forms and proposed the following eight basic dimensions:

- *Union* is a type of behavior which takes something from the outside world into its own sphere. The unified stimuli are generally pleasant and beneficial.
- *Refusal* is a type of behavior which removes harmful things, i.e., excretion and vomiting.
- *Destructiveness* is a type of behavior generated by pain, destruction, or the threat of either.
- *Reproduction* is a type of behavior related to sexual activity. It is considered connected to emotions like "pleasant" to maintain contact. All behavior types related to sexual activity are considered connected to "pleasant."
- *Protection* is related to confusion, fear, timidity, and anxiety.
- *Loss* is a type of behavior exhibited when a pleasant object once acquired by contact and union is lost.
- *Disorientation* is a type of behavior generated when encountering a new and strange object. When it occurs, it is not known whether an object is beneficial of harmful, or whether an object is pleasant or unpleasant. This behavior generally exists for a short period of time.
- *Search* is a type of behavior which involves random exploration of the environment. Search activity is spontaneous and continuous. It can also be called curiosity or play when linked to humans.

When two of these eight basic behavior dimensions are paired, their function becomes even clearer: destruction/protection, reproduction/loss, union/refusal, and disorientation/search are behavior dimensions which represent opposite functions.

Table 9. Intensities of basic behavior dimensions

Destructiveness	Reproduction	Union	Disorientation	Protection	Loss	Refusal	Search
rage (9.90)	ecstasy (10.00)	admission (4.61)	amaze (9.30)	shudder (10.13)	grief (8.83)	detest (9.10)	expectation (7.30)
anger (8.40)	joy (8.10)	acceptance (4.00)	astonish (8.30)	confusion (9.75)	sadness (7.53)	hatred (7.60)	anticipation (6.76)
perplexity (5.00)	happiness (7.10)	union (3.30)	surprise (7.26)	fear (7.96)	discouragement (6.26)	dislike (5.50)	careful (5.86)
	pleasant (5.70)			anxious (6.40)	gloominess (5.50)	boredom (4.70)	posture (3.56)
	quiet (4.36)			timid (4.06)	meditation (4.40)	trouble (4.50)	
	calm (3.30)						

Concrete model of emotions

Plutchik also proposed a concrete model for analogizing emotions in terms of solid colors and mixed emotions in terms of mixed colors. He proposed the following six postulates to construct such a model.

Postulate 1. All other emotions are mixed, that is, they can be synthesized by various combinations of primary emotions.

Postulate 3. There are a small number of pure or primary emotions.

Postulate 2. Primary emotions differ from each other, both with regard to physiology and behavior.

Postulate 4. The emotions of daily life are mixed.

Postulate 5. Primary emotions can be conceptualized in terms of a pair of polar opposites.

Postulate 6. Each emotion can exist in various degrees of intensity.

Appendix B

Outline of Young's theory

Young proposed that emotional transition occurs depending on three factors: sign, intensity, and duration [8].

1. *Sign:* We can find two phases in our activities, i.e., approach and avoidance for the concerned object, corresponding to the signs + and -, respectively.
2. *Intensity:* The emotional process is affected by the intensity of the inputted signal, and the intensity can be drawn on a continuous coordinate with two poles, + and -.
3. *Duration:* Emotion varies, and is evoked depending on the duration of expectation on the object.

References

[1] Yanaru, T. and Hirota, T., Basic theory for subjective observation model and its applications, *Proc. of Inter. Symposium on Fuzzy Systems* (ISKIT'92), pp. 5-8, 1992.

[2] Yanaru, T., Basic concept and theory for subjective observation model, and the applicability to create a new machine equipped with emotional functions, *Fifth IFSA World Congress*, pp. 50-53, 1993.

[3] Yanaru, T., Hirota, T., and Kimura, N., An emotion-processing system based on fuzzy inference and its subjective observations, *International Journal of Approximate Reasoning*, 10, 1, pp. 99-122, 1994.

[4] Yanaru, T., Hirota, T., and Kimura, N., An emotion-processing system based on fuzzy inference and its subjective observations, *International Journal of Approximate Reasoning*, 10, pp. 99-122, 1994.

[5] Yanaru, T., Shirahama, N., Tamaki, A., and Hirota, T., Expression of emotions based on subjective observation model theory, *Japanese Journal of Fuzzy Theory and Systems*, 5, 4, 1993.

[6] Plutchik, R., The multifactor-analytic theory of emotion, *Journal of Psychology*, 50, pp. 153-171, 1960.

[7] Matuyama, Y. and Hama, H., *Emotion Psychology* (in Japanese), Seisin Syobou Inc., 1974.

[8] Young, P. T., Affective arousal, *American Psychologist*, 22, pp. 32-40, 1967.

[9] Kawata, T., *Affine geometry/projection geometry* (in Japanese) (Iwanami Kouza Kiso Sugaku Senkei Daisu 5), Iwanami Syoten Inc., 1976.

[10] Parzen, E., *Stochastic Processes*, Holden-Day, Inc., 1962.

[11] Satoh, H., *Kokoro no uta,* San-rio Inc. (in Japanese), 1989.

Remarks on the use of fuzzy logic and soft computing in psychology

H.N. Teodorescu

Some of the concepts presented in this chapter were used by the authors in cooperation with T. Kato in the development of a multimedia image retrieval system. The system is able to learn and make use of the user subjective interpretation of images and to help users retrieve images from a database, based on similarity of interpretation of the images as a searching tool. The learning is interactive and progressive. The system was used to construct an intelligent *Art Museum* system which helps the user select images from a database of impressionist pictures.

Interested readers are referred to

Youshida, K., Kato, T., and Yanaru, T., Image retrieval system based on subjective interpretation, *J. Biomedical Soft Computing and Human Sciences,* 4, 1, pp. 65-74.

Early papers and volumes on psychological interpretation of vagueness in the frame of experimental psychology (vagueness in memory processes, perception, language, image recognition, behavior, psychological interpretation of membership functions) as well as interpretation of psychological facts by fuzzy theory are

Oden, G.C., Integration of fuzzy logical information. *J. of Experimental Psychology: Human Perception and Performance,* 4, pp. 565-575, 1977.

Hersh, H.M. and Caramazza, A., A fuzzy set approach to modifiers and vagueness in natural language, *J. Experimental Psychology: General,* 105, pp. 254-276, 1976.

Horvath, M.J., Kass, C.E., and Ferrell, W.R., An example of the use of fuzzy concepts in modeling learning disability, *American Educational Research Journal,* 17, pp. 309-324, 1980.

The first edited volumes in this field, or significantly related to it, are

Karwowski, W. and Mital, A. (Eds.), *Applications of Fuzzy Set Theory in Human Factors*, Elsevier, pp. 395-446, 1986.

Smithson, M., *Fuzzy Set Analysis for Behavioral and Social Sciences*, New York, Springer, 1987.

Zentenyi, T. (Ed.), *Fuzzy Sets in Psychology*, North-Holland, 1988.

(This last volume includes a good review of the field before 1988 and represents a consistent reference on early developments.)

A recent chapter dealing with the interpretation of the neural activity and of taste in the frame of fuzzy logic is

Erickson, R.P., Chelaru, M.I., and Buhusi, C.V., The brain as fuzzy machine: a modeling problem, *Fuzzy and Neuro-Fuzzy Systems in Medicine*, Chapter 2, pp. 17-54, H.N. Teodorescu, A. Kandel, L.C. Jain (Eds.), CRC Press, FL, 1998.

A good source for new articles in the field, mainly contributed by Japanese researchers, is

Biomedical Soft Computing and Human Sciences, Official Journal of the Biomedical Fuzzy Systems Association (http://www.kct.ac.jp/BMFSA/).

The reader may find of interest several chapters in the volume

Teodorescu, H.N., Kandel, A., and Jain, L.C. (Eds.), *Fuzzy and Neuro-Fuzzy Systems in Medicine*, CRC Press, FL, 1998.

Other than interest for psychologists, the interpretation of emotions by machines is an essential topic in the development of man-machine communication, computer-aided education, decision-support systems, and other related applications.

Chapter 10

Fuzzy methods in nutrition planning and education and in clinical nutrition

Bernd Wirsam and Andreas Hahn

The recommended dietary intakes for nutrients are usually stated as crisp ranges (intervals) of allowances. This crisp representation can be transformed to a fuzzy set, describing the optimal intake of a nutrient. Together with a fuzzy set for the Hamming distance, these sets allow us to improve education in nutrition even in both normal and special diet cases.

With the knowledge of the correlation of nutritional intake and biochemical changes, both setting recommendations for nutrients and nutrition controlling for individuals are possible.

1. Introduction

Nutrition is defined as the science of food, the nutrients and other substances in food; their action, interaction, and balance in relation to health and disease; and the processes by which the organism ingests, absorbs, transports, uses (metabolizes), and excretes food substances [1] [1]. Today more than ever, the interactions between nutrition and disease are important. The U.S. Department of Health and Human Services and the Department of Agriculture suggests that nutritional intervention can reduce morbidity and mortality that result from cardiovascular diseases by 25%, from respiratory and infectious diseases by 20%, from cancer by 20%, and from diabetes by 50% [2]. If this is considered, the economical relevance of healthy nutrition is obvious.

The frequency of different diseases (heart attack, cancer, hypertension, diabetes mellitus, gout) in developed western countries is in direct relationship with the alternations of diet in the past centuries. The main component of diet used to be carbohydrates (potatoes, bread) with a large amount of vegetables and fruit and thus the diet was high in vitamins and minerals. Consequently, the diet was low in fat and protein-rich foods, e.g., meat and products of animal origin. Over the centuries, the diet has altered, and today's diet is rich in protein and fat, and low in fruit and vegetables. These changes also reduced the daily consumption of dietary fiber, while the total energy intake was increased. Through epidemiological and clinical studies, it has been shown that these dietary habits increase the risk of the mentioned diseases. It is the goal of today's nutritionists to change the present dietary habits back to an increased consumption of fruit and vegetables.

Many countries and organizations, such as the United States, Germany, and the European Community, release nutritional recommendations in forms suitable for the public. The first set of Recommended Daily Allowances (RDAs) in the U.S.A. was established in 1941 and has been revised approximately every 5 years. RDAs are intended to prevent nutrient deficiencies and are often called "safe levels" recommendations. The RDAs include a safety margin, so the daily allowances are more than the human body actually needs [3]; yet, the RDAs are merely abstract numbers for a large part of the population. A further problem is that a high intake of minerals and vitamins is desirable, but at the same time, the intake of fat and energy should be limited. The conflict can be solved only if food items are selected and precisely combined. Even then, the exact RDAs of all nutrients would hardly be met. It is necessary to find a compromise between this very healthy diet and the diet consumed by most people today. Radical changes would be preferable but are not realistic. Variations of the diet must be accepted and understood by the population, and most of all, they must be compatible with the modern life style [4, 5]. This is where fuzzy logic can be applied in the field of nutrition.

---

[1] In this chapter, the word *nutrition* may be used with its various partial meanings, or with the general meaning, depending on the context.

In this chapter, the application of fuzzy methods in the field of nutrition education is discussed. The use of fuzzy evaluation and fuzzy decision making in nutrition education is well established in practice. The applied methods are based on fuzzy sets describing the degree of health when varying the intake of a specific nutrient. The corresponding curves are derived by setting the optimal intake equal to the recommended dietary allowances and by describing the degree of health when deviating from the RDAs. For special diets, these fuzzy sets have to be modified by simple operators, like shift and scale. A method to derive RDAs from biochemical correlations is explained. The purpose of RDAs is to give a safe recommendation for nearly all (98%) people within a certain population. Therefore, nearly all recommendations establish values much higher than the average requirement, and in nearly all cases, much higher than the individual needs. A nutrition education based on the RDAs usually results in unnecessary changes in nutrition behavior. To avoid this and to improve individual nutrition education, the inclusion of personal indicators is necessary. With these indicators, classical fuzzy control in nutrition is possible.

2. Crisp and fuzzy interpretation of RDAs

In U.S.A., the recommended dietary intakes for nutrients are given as a range of allowances described by numbers, RDAs, or an interval of estimated safe and adequate daily dietary intake (ESADDI). In nutrition education practice, these numbers are often interpreted as crisp values. In this case, the range of allowed intake x_a of a nutrient "a" could be described by

$$x_{a,min} \leq x_a \leq x_{a,max}$$

This is the crisp formulation of allowances and can be used, for example, as restrictions in linear optimizations. The corresponding set "allowed intake" can be defined by a characteristic function $\mu(x_a)$.

$$\mu(x) = \begin{cases} 1 & \text{for allowed range (acceptable intake)} \quad x_{a,\min} \leq x_a \leq x_{a,\max} \\ \\ 0 & \text{for not allowed range (unacceptable intake)} \end{cases}$$

This characteristic function can be plotted as shown in Figure 1 (dotted line). The characteristic function in a crisp set $[\mu(x_a) = 0$ or $1]$ corresponds to the membership function in a fuzzy set $[0 \leq \mu(x_a) \leq 1]$.

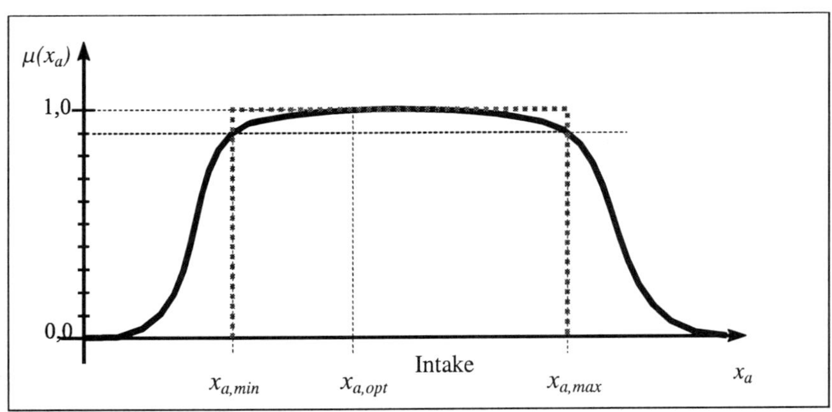

Figure 1. The crisp set "allowed intake" of a nutrient (dotted line). The fuzzy set "optimal intake" of a nutrient (solid line).

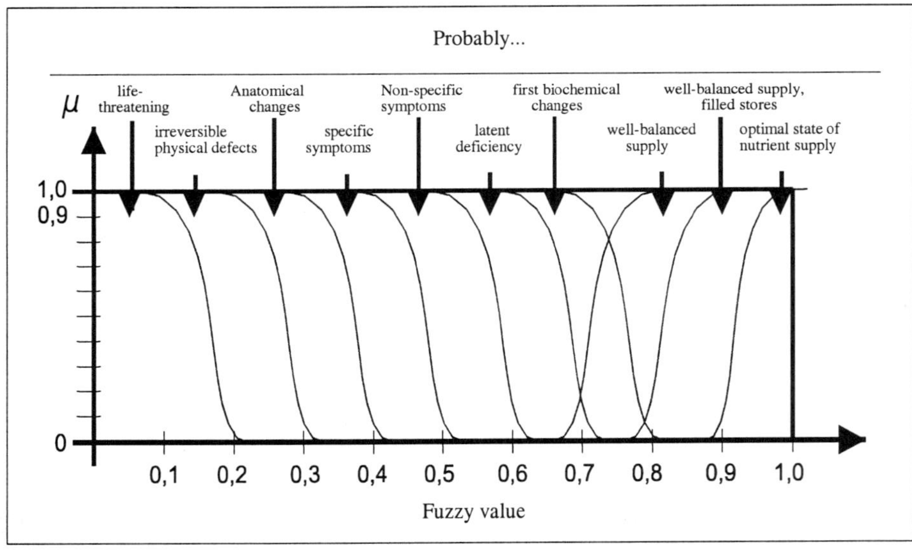

Figure 2. The membership function for linguistic variables.

The membership function defines the fuzzy set. Fuzzy sets were developed to describe systems that cannot be satisfactorily explained in a "crisp" way. The dose-response curve, which shows the degree of health against varying intake of a single nutrient, describes such a vague system. It can be interpreted as a fuzzy set "optimal intake" and can be defined by a curve as shown in Figure 1 (solid line). Optimality is now an integral feature of the set and is reached with the fuzzy value 1, which represents the maximum value. Each x_a has a corresponding membership value μ which can vary between 0 and 1, inclusive; the membership function is thus $\mu(x_a)$. The value 0 corresponds to no membership and 1 to full membership. All values between 0 and the value 1 represent degrees of membership and can be interpreted verbally. In fuzzy logic this is done by the use of linguistic variables. Note that we use type-2 fuzzy sets; their arguments are fuzzy values of type-1-fuzzy sets [6]. Some linguistic variables are shown in Figure 2. These variables have to be the same for all nutrients in order to allow comparisons and combinations.

Using these verbal interpretations, every intake value can be assigned a linguistic evaluation. Intakes which do not meet the RDAs are "not allowed" but are attached to verbal statements like "this intake can possibly lead to biochemical changes" or "this intake is possibly life-threatening". The overlap of the fuzzy sets for the linguistic variables causes continuous progression in interpretation and a modification of the verbal statements like "more or less" (true).

3. Principles of assessing RDA-oriented nutrition by fuzzy methods

Almost all countries and many international agencies have published nutrition recommendations for healthy (normal) people. The general policy is to recommend an intake that covers the needs of all or almost all members of a certain population group. Adding the standard deviations information to the mean requirements helps provide the range corresponding to the need of most (i.e., 98%) healthy individuals. In the USA, the National Research Council publishes these values as the recommended dietary allowances (RDAs) [7]. The mean requirement minus two standard deviations gives the lowest threshold intake. Below this value of the intake, almost all individuals will be unlikely to maintain metabolic integrity. For some nutrients, however, undesirable effects can also occur at amounts above the recommendations, even relatively close to the recommendations. Sometimes, the safe upper limits or the toxic area of intake is listed in official committees' publications. All of these numbers do not represent full reality, which is a continuous transition from critical low intake to adequate intake to excess or even toxic amounts.

Using fuzzy methods, the recommendations are no longer represented as fixed numbers but as fuzzy sets. With the help of these sets, an evaluation of nutrient intake as well as an optimization of food consumption in nutrition education is possible.

On the basis of the above mentioned verbal interpretations, fuzzy sets were developed for those nutrients for which RDAs exist and for which data may be found in the national and international nutrition data bases. For the construction of the fuzzy sets, five points are used: (a) the fuzzy value for zero intake, (b) safe minimum limit, (c) optimal intake, (d) safe upper limit, (e) the toxic perilous area. These points were fitted, segment by segment, by parabolas to get smooth curves.

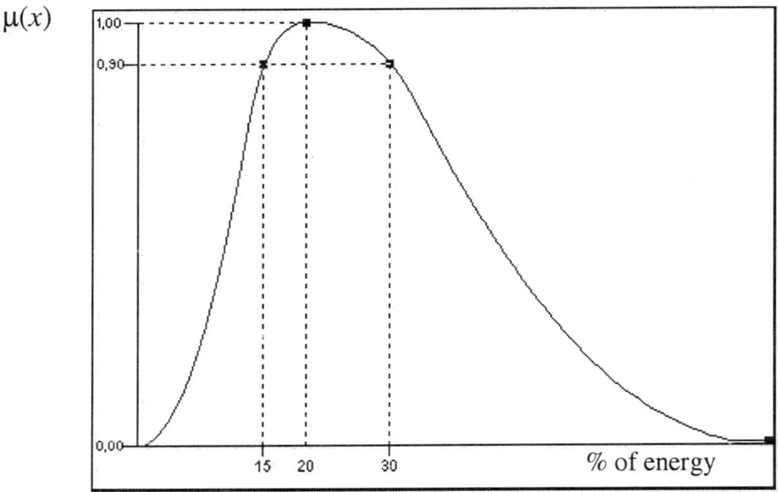

Figure 3. The fuzzy set "optimal intake of fat."

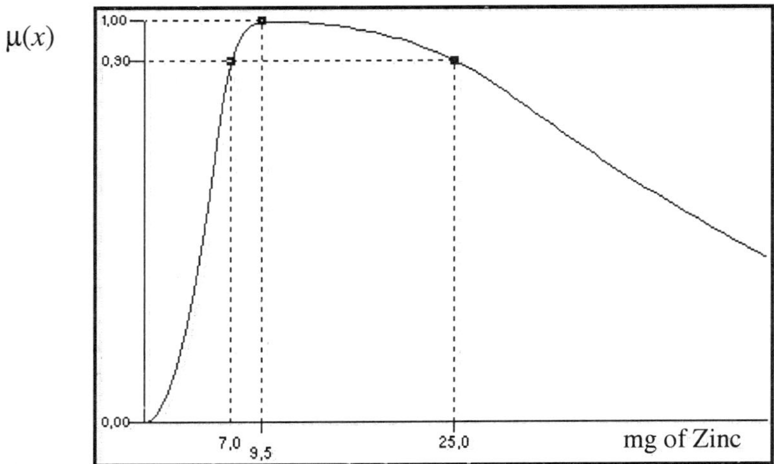

Figure 4. The fuzzy set "optimal intake of zinc."

For example, the total fat intake should not exceed 25-30% of caloric intake. The fuzzy set for fat is therefore constructed as shown in Figure 3, with safe minimum limit 15%, optimal intake 20%, and safe upper limit 30%. As a further example, Figure 4 shows a fuzzy set for a mineral (zinc).

In addition to the fuzzy sets for essential nutrients, fuzzy sets for some other dietary substances can be defined, e.g., cholesterol, alcohol, or sucrose. As they are not essential, the membership functions for zero intake do not start at the zero point. Moreover, as they are generally not considered beneficial to health, they start with a fuzzy value of 1, as shown for cholesterol in Figure 5. This means the optimum is reached with zero intake, which classifies such substances as more or less critical.

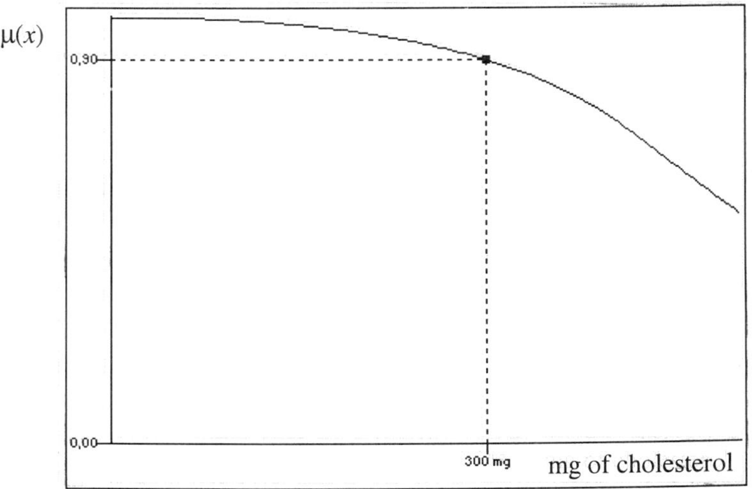

Figure 5. The fuzzy set "optimal intake of cholesterol."

For economic applications, fuzzy sets of this type can even be used to define problems associated with the cost of food. This is essential in planning, as the uncertainty of the cost of food from region to region and the uncertainty of the evolution of the prices can be high.

In nutrition education, it is always important to make acceptable and realizable recommendations. A nutritionist or dietitian has to start with the actual nutritional situation of a certain person or group and only recommend nutritional changes that are not too large. To achieve this by using a computerized decision support system, the Hamming distance was applied. This distance between two nutritional situations is measured in kitchen units. The fuzzy set defined, based on these units, describes the degree of acceptance of the number of necessary changes, as shown in Figure 6.

In practical nutrition education, single nutrients cannot be optimized. Instead of nutrients, we have to deal with foodstuffs, which contain a set of different nutrients. Very frequently, conflicts occur between varying foodstuffs. For example, if there is too little dietary fiber and too much energy in the diet, adding whole meal bread gives more dietary fiber, but more energy too.

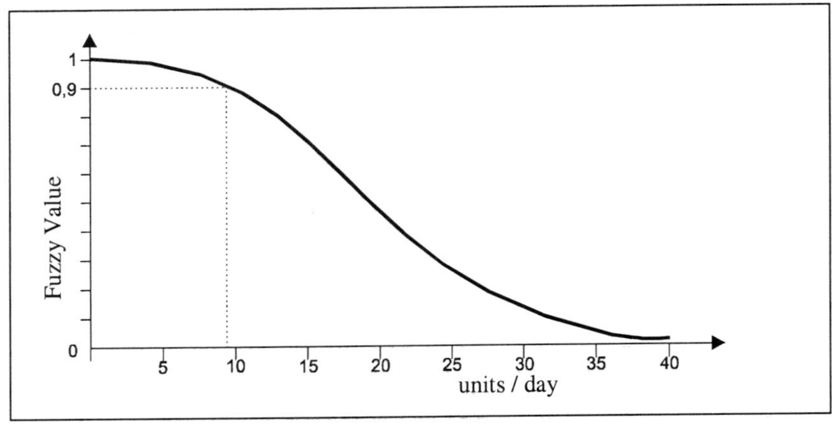

Figure 6. The fuzzy set "degree of acceptance when varying the Hamming distance."

To solve this conflict and to represent the logic *"and"* (because the goal is to reach good intakes for both dietary fiber *and* energy), compromises have to be made. In fuzzy logic, this is done with special operators.

The operator used is the minimum operator corrected by the harmonic mean for all other fuzzy values $\mu(x_i)$. Its application to the fuzzy sets of all nutrients for which recommendations exist and for which data are to be found in nutrition data banks gives the so-called *"Prerow value"* (PV) [8, 9].

$$PV = \min\left(\mu(x_i)\right) \cdot \frac{1}{\dfrac{1}{n-1} \displaystyle\sum_{i \neq \min}^{n} \dfrac{1}{\mu(x_i)}}$$

The "Prerow value" so defined is a measure of how closely nutrition recommendations are reached or how healthful the food is. With the Prerow value, a decision whether a certain nutrition situation is better or worse than another can be made. Within a certain nutrition situation, answers can be obtained to questions like "what happens if less or more of one foodstuff is eaten while the others remain constant?" The resulting curve describes an improvement or deterioration. If two foodstuffs are varied, instead of a curve a response surface is the result when the Prerow value is plotted. In reality, of course, this will be an *n*-dimensional discrete decision space, because only changes in kitchen units are made. Such an *n*-dimensional surface cannot be plotted, but a computerized decision support system can be developed to calculate the gradient and thus find points in the "nutrition landscape" near the starting point but in good agreement with the recommendations. Experience with many nutrition consultations shows that the acceptance of such recommendations is good, because this method tries to make only small changes in nutritional behavior. This is because the operator also operates on the fuzzy set for the Hamming distance. In this way, the optimization tries to reach a favorable nutrition situation with the smallest possible changes.

4. Modifiers for special diets

In some cases, changes in the official recommendations have to be made to fulfill specific goals. For example, in high-performance sports, the value for magnesium is two times the RDA value. For smokers, consumers of special drugs (e.g., diuretics), people with food intolerance, or in the case of some diseases the recommendations for some nutrients change. The corresponding diet is called a special diet.

To represent special diets by using fuzzy sets, modifications of the original fuzzy sets are necessary. This can be done by simple operators like scaling or shifting, which work only on the fuzzy set of the nutrient under consideration. To reach, for example, a Dean Ornish diet [10] (low in fat, cholesterol, and sodium, but high in carbohydrate), the fuzzy sets for fat, carbohydrates, sodium, and cholesterol have to be modified accordingly.

5. Setting recommendations by fuzzy methods

To develop fuzzy sets for the intake of one nutrient based on biochemical correlations, it is necessary to find one or more biochemical indicators (*i*) which are clearly dependent on the intake of a nutrient (*a*) and which are a measure of health status. The indicator is measured by $y_{a,i}$. There are several indicators, e.g., the body mass index (weight in kg divided by the square of the height in m), or the nutrient dependent concentration of an enzyme or other substances in plasma or erythrocytes (in μmol/l.) Here, $y_{a,i}$ should be a function of the intake (x_a) of the nutrient a: $y_{a,i} = f_i(x_a)$. Such functions are derived from long-term experiments with healthy people who have no deficiencies related to other nutrients. In other words, the intake of all other nutrients is assumed to be optimal. The function can be plotted as a curve as shown in Figure 7 (for example, zinc intake and erythrocyte zinc [11]).

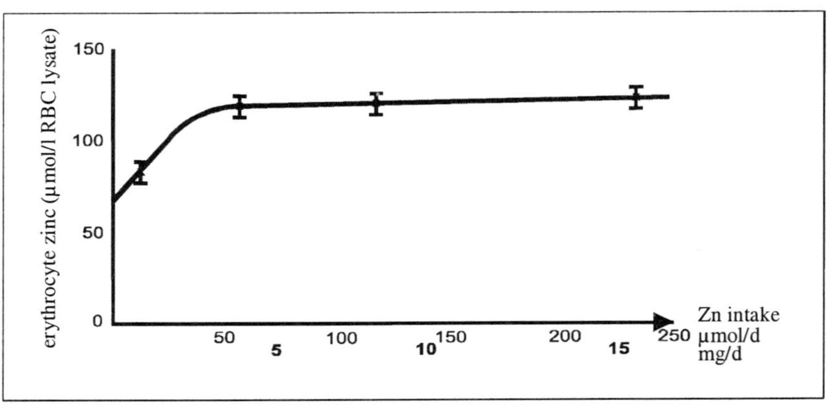

Figure 7. The correlation between nutrient intake and an indicator (zinc intake and erythrocyte zinc).

The indicator should be a measure of health status when regarding long time intervals. Using the same verbal interpretation as shown in Figure 2, $y_{a,i}$ can be correlated to the degree of health by a membership function $\mu(y_{a,i})$ and can be plotted as a curve (Figure 8).

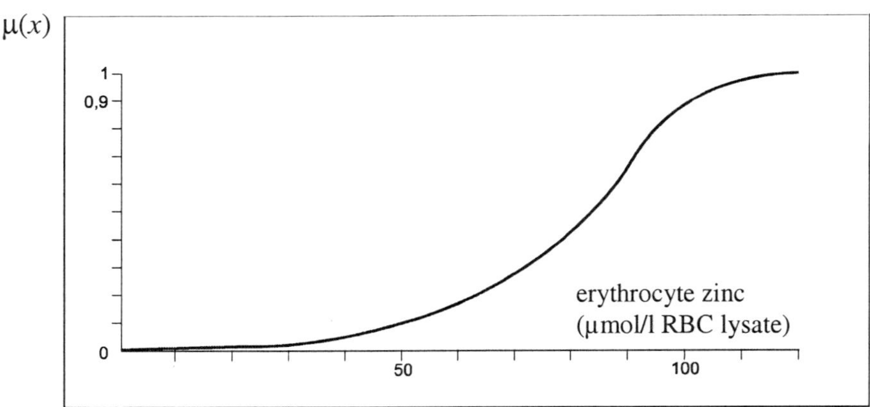

Figure 8. The fuzzy set "degree of health when varying the amount of the indicator" (erythrocyte zinc).

This curve can be used to transform the experimentally derived correlation $y_{a,i} = f_i(x_a)$ to a fuzzy set in order to provide a unitless (and hence more easily compared and combined) evaluation of nutrient intake. This fuzzy set relates the dietary intake to the degree of health as outlined in the following steps:

$$\mu(y_{a,i}) = \mu(f_i(x_a))$$

With this formula, the membership function becomes a direct function of the intake x_a with respect to the indicator i.

$$\mu_i(x_a) = \mu\,(f_i(x_a))$$

This can be plotted as shown in Figure 9.

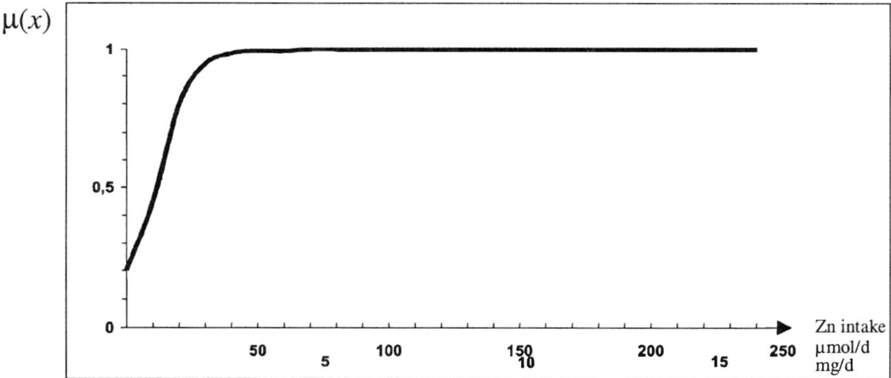

Figure 9. The partial fuzzy set *"degree of health when varying the intake of one nutrient with respect to one indicator"* (zinc with respect to erythrocyte zinc).

In general, there exist n different independent indicators. They describe different health problems. Therefore, there exist n different correlations, n different transformations, and thus n different fuzzy sets μ_i which can be considered as "partial fuzzy sets," because they describe only one partial aspect of health related to the intake of the regarded nutrient or other substances. For the intake of a certain nutrient, the indicator which has the smallest, most dominant fuzzy value describes the health status. This means that for a first approximation, the minimum of all fuzzy values has to be taken to describe health status. However, there must be a mechanism to account for all the other indicators. For example, if other indicators are nearly as bad as the indicator with the smallest fuzzy value, the status must be worse than the status described by only the smallest fuzzy value. Hence, the summarized status must be described by values down correcting the minimum. The operator defining the Prerow value has this feature. Thus, the following aggregation was chosen:

$$\mu(x_a) = \min(\mu_i(x_a)) \cdot \frac{1}{\dfrac{1}{n-1} \displaystyle\sum_{i \neq \min}^{n} \dfrac{1}{\mu_i(x_a)}}$$

In the case of zinc, a second indicator (Cu-Zn ESOD) was used to describe the problems with excess intake of zinc. The RDAs should be valid for most people within a population. To satisfy this condition, all the above mentioned correlations and transformations are not derived from average values. Instead, those values that represent the 98th percentile are taken. The inclusion of the statistical safety margin gives a fuzzy set similar to that shown in Figure 4. Maximizing the membership function gives an RDA for nutrient a

$$\text{RDA}(a) = \max(\mu(x_a)) \qquad 0 \leq x_a \leq \infty$$

In the example of zinc, this gives an RDA of about 9 mg, which is in good agreement with the newest European recommendations [12], but not with the American recommendation of 15 mg for males.

6. Nutrition control

The RDAs do not necessarily represent the optimum intake for every nutrient for either individuals or populations because that is not their purpose. Thus RDA orientated nutrition education is limited in application for individual nutritional consultations. For an individual, a nutrition, which meets the RDA, is surely healthy, but very often it is far from actual nutrition behavior. Needs in energy and nutrients vary from person to person. To come closer to the individual requirements for energy and nutrients, which in most cases lie below the RDA, more information about personal indicators are necessary. In 2% of a population the individual requirement can lie above the RDA. These indicators have to be clearly dependent on the intake of a nutrient and they have to be a measure of health status. For energy, for example, a good indicator is the body mass index. For other nutrients, these indicators can be the same as used for setting RDAs. With the help of these indicators, classic fuzzy control can be used as demonstrated on the base of the body mass index.

For an average person, a body mass index (kg/m^2) of 20 to 25 is recommended. A value of more than 25 is called overweight, more than 30 obese, and under 20 underweight. The further the body mass index is removed from the recommended area, the less the degree of health. Therefore, the degree of health can be plotted against body mass indices as a fuzzy set as shown in Figure 10. This curve can be modified for individual purposes.

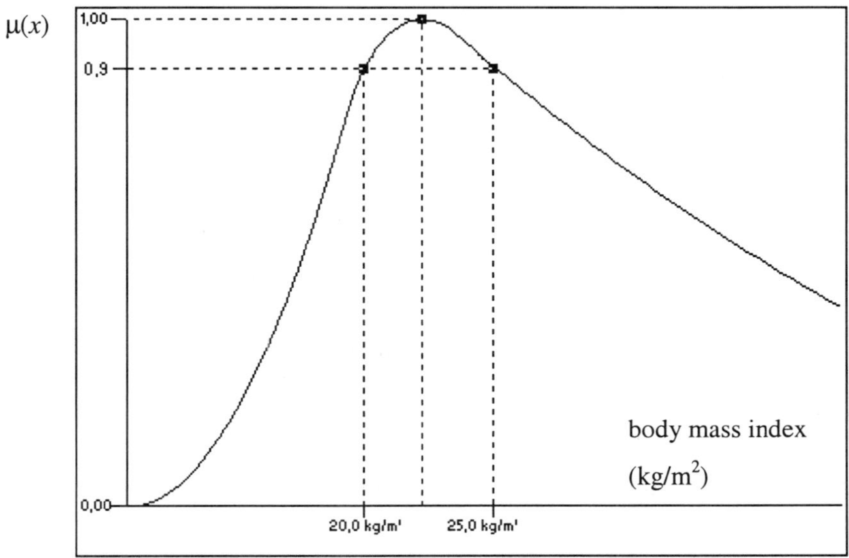

Figure 10. The fuzzy set "optimal body mass index."

Using the body mass index, the fuzzy control will not recommend changing the total energy intake if the measured body mass index is within the recommended interval.

In the case of a too high body mass index, less energy than the actual intake is recommended; in the case of too low an index, more energy is recommended. In order to reach the recommended body mass index, rules about the procedure are necessary. These rules are derived in discussions with nutritionists, dietitians, and physicians. The body mass index only varies as a function of the weight. Therefore, rules like, *"If a person wishes to lose 1 kg weight within a week, he has to reduce energy intake by 1000 kcal per day"* were used. These rules are translated into modifiers for the corresponding fuzzy sets for energy. In a similar way, modifier fuzzy sets can be derived for other nutrients on the basis of suitable individual indicators. With these fuzzy sets, nutrition evaluation, decision-making, and optimization can be made with the same methods as described above. In this way, nutrition education may be individualized.

7. Applications

By using the RDAs to describe the nutritional situation of a population, only two options are possible: either the RDAs are met or they are not. Using fuzzy sets, the situation can be looked at more closely. The degree by which the intake differs from the RDA can be determined. The deviation can be described continuously and thus the nutritional situation can be assessed to a better extent. Furthermore, through the Prerow value, the single nutrients are not only observed one by one, but an overall statement of the complete nutritional situation of one individual, as well as of a complete population, can be made.

Besides a better description of the nutrition status, fuzzy sets can contribute to better nutritional advice. With the help of fuzzy sets and fuzzy decision making, the best compromise to optimize the nutrition of an individual can be established. Realistic changes can be determined so that healthy nutrition is possible for a great part of the western population.

In the following, a few applied examples for fuzzy sets and evaluations are given. The methods of fuzzy decision making described above were applied in nutrition education for 15,000 people, who were members of a German Health Insurance group (Kaufmännische Krankenkasse). The nutrition behavior was typically German. The main problems arise from the unfavorable relation between fat and carbohydrate intake and the high intake of alcohol. Some smaller problems were also found, related to too little dietary fiber and too much sodium.

The mean Prerow value of about 0.6 indicates that the health status on average will deteriorate if this nutrition behavior continues. After optimization, the Prerow value of about 0.9 indicates a desirable diet. The fuzzy values obtained for each nutrient are of course above 0.9 also, which corresponds to a verbal interpretation of a good supply of all nutrients. This was reached with an average change of only about two kitchen units per day. The main recommendation for foodstuffs was less meat and sausage and more bread, rice, and vegetables.

In a study of population nutritional state we performed for the WHO, the situation in Bangladesh was analyzed using the above-described methods. Starting with the average intake of food consumption, the analysis showed a Prerow value of only 0.3. Big problems occurred in supply of energy, protein, some minerals, and the vitamins A, B_1, and B_2. After optimization, a Prerow value of about 0.8 indicates a satisfactory supply. The recommendation for foodstuffs was: *more of everything, especially more meat.*

Nutrition control with fuzzy methods as described above is applied to high-performance sports at the Olympic level, with great success. In this case, the body-mass index, lipoproteins, serum concentration of ferritin, magnesium, potassium, sodium, and some vitamins are used as indicators. Last but not least, fuzzy sets and fuzzy evaluation are used in nutrition education software by the German Nutrition Society, DGE (Deutsche Gesellschaft für Ernährung), called DGE-PC professional.

8. Discussion and conclusions

A human being does not eat single nutrients but consumes a diet prepared out of a series of food items, which are mixed into meals and menus. The goal of an optimization is to combine different foodstuffs over a period of time (e.g., a week) so that the result represents an optimal intake of nutrients. The possible combinations of all food items in different amounts cannot be determined without the help of a computer program. With its help, the nutrient value of meals can be calculated quickly and thus the effect of changes within the meal components can be recognized. With the traditional optimization method, it was not possible to determine an optimal nutrition due to the complex task of fulfilling all RDAs exactly. If a diet has to be improved in a conventional way, single food items should be exchanged and a complete new calculation of the diet is necessary.

A common conflict is bound to appear: the exchange of one food item would surely change one nutrient, but at the same time it might alternate a different nutrient to such an extent that the other nutrient is not equivalent to the corresponding RDA. Up to now, an optimal compromise was sought for each individual. Needless to say, few compromises are near optimal. Using fuzzy sets and fuzzy decision making [13], it is possible to calculate a diet optimally fulfilling the criteria of different goals. These can be nutritional as well as economic goals. The main criterion is to reach the highest possible Prerow value with minimal changes. Nutrients with higher deviation from the set RDAs (low fuzzy value) are primarily considered.

Fuzzy logic and fuzzy decision making allow a new assessment of nutritional intake. If each RDA is formulated as a fuzzy set and the Prerow-value represents a "physiologic value" of the complete nutritional intake, a quick judgement of a nutritional situation is possible. This also shows that rigid RDAs do not correspond with the real situation. It is not the fulfillment or nonfulfillment of the RDAs, but a transitional stage which can be described continuously.

References

[1] Guthrie, H.A. and Picciano, M.F., *Human Nutrition.* Mosby, St. Louis, Missouri, 1995.

[2] *U.S. Department of Health and Human Services: The surgeon general's report on nutrition and health*, U.S. Public Health Service Pub No. 88-50210, Washington DC, Government Printing, 1988.

[3] Ziegler, E.E. and Filer, L.J. (Eds.), *Present Knowledge in Nutrition*, ILSI Press, 7th. Edition, Washington DC, 1996.

[4] Hahn, A., Pfeiffenberg, P., Wirsam, B., and Leitzmann, C., Bewertung und optimierung der nährstoffzufuhr mit hilfe der fuzzy-logik. *Ernährungsumschau*, 442, 367-714, 1995.

[5] Wirsam, B., Fuzzy-sets - ein neuer weg zu einer optimierten ernährung, *Ernährungsumschau* 42, 95-96, 1995.

[6] Zadeh, L.A., *The concept of a linguistic variable and its application to approximate reasoning*, Memorandum ERL-M 411, Berkeley, CA, 1973.

[7] *NRC: Recommended Dietary Allowances*, 10th edition, NRC, Washington, DC, 1989.

[8] Wirsam, B. and Uthus, E.O., The use of fuzzy logic in nutrition, *J. Nutr.* 126, 2337S-2341S, 1996.

[9] Wirsam, B., Hahn, A., Uthus, E.O., and Leitzmann, C., Fuzzy sets and fuzzy decision making in nutrition, *Eur. J. Clin. Nutr.*, 51, 286-296, 1997.

[10] Ornish, D., Brown, S.E., Scherwitz, L.W., Billings, J.H., Armstrong, W.T., Ports, T.A., McLanahan, S.M., Kirkheeide, R.L., Brand, R.J., and Gould, K.L., Can lifestyle changes reverse coronary heart disease?, *Lancet*, 336, 129-133, 1990.

[11] Thomas, E.A., Bailey, L.B., Kauwell, G.A., Lee, D., and Cousins, R.J., Erythrocyte metallothionein response to dietary zinc in human, *J. Nutr.* 122, 2408-2414, 1992.

[12] SCF: Commission of the European Communities: Nutrient and energy intakes for the European Community. *Reports of the Scientific Committee for Food* (31st Series), EC: Brussels, 1993.

[13] Mayer, A., Mechler, B., Schindwein, A., and Wolke R., *Fuzzy-Logic*, Addison-Wesley Publishing Company, Bonn, Paris, Reading, Mass., 1993.

Chapter 11

Designing experiments for medical diagnosis evaluation using membership functions

José Luis Verdegay and Alejandro Sancho-Royo

Training is an important issue in all professions and it is specifically essential in medicine. The ability to make a correct diagnosis has to be assessed as a part of training. The evaluation of the diagnosis ability is usually performed based on senior physician diagnosis.

Medical diagnosis evaluation in a clinical context is the focus of this chapter. To solve this problem, one proposes a fuzzy set-based experiment design. The membership functions are built based on the Theory of Psychological Measurement, using scaling methods. The main tasks related to the scaling methods are analyzed, and conditions for extracting the membership functions are derived. The proposed method and the related experiments that can be built upon are aimed to allow the acquisition of medical experience in diagnosis. Although initially the hypotheses are informally stated, by using the framework of the proposed methodology here, they can be precisely determined and then validated.

1. Introduction

A good diagnosis based on the symptoms that a patient displays is of great importance. In addition, in the field of medicine, the very definition and classification of the upheavals are in themselves an object of analysis that is difficult to solve except for some specific experimental purposes. For example, in the case of Primary Care, several difficulties in detecting various mental disorders have been encountered [1]. In particular, the study of the diagnosis capability of these disorders by the physicians is highly important [2]. We may find that medical diagnosis is difficult in two ways: first, in the definition of the classification itself and second, during the process of diagnosing. We should also emphasize that the prognosis is an important element in medical decision making; moreover, it is mandatory to communicate it to the patient and her/his relatives. When reporting the prognosis to the patient and her/his relatives, the prognosis has to be described using vague attributes. According to the established conventions, it is understood that all patients diagnosed with mental disorders with the attribute *"serious"* have the same state of gravity. However, it is well known that although a patient state is still serious, various degrees may be assigned to this state. It therefore makes sense to study these problems of diagnosis in the context of fuzzy sets.

The first task involved is the construction of membership functions associated to the different characteristics to be evaluated. Based on them, one can extend the use of fuzzy sets and systems in a medical context, and sentences such as "patient A's condition is serious to degree x," or "A shows symptoms of X to degree y" can be represented.

When the characteristic to be evaluated relates to a direct measurement on a continuum (e.g., age, body temperature, etc.), methods to construct the membership functions exist. When this is not possible, we have to resort to other methods to construct the associate membership functions. In this last case, the characteristic or adjective that is evaluated cannot be put into a direct form in relation to a measurement continuum (e.g., the prognosis, the severity of disease, the risk of contracting it, the capacity of recovery, etc.). From this point of view, several methods for constructing membership functions based on the Theory of Psychological Measurement, will be introduced. These methods are associated to specific circumstances. This objective will be achieved in Section 2.

In Section 3, a general framework for using the membership functions developed by comparative tools is proposed. Moreover, the design of an experiment will be considered which, in a clinical context, allows us to compare the diagnosis proposed by junior specialists with the diagnosis of experienced physicians. A discussion of the methods presented in this chapter is given in Section 4.

2. Membership functions built using measurement theory

Let X be the set of elements (objects) to be evaluated. All existing methods for constructing membership functions assume a function $V : X \to U$, from the element set, X, to a numerical referential U. Generally, U is an interval in the wider sense of a real straight line, that is, an interval with finite or infinite limits.

When dealing with linguistic terms in relation to attributes that cannot be directly measured, for example, *gravity*, *severity*, *risks*, ... the usual methods for constructing membership functions are not valid as they appear.

The scaling methods in the Theory of Psychological Measurement are appropriate tools for these kinds of problems. In this section, we describe the techniques to extract the membership functions for the fuzzy characteristics or attributes of an object, using the classic scaling methods.

We want to clarify the meaning of the word *"object"* in this context. Generally, what is evaluated in the medical scope is not the patient as a person but a medical corpus of data such as: a given clinical history, a diagnostic test, etc. In this sense, we reason about "objects" or "evaluated elements" instead of referring to the patients themselves.

Given a finite object set, any scaling method can produce a scale. If this scale is an interval scale, it has a map on an interval I. Moreover, this map associates to each object a real value on this interval. The scale can be understood as the valuation (for a subject or for an assembly of subjects) of a certain characteristic of the object. Nevertheless, a measurement interval does not itself guarantee the existence of a fuzzy set at such an interval. In this respect, the works of Norwich and Turksen, and Turksen [3, 4, 5, 6, 7] have based the construction of membership functions of fuzzy sets on the Theory of Psychological Measurement [8].

Assume that an empirical structure of membership for the object sets can be established and based on it and on the comparison of pairs of objects, a structure can be constructed. Then, the scale obtained can be interpreted as a fuzzy set on X by making a transformation of I in the unit interval [0, 1].

The permissible transformations in scales of intervals are linear transformations. Therefore, if the scale is an interval scale and this structure of membership exists, the associated membership function must be unique, because there is only one positive linear transformation of $I = [\alpha, \beta]$ to [0, 1], namely,

$$y = \frac{x}{\beta - \alpha} - \frac{\alpha}{\beta - \alpha}.$$

The methods of information gathering can be classified generally according to the following categories [9]: simple "stimuli" tasks, alternatives choice tasks, stimuli comparison tasks, and stimuli arrangement tasks. Here, we consider judgement tasks. In a judgement task, the subject emits a judgement about the considered stimuli. In the following section, we will describe several types of tasks.

2.1. Various tasks for information gathering

Since these tasks of information gathering were born in a psychological context, we maintain the stimulus concept referring to each of the objects set out for their evaluation. In this context, we are talking about each of the clinical histories, tests of diagnosis, etc., whose fuzzy characteristics are going to be evaluated by specialists. For this reason, the terms *stimulus* and *object* are considered synonymous. Also, remember that the subjects here are specialists (doctors).

2.1.1. Simple stimuli task

In a simple stimuli task, a dichotomizing answer in relation to a stimulus is requested of the subject. Let us introduce an example. Consider the stimulus is a chest X-ray, and the question asked the subject is "Can the situation of the patient be considered serious?" This sentence has two possible answers: "Yes/No." For this task, a collective membership function is obtained (from the set of specialists). If we want to obtain an individual membership function, we have to make repeated measures for each subject.

2.1.2. Alternative choice task

In this case, the task consists of the selection of an answer among a small number of possibilities, generally ordered linguistics expressions in increasing order, e.g., $1 \leftrightarrow$ Very Low; $2 \leftrightarrow$ Low; $3 \leftrightarrow$ Medium; $4 \leftrightarrow$ High; $5 \leftrightarrow$ Very high. Generally, the number of linguistic degrees is an odd number: 3, 5, 7, and less frequently 9 or higher [10, 11].

It is interesting to make a distinction among these alternatives – as proposed to the subject – and other verbal labels that can be used within a data processing model in the context of fuzzy sets. The use of ordered strings of linguistic expressions is common. Many authors analyzed the use of connectives and the relationships established among linguistic expressions. Bonisonne and Decker [12] essentially contributed to this topic. These linguistic alternatives are not designed for their use with experimental subjects. The linguistics alternatives in this last case are designed for their use in expert systems that operate in conditions of uncertainty.

Maintaining the previous example, the difference consists of the number of alternative answers. That is, once the said X-ray has been shown, the specialist would be asked the following question, "How do you consider the patient's gravity?" The answer may be

1. Not serious
2. A bit serious
3. Serious (Fairly serious)
4. Rather serious
5. Very serious (Extremely serious)

Several sets of alternatives are possible. Some classical methods for obtaining scales start from choices with verbal [10] or numerical alternatives [13].

2.1.3. Stimuli comparison task

Let us assume that we form all the possible groups of m objects. We show these groups to the subjects and we ask them to state which group has the fuzzy quality that is evaluated to the greatest extent. Its application for the previous example is as follows: the subject is asked to choose from each group of images shown the one he/she feels is representative of the most "serious" case.

2.1.4. Stimuli arrangement task

The task consists of ordering groups in the object set according to the characteristic to be evaluated. An arrangement task is simply a task of successive comparisons. One chooses the best one, then the best one from the rest, and so on.

2.2. Membership functions for various tasks

Once we have described the elementary tasks on which the scaling methods are based, our intention is to find under what conditions it is possible to associate a model for the construction of membership functions to these methods. Norwich and Turksen [7] demonstrate that for this purpose we need the existence of an empirical structure to which a scale can be associated. This scale must be at least ordinal. This means that it will be unique up to monotonous transformations. However, this is not enough if we want the membership function obtained by means of the task studied to be unique.

To obtain the uniqueness, it is necessary to extend the empirical structure to pairs of stimuli (i.e., to the Cartesian product of the set of stimuli by itself). Furthermore, it is necessary to build a structure of comparable differences [6].

According to the results reported in [5], this structure generates a unique scale of intervals except for positive linear transformations. Because the scale obtained is on the [0,1] interval, the membership function is unique.

When we state that the membership function is unique, we mean that there is no other membership function associated to the empirical structure; moreover, we assume that the structure of comparable differences is defined. Possibly, given an information-gathering task there is more than one way to define the membership structures. Nevertheless, we think that those that are going to be proposed for each task here are the simplest and most intuitive ones, when the average (arithmetic mean) is being used as an operator for the aggregation of each one of the answers from the subjects.

The structures mentioned in the previous paragraph can be constructed for these classic scaling methods [9, 14]. We introduce the definitions of the membership functions associated to these tasks. The details, including the definition of the constructed structures and the demonstration of their properties are omitted here. (These details and demonstrations can be found in [14].)

We use the following notations. Let $X = \{x_1,..., x_m\}$ be a finite set of m stimuli. Let A be a fuzzy quality to be evaluated for these objects (e.g., "*serious*"). Let $S = \{e_1,..., e_n\}$ be a set of experts (specialists). Let $\mu_A(x_j)$ represent the degree to which the object x_j is evaluated with respect to the quality, A. Then, $\mu_A(x_j) \in [0,1]$ for all j, since μ is a membership function on X.

2.2.1. Simple stimuli task

In this task, each specialist is asked, for each x_j, the question: "Is x_j in state A ('*serious*')?"

Let l_{ij} ($i = 1,..., n$, and $j = 1,..., m$) be the answer of the subject i to the question relating to object j, coded with 1 for a positive answer and 0 for a negative answer.

We define

$$\mu_A(x_j) = \frac{\sum\limits_{i=1}^{n} l_{ij}}{n} \tag{1}$$

Notice that $\mu_A(x_j) = 0$ if and only if all the specialists answer negatively. Moreover, $\mu_A(x_j) = 1$ if and only if all the experts answer in the positive way. In this type of task, the membership function obtained is collective, unless we resort to repeated measures.

2.2.2. Alternative choice task

Using the same notation as in the previous section, let the possible answers be: $\{a_0, a_1,..., a_h\}$ (for example, *very little, little, average, enough, a lot*).

Let l_{ij} be the i-th specialist's answer to the question relating to the object j, coded as 0 for the answer a_0, 1 for $a_1,...,$ and h for a_h.

We define

$$\mu_A(x_j) = \frac{\sum_{i=1}^{n} l_{ij}}{n \cdot h} \tag{2}$$

Here, $\mu_A(x_j) \in [0,1]$ for all j. We can see that $\mu_A(x_j) = 0$ if and only if all the subjects answer with the alternative a_0 for stimulus j, whereas $\mu_A(x_j) = 1$ if and only if all the subjects answer a_h for this stimulus. (Only in the case that all experts select the last response alternative a_h, coded by h the membership function has value 1; the formula assumes the response alternatives are ordered accordingly.) In the same way as before, the resulting function μ_A is referred to as the specialist set. We say that μ_A is a collective function. For constructing a membership function that represents an individual response, we have to resort to repeated measures as before.

2.2.3. Stimuli comparison task

Let $\sigma_1,..., \sigma_k$ be groups ($t \le m$) of t objects of X. Let us remember that the specialist has to choose, for each group, the most representative object for the characteristic to be evaluated. Let $l_{ij} = 1$ if the stimulus x_j is chosen in group σ_i and 0 in another case (here $i = 1..., k$ and $j = 1..., m$).

We define

$$\mu_A(x_j) = \frac{\sum_{i=1}^{k} l_{ij}}{k} \tag{3}$$

In the two previous tasks, membership functions for the stimuli were obtained for a group of specialists. Now, we obtain them for a single subject. In the definition of the membership function in Equations (1) and (2), the addition is extended to the specialist set. For the case in Equation (3), the addition is extended to the groups. By construction, the following situation occurs: $\mu_A(x_j) = 0$ if and only if the object x_j is not chosen in any group, whereas $\mu_A(x_j) = 1$ if and only if this object is chosen in all the groups, when it appears.

2.2.4. Stimuli arrangement task

Let $\sigma_1,..., \sigma_k$, be groups ($t \leq m$) of objects from X. The specialist is asked to order these groups from a greater to a smaller degree, in relation to the evaluated characteristic.

Let l_{ij} ($i = 1..., k$ and $j = 1,..., m$) be the order that x_j takes in group σ_i ; we assume $l_{ij} = 0$ if x_j does not appear in σ_i.

If

$$\Gamma(x) = \begin{cases} 1 & if \quad x \neq 0 \\ 0 & if \quad x = 0 \end{cases} \tag{4}$$

we define

$$\mu_A(x_j) = \frac{\dfrac{\sum\limits_{i=1}^{k} l_{ij}}{\sum\limits_{i=1}^{k} \Gamma(l_{ij})} - t}{1 - t} \tag{5}$$

If $x_{min} = x_r$ is the last object in all groups when it appears, then

$$\mu_A(x_{min}) = \mu_A(x_r) = \frac{\dfrac{M \cdot t}{M} - 1}{1 - t} = 0 \tag{6}$$

Moreover, if $x_{max} = x_r$ is the first object in all groups when it appears, then

$$\mu_A(x_{min}) = \mu_A(x_r) = \frac{\dfrac{M \cdot t}{M} - 1}{1 - t} = 1 - t \tag{7}$$

2.2.5. Example

Let us assume that $X = \{a, b, c, d, e\}$ represents the object set to be evaluated. Groups of four of these stimuli are shown to five subjects and they are asked to arrange the groups from greater to smaller with respect to their seriousness. Let us assume that the arrangements offered the five specialists are those shown in Table 1.

<table>
<tr><td colspan="6" align="center">Table 1
Stimuli Arrangement</td></tr>
<tr><td>SUBJECT</td><td>t-uple #1</td><td>t-uple #2</td><td>t-uple #3</td><td>t-uple #4</td><td>t-uple #5</td></tr>
<tr><td>1</td><td>bcad</td><td>bcde</td><td>bcea</td><td>bead</td><td>cead</td></tr>
<tr><td>2</td><td>cbda</td><td>bced</td><td>bcea</td><td>beda</td><td>ceda</td></tr>
<tr><td>3</td><td>bcad</td><td>bced</td><td>bcea</td><td>bead</td><td>cead</td></tr>
<tr><td>4</td><td>bcad</td><td>becd</td><td>bcea</td><td>bead</td><td>ecad</td></tr>
<tr><td>5</td><td>cdba</td><td>cbed</td><td>cbae</td><td>ebad</td><td>cead</td></tr>
</table>

By means of the membership function defined in Section 2.2.4, for $m = 5$ and $t = 4$, we obtain the membership values as in Table 2.

<table>
<tr><td colspan="6" align="center">Table 2
Membership values</td></tr>
<tr><td>SUBJECT</td><td>OBJECT a</td><td>OBJECT b</td><td>OBJECT c</td><td>OBJECT d</td><td>OBJECT e</td></tr>
<tr><td>1</td><td>0,25</td><td>1,00</td><td>0,75</td><td>0,08</td><td>0,42</td></tr>
<tr><td>2</td><td>0,00</td><td>0,92</td><td>0,83</td><td>0,25</td><td>0,50</td></tr>
<tr><td>3</td><td>0,25</td><td>1,00</td><td>0,75</td><td>0,00</td><td>0,50</td></tr>
<tr><td>4</td><td>0,25</td><td>1,00</td><td>0,58</td><td>0,00</td><td>0,67</td></tr>
<tr><td>5</td><td>0,25</td><td>0,58</td><td>1,00</td><td>0,17</td><td>0,50</td></tr>
</table>

The table can be easily interpreted: the values indicate the level of gravity of the state of each of the patients to whom the objects refer. The table must be understood within the present context, i.e., an object with degree 0.00 means that the one amongst the stimuli shown is, for the specialist, the one with the least gravity, without any doubt. The membership functions obtained are, by their very nature, contextual to the stimuli set considered.

2.3. Aggregation of evaluations

When we have a collection of individual membership functions, the construction of a collective membership function may be necessary, i.e., adding the evaluations of the different subjects.

We could formulate the problem in the following way. Let $X = \{x_1, ..., x_m\}$ be the finite set that represents m stimuli, let $A_1,..., A_n \in P^f(X)$ be n fuzzy subsets, corresponding to the same amount of evaluations of a characteristic A carried out by n subjects.

What is the total evaluation $A_T \in P^f(X)$ that represents the joint evaluation of the n subjects?

If we want the membership function of A_T to be consistent with the membership empirical structure, it is necessary that the construction method for A_T be the same as that for $A_1,..., A_n \in P^f(X)$. In [14] it may be seen that, for the tasks discussed, the membership function A_T is constructed by means of the average of $A_1,..., A_n \in P^f(X)$.

$$\mu_{A_T}(x_j) = \frac{\sum_{k=1}^{n} \mu_{A_k}(x_j)}{n} \tag{8}$$

In fact, this result is the only compatible one with the definitions of membership functions for the different tasks given in this chapter. Details on the meaning of this compatibility can be found in [14].

3. A general framework for applications

In any judgement task, we can distinguish among three types of elements: the subjects, the stimuli or objects, and the characteristic that is judged. This characteristic may be assumed to be described by an adjective or equivalent linguistic construction.

Given a stimuli set $X = \{e_1, ..., e_n\}$, an adjective set $A = \{A_1, ..., A_m,\}$, and a subject set $S = \{s_1, ..., s_l\}$, we call $A^k_j(e_i)$ the membership degree of the stimulus e_i ($i = 1, ..., n$) according to the adjective A_j ($j = 1, ..., m$) evaluated by the individual s_k ($k = 1, ..., l$). We call the sets X, A, and S element sets.

Coherence measures were defined and constructed that allow us to compare different fuzzy evaluations, like those we are dealing with here [14]. Also, a method for the construction of partitions was developed for various index sets, based on coherence among the evaluations [14]. These tools and the aggregation of evaluations (Section 2.3.) allow us to obtain the objectives described in the next section.

3.1. Objectives

3.1.1. Individual objectives

Objective 1. Case of subjects not separated into groups. Classify the subjects into homogeneous groups in relation to $A^k_j(e_i)$ in each $s_k \in S$. If the subjects are grouped, compare these groups for two criteria:

1) the total evaluations of the groups for each A_j and each e_i, and
2) the coherence of the subjects among themselves (intra-subject), among the individuals in the same group (intra-group), and coherence among the individuals in different groups (inter-groups).

Objective 2. Relate these subjects and groups of subjects to other subject variables. These variables may be fuzzy or classical (crisp).

3.1.2. Stimuli objectives

Objective 1. Case of stimuli not separated into groups. Classify the stimuli into homogeneous groups in relation to $A^k_j(e_i)$ in each $e_i \in X$.
Case of grouped stimuli. Compare these groups for two criteria:

1) the total evaluations of the groups for each A_j and each s_k, and
2) the coherence among the stimuli with themselves (intra-stimuli), of the stimuli in the same group (intra-group), and coherence among the stimuli of different groups (inter-groups).

Objective 2. Relate these stimuli and groups of stimuli to other stimuli variables. Again, these variables may be fuzzy or classical.

3.1.3. Characteristic-related objectives

Objective 1.
Case 1. The adjectives are not separated into groups. Classify the adjectives into homogeneous groups in relation to $A^k_j(e_i)$ in each $A_j \in A$.
Case 2. The adjectives are grouped. Compare these groups for two criteria:
1) the total evaluations of the groups for each e_i and each s_k, and
2) the coherence of the adjectives amongst themselves (intra-adjective), of the adjectives in the same group (intra-group), and the coherence among the adjectives in different groups (inter-groups).

Objective 2. Relate these adjectives and groups of adjectives to other adjective variables. The variables may be fuzzy or classical.
The objectives described are among the most general ones in any methodology for the investigation and processing of data: classify, compare, and group the information. Objective 1 considers the classification of the subjects, stimuli, and adjectives, respectively. Sometimes that classification is *a priori* data, while in other cases, it is exactly the result of the analysis. Here, we assume that the classifications of element sets (X, A, S) are given previously. Otherwise, it is possible to resort to classic or fuzzy methods of classification.

In addition to these, in [14] a classification tool was developed for element sets based on the coherence measures. The presentation of this method is not in the scope of this chapter.

In any case, once given a classification of the elements (subject, stimuli or adjectives), the immediate question is whether these groups differ from each other and to what extent. The measures of coherence defined in [14] allow us to make this comparison in a way that, we think, is sensitive to the evaluated adjectives semantic. As may be seen, the proposed formal processing is symmetrical in relation to the role played by subjects, stimuli, and adjectives in the framework of applications. Nevertheless, in each context of application, as may be seen later, this symmetry may or may not be significant. Indeed, for each $i = 1, ..., n$; $j = 1, ..., m$; $k = 1, ..., l$ indices that represents the stimuli, adjectives, and subjects, respectively, there is a value $A^k_j(e_i) \in [0,1]$. This is why for each application (at least formally) we have a matrix **M** with $n \times m \times l$ elements in the interval unit.

Given *X, A,* and *S,* as they were previously defined, any tasks of psychological measurement, along with the construction methods developed for membership functions in this work, will produce the matrix **M**.

From a formal point of view, the definition of coherence measures for $P^f(X)$, may also be defined for $P^f(A)$ and for $P^f(S)$, immediately, when applying the processing to rows, columns, or lists from the matrix [14]. Formally, we can consider $A^k_j(e_i) \in [0,1]$ having m times l elements (with n components) of $P^f(X)$, having n times m elements (with l components) of $P^f(S)$, or having n times l elements (with m components) of $P^f(A)$. In all these cases, we can calculate coherence measures for each of the indices considered.

Example:

<table>
<tr><td colspan="4" align="center">Table 3
Example: Evaluations Data</td></tr>
<tr><td rowspan="4">M_{A1}</td><td>0.42</td><td>1.00</td><td>0.75</td></tr>
<tr><td>0.33</td><td>1.00</td><td>0.75</td></tr>
<tr><td>0.33</td><td>1.00</td><td>0.75</td></tr>
<tr><td>0.08</td><td>1.00</td><td>0.75</td></tr>
<tr><td rowspan="4">M_{A2}</td><td>1.00</td><td>0.00</td><td>0.42</td></tr>
<tr><td>0.83</td><td>0.00</td><td>0.42</td></tr>
<tr><td>1.00</td><td>0.08</td><td>0.67</td></tr>
<tr><td>0.58</td><td>0.50</td><td>0.92</td></tr>
</table>

Let $X = \{e_1, e_2, e_3\}$ be the set of the evaluated stimuli, $A = \{A_1, A_2\}$ the characteristics that in this example can be "*seriousness*" and "*capacity of recovery*", and $S = \{s_1, s_2, s_3, s_4\}$ the set of subjects. The matrix formed by M_{A1} and M_{A2} is **M**, where these represent the results of the evaluations (membership functions) relating to both adjectives of A. **M** can be considered as a 2×3×4 matrix (Table 3).

We consider here, for the sake of simplicity, Yager's measure of coherence (Y_{max}). This measure comes from Yager's work on the measurement of ambiguity [15, 16, 17, 18] and using the extension theorem shown in [14]. This theorem allows us to extend a wide range of measures of ambiguity to measures of coherence between evaluations. In this theorem for each measure of ambiguity, one can produce two measures of coherence by using the operators *max* and *min*. A formulation of the measure of coherence Y_{max} is given by [14].

$$\beta_{Y_{max}}(A, B) = \sum_{i \in J_{11}} \left(\frac{1}{m} - \left(\frac{1}{m} \cdot \max(a_i, b_i) \right) \right) +$$

$$+ \sum_{i \in J_{12}} \left(\frac{1}{m} - \left(\frac{1}{m} \cdot \max(a_i, 1 - b_i) \right) \right) + \sum_{i \in J_{21}} \left(\frac{1}{m} - \left(\frac{1}{m} \cdot \max(1 - a_i, b_i) \right) \right) + \quad (9)$$

$$+ \sum_{i \in J_{22}} \left(\frac{1}{m} - \left(\frac{1}{m} \cdot \max(1 - a_i, 1 - b_i) \right) \right)$$

Next we will develop all possible coherence measurement values to be computed with these data and the measure of coherence Y_{max}.

<table>
<tr><td colspan="8" align="center">Table 4
Example: Coherence matrices among subjects by adjectives</td></tr>
<tr><td colspan="4" align="center">Adjective #1</td><td colspan="4" align="center">Adjective #2</td></tr>
<tr><td>0.78</td><td>0.78</td><td>0.78</td><td>0.78</td><td>0.86</td><td>0.80</td><td>0.76</td><td>0.50</td></tr>
<tr><td>0.78</td><td>0.81</td><td>0.81</td><td>0.81</td><td>0.80</td><td>0.80</td><td>0.75</td><td>0.50</td></tr>
<tr><td>0.78</td><td>0.81</td><td>0.81</td><td>0.81</td><td>0.76</td><td>0.75</td><td>0.88</td><td>0.58</td></tr>
<tr><td>0.78</td><td>0.81</td><td>0.81</td><td>0.81</td><td>0.5</td><td>0.5</td><td>0.58</td><td>0.67</td></tr>
</table>

Coherence among the subjects (intrasubject) can be computed using adjectives (and they are given by two symmetrical matrices 4×4, one for each adjective, Table 4) or by stimuli (three symmetrical matrices 4×4, one for each stimulus, Table 5).

<table>
<tr><td colspan="4" align="center">Table 5
Example. Matrices of coherences among subjects by stimuli</td></tr>
<tr><td colspan="4" align="center">Stimulus #1</td></tr>
<tr><td>0.79</td><td>0.70</td><td>0.79</td><td>0.58</td></tr>
<tr><td>0.70</td><td>0.75</td><td>0.75</td><td>0.63</td></tr>
<tr><td>0.79</td><td>0.75</td><td>0.83</td><td>0.63</td></tr>
<tr><td>0.58</td><td>0.63</td><td>0.63</td><td>0.75</td></tr>
<tr><td colspan="4" align="center">Stimulus #2</td></tr>
<tr><td>1</td><td>1</td><td>0.96</td><td>0.75</td></tr>
<tr><td>1</td><td>1</td><td>0.96</td><td>0.75</td></tr>
<tr><td>0.96</td><td>0.96</td><td>0.96</td><td>0.75</td></tr>
<tr><td>0.75</td><td>0.75</td><td>0.75</td><td>0.75</td></tr>
<tr><td colspan="4" align="center">Stimulus #3</td></tr>
<tr><td>0.67</td><td>0.67</td><td>0.59</td><td>0.59</td></tr>
<tr><td>0.67</td><td>0.67</td><td>0.59</td><td>0.59</td></tr>
<tr><td>0.59</td><td>0.59</td><td>0.71</td><td>0.71</td></tr>
<tr><td>0.59</td><td>0.59</td><td>0.71</td><td>0.84</td></tr>
</table>

<table>
<tr><td colspan="6" align="center">Table 6
Example: Matrices of coherence values among stimuli by adjectives</td></tr>
<tr><td colspan="3" align="center">Adjective #1</td><td colspan="3" align="center">Adjective #2</td></tr>
<tr><td>0.72</td><td>0.29</td><td>0.29</td><td>0.85</td><td>0.19</td><td>0.52</td></tr>
<tr><td>0.29</td><td>1</td><td>0.75</td><td>0.19</td><td>0.86</td><td>0.5</td></tr>
<tr><td>0.29</td><td>0.75</td><td>0.75</td><td>0.52</td><td>0.5</td><td>0.69</td></tr>
</table>

Finally, coherence among the adjectives can be computed for each stimulus (three matrices 2×2, Table 8) or for each subject (four matrices 2×2, Table 9).

Table 7					
Example: Matrices of coherences among stimuli by subjects					
Subject #1			Subject #2		
0.79	0.34	0.42	0.75	0.3	0.38
0.34	1	0.67	0.3	1	0.67
0.42	0.67	0.67	0.38	0.67	0.67
Subject #3			Subject #4		
0.83	0.21	0.5	0.75	0.29	0.29
0.21	0.96	0.54	0.29	0.75	0.63
0.5	0.54	0.71	0.29	0.63	0.84

Table 8					
Example: Matrices of coherence values among adjectives by stimuli					
Stimulus #1		Stimulus #2		Stimulus #3	
0.72	0.38	1	0.145	0.75	0.57
0.38	0.85	0.145	0.86	0.57	0.69

We briefly comment on this example to provide an interpretation of its meaning. In relation to the subjects, the three first subjects are very coherent to each other; nevertheless, subject #4 interprets the characteristic *"capacity of recovery"* in a different way than the rest of the subjects; for the other adjective, *"seriousness,"* this difference is not observed.

Table 9			
Example: Matrices of coherence values among adjectives by subjects			
Subject #1		Subject #2	
0.78	0.24	0.81	0.25
0.24	0.86	0.25	0.80
Subject #3		Subject #4	
0.81	0.36	0.89	0.56
0.36	0.88	0.56	0.67

In relation to the stimuli, the stimuli are distinguished among themselves very well, with the difference between stimuli #1 and #2 being more noticeable. For example, for the second adjective, stimuli #1 and #2 may be considered to be opposite.

In relation to the adjectives, the adjectives can be considered as almost the opposite meaning for all the subjects except for #4. The stimulus that best separates these adjectives is two.

The fact that a certain calculation of coherence may be formally settled does not mean that it is significant for all applications. In fact, hardly any combination of indices for the calculation of coherence among evaluations could be significant. What was stated in the previous paragraphs is the possibility of making this formal calculation. The sense of the calculation will give the concrete application for it, that is, the context in which this one is located. In certain situations, the computation of coherence is not of interest; in other cases, it could be the object of the study.

3.2. An experimental design for medical diagnosis evaluation

Next we design an experiment that tries to recognize the acquisition of medical experience in diagnosis. As a starting point, we can raise the fact that in a certain medical service we can find specialists with different degrees of experience. An experiment similar to this one has been carried out in the context of an educational institution [14]. The results of the experiment confirmed the possibility of recognizing the transmission of knowledge within a scant structure and by means of the exclusive use of fuzzy adjectives. In this experiment, 29 adjectives were studied. We could find that some adjectives separate well the individuals among themselves: the teachers from the more experienced students, and these from the beginners. Other adjectives do not separate the individuals into groups. We can, therefore, find verbal labels (adjectives) that "transmit" a greater amount of information, and we can study the agreement on their meaning among the subjects.

In this context, an experimental design for medical diagnosis is aimed at
a) Contrasting if the effective acquisition of experience occurs in the service,
b) Contrasting the predictive capacity of the medical staff,
c) Distinguishing the agreement among the specialists in the use of adjectives.

With the purpose of approaching these objectives, we raised the following elements:

3.2.1. Experimental elements: individuals, stimuli, characteristics

Individuals are doctors from the same service and working in the same specialty. As a hypothetical example, we assume that they are medical staff in an emergency care service. These specialists can previously be classified (e.g., consultants, residents, interns, students...), with which we would form different groups of subjects. Again, to establish our ideas, we assume that we have four groups G_1, G_2, G_3, and G_4 of specialists in decreasing order as far as their experience in the service is concerned.

Stimuli or objects to evaluate: X-rays of fractures or traumas along with a standardized description of the patient: age, sex, height, weight, etc. Let us assume that we have six stimuli of this type. Each stimulus is a set of data, of course. The data shown for the patient are those that correspond to the date on which the accident took place. Nevertheless, in order to be able to analyze the specialists' predictive capacity in the experiment, each one of these stimuli should take on an associated description (that, obviously, should not be shown to the specialists) of their evolution, recovery, etc.

The different fuzzy adjectives for medical use or for communication with relatives, nonmedical institutions, etc. would be the characteristics to be evaluated. In this case, we can select "seriousness," "capacity of recovery," "need for medical care," "possibility of complications," etc.

We start with the fact that this description is hypothetical and that, in each case, the professionals should understand which is the fuzzy adjective whose study arouses the highest interest that is most required in a health environment.

3.2.2. Tasks

Any studied task can be exposed to the subjects. We propose for this experiment a task for arranging stimuli into groups. Here, we set groups of five stimuli, with which we have 5 stimuli in each of 6 groups. For each one of these groups of five stimuli, we ask the specialist to arrange them from the greatest to the lowest with respect to each of the characteristics being evaluated. Therefore, the following questions or propositions can be asked for each group of five stimuli:

a) Could you order the X-rays starting with the most serious one and ending with the least serious one?

b) Please order the X-rays starting with the one showing the highest capacity of recovery and ending with the one showing the lowest capacity of recovery.

c) Please order the X-rays starting with the one showing the highest need for care and ending with the one showing the lowest need for care.

d) Could you order the x-rays starting with the one showing the highest possibility of complications and ending with the one showing the lowest possibility of complications?

In order to avoid the effect of memory as far as possible, we need to effectively separate each group of stimuli. This can be done in two ways: separating the sessions in time or introducing spurious stimuli among each group of stimuli in the experiment.

3.2.3. Hypotheses and objectives

With respect to objective a) "Contrasting whether the effective acquisition of experience occurs in the service," we can raise the following informal hypotheses:

H1: The doctors' answers are more coherent as their experience in the service increases.

H2: The differences with respect to coherence will be more noticeable at the beginning than at the end of the process of experience acquisition.

With respect to the objective b) "Contrast the doctors' predictive capacity," we can assume the informal hypothesis,

H3: The medical predictive capacity increases with experience.

If we deal with the objective c) "Distinguish the agreement among the specialists in the use of the adjectives," we will assume the hypothesis,

H4: The agreement among the specialists increases with experience.

In addition to the hypotheses presented above, the experiment will offer information on each one of the studied characteristics and, of course, on the valuation of each stimulus shown.

3.2.4. Formalization

We are going to determine the hypotheses formulated in the previous section with respect to the tools for the comparison of evaluations [14]. To do so, we define different types of averages or means.

First approach: Total evaluation comparison.

Let us assume that we have two groups: G_1 and G_2, with g_1 and g_2 individuals, respectively, let A_j be any adjective. If we call, for simplicity's sake, $A1_j$ the total evaluation of group 1 with respect to A_j and $A2_j$ to the one in group #2 with respect to this same adjective, we obtain, according to Section 2.3,

$$A1_j(e_i) = \frac{\sum_{x_k \in G_1} A_j^k(e_j)}{g_1}$$

and

$$A2_j(e_i) = \frac{\sum_{x_k \in G2} A_j^k(e_j)}{g_2} \tag{10}$$

Let us denote by *cohe* coherence measure. We can calculate *cohe* $(A1_j, A2_j)$ that provides a way to compare attributes by means of this criterion. Thus, we can define

- Mean of Coherence among total Evaluations of a group (MCEG).

$$MCEG(G) = \frac{\sum_{j=1}^{m} cohe(AT_j, AT_j)}{m} \tag{11}$$

where AT_j represent the total evaluation of group G for adjective j.

- Mean of Coherence among total Evaluations of two groups (MCEEG) .

$$MCEG(G_1, G_2) = \frac{\sum_{j=1}^{m} cohe(A1_j, A2_j)}{m} \tag{12}$$

where $A1_j$, $A2_j$ represent the total evaluations of groups G_1 and G_2, respectively, for adjective j.

In this approach, the total evaluations of each group for a given adjective are compared. This does not seem suitable if we want to compare the subject's criterion coherence. Otherwise, if we want to know the coherence among the evaluations of two groups of subjects without comparing the coherence among the individuals that compose both groups, this approach is then appropriated. In the following approach, coherence among evaluations are compared.

In the second approach, given both groups indicated above, we can calculate and compare, given to an A_j any adjective, three types of averages of coherence among evaluations. We define, in order to simplify, the first two averages for group #1 and the last one for groups #1 and #2.

- Mean of Coherence intra-subject for the adjective j (MCISj).

$$MCIS_j(G_1) = \frac{\displaystyle\sum_{x_k \in G_1} cohe\left(A_j^k, A_j^k\right)}{g_1} \tag{13}$$

- Mean of Coherence intra-group for the adjective j (MCIG$_j$) .

$$MCIG_j(G_1) = \frac{\displaystyle\sum_{\substack{x_k, x_{k'} \in G_1 \\ k < k'}} cohe\left(A_j^k, A_j^{k'}\right)}{\dfrac{g_1 \cdot (g_1 - 1)}{2}} \tag{14}$$

- Mean of Coherence among groups for the adjective j (MCEG$_j$) .

$$MCIS_j(G_1) = \frac{\displaystyle\sum_{\substack{x_k \in G_1 \\ x_{k'} \in G_2}} cohe\left(A_j^k, A_j^{k'}\right)}{g_1 \cdot g_2} \tag{15}$$

Of course, these comparisons can be done considering the total of the adjectives by means of the aggregation of the measures defined for the adjective set, A. Using the average as an aggregation operator, we can define for a given experiment

- Mean of Coherence intra-subject (MCIS).

$$MCIS(G_1) = \frac{\sum_{j=1}^{m} MCIS_j(G_1)}{m} \qquad (16)$$

- Mean of Coherence intra-group (MCIG) .

$$MCIS(G_1) = \frac{\sum_{j=1}^{m} MCIG_j(G_1)}{m} \qquad (17)$$

- Mean of Coherence among groups (MCEG) .

$$MCIS(G_1) = \frac{\sum_{j=1}^{m} MCES_j(G_1,G_2)}{m} \qquad (18)$$

With these definitions, and since we have four groups of individuals labeled as G_1, G_2, G_3, and G_4, the informally raised hypotheses can be formulated as follows:

H1: The medical answers are more coherent as experience in the service increases.

This hypothesis can be reformulated as: the average of the coherence intra-subject increases with service experience,

$$MCIS(G_1) \geq MCIS(G_2) \geq MCIS(G_3) \geq MCIS(G_4)$$

H2: The differences with respect to the coherence will be more noticeable at the beginning than at the end of the experience acquisition process,

$$MCIS(G_4) - MCIS(G_3) \geq MCIS(G_3) - MCIS(G_2) \geq MCIS(G_2) - MCIS(G_1)$$

H3: The medical predictive capacity increases with experience.

To formalize this hypothesis, we must add some terms to the denotation. Let F_j be the final evaluation with respect to the adjective j resulting from ordering the stimuli according to the final data known for each patient. Let us call MCEF(G_v) (v =1,...,4) the average of coherence among the final evaluations and the evaluations of the subjects in the group v. The MCEF definition is equivalent to those given previously. Using this notation, the formalization of this hypothesis reads

$$MCEF(G_1) \geq MCEF(G_2) \geq MCEF(G_3) \geq MCEF(G_4)$$

H4: The agreement among the specialists increases with experience.

One formulation is the coherence intra-group increases with experience,

$$MCIG(G_1) \geq MCIG(G_2) \geq MCIG(G_3) \geq MCIG(G_4)$$

But this hypothesis can also be interpreted as an agreement among groups and not within each group, hence this interpretation gives rise to the formal hypothesis,

$$MCEG(G_4, G_3) \geq MCEG(G_4, G_2) \geq MCEG(G_4, G_1)$$

In addition to these hypotheses, the experiment provides information on the adjectives and stimuli by means of the different matrices of coherence obtained. The approach in this experiment is aimed at extracting and handling information based on linguistic expressions with a vague meaning and therefore, highly context sensitive. Using the formalization of the initial hypotheses, we may effectively compare them. Consequently, we can recognize those individuals who do not agree with the use of the said adjectives according to the majority use. Therefore, for example, for an individual x, we can offer a report of the kind shown in Table 10. The average of the intra-subject coherence for the group of subjects for each adjective is located in the center of the scale. The values in each row refer to the average intra-subject coherence for the subject x and the adjective to which the row refers.

With this report, the subject can recognize his or her degree of ambiguity in the use of certain adjectives: more ambiguous than the average (in Table 10, Adjective #1), more precise than the average (in Table 10, Adjective #5), or about average (gray area).

Similarly, consider we use *MCIG* (for the group to which the subject belongs or for the total group of subjects), instead of the *MCIS*. Then, the subject can recognize those adjectives in which disagreement arises (when under *MCIG*) or a high degree of agreement (when above *MCIG*) with the evaluation of the group considered.

We believe that among other uses these reports may provide interesting feedback to the doctors who have just joined the service in their process of acquiring experience.

Adjective	**MCIS$_j$**	
	- *MCIS$_j$*	+ *MCIS$_j$*
Adj. 1		
Adj. 2		
Adj. 3		
Adj. 4		
Adj. 5		
....		

Table 10

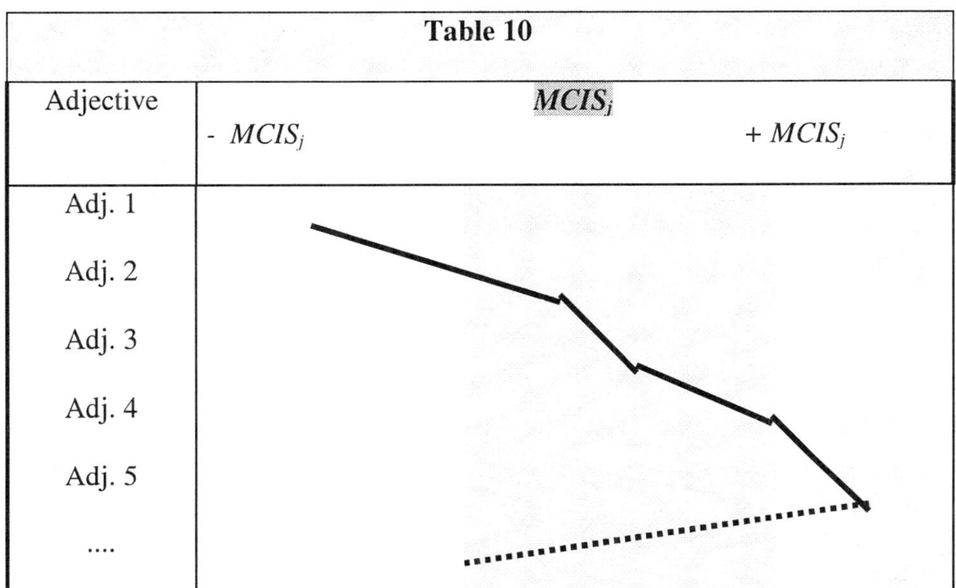

We assume the symmetry among the different elements in the general framework is known. Then, this type of report may be generated for each pair of elements considered and make an average with the remaining elements (after all, it is a way of graphically expressing the columns or rows of the matrices presented earlier). A large amount of information may be extracted from these reports for the experiment. This information may play a relevant role in the evaluation of the service.

4. Conclusions

In this chapter, a method for designing experiments for medical diagnosis evaluation using fuzzy sets has been shown. Fuzzy sets stand for vague characteristics that the specialists use. Several fuzzy adjectives for medical use or for communication with relatives, nonmedical institutions, etc. have been considered.

We showed why and how to use the scaling methods of Psychological Measurement Theory in order to build membership functions for fuzzy sets that are not in direct relation to a measure continuum.

The task of information gathering can be classified generally according to the following categories: simple stimuli tasks, alternative choice tasks, stimuli comparison tasks, and stimuli arrangement tasks. Based on this classification, a method of construction membership functions for these tasks has been built. It has been shown that the obtained membership function is unique for each experiment.

In order to assemble individual membership functions, a method of aggregation of membership functions has been shown. This method is the only one compatible with the definition of membership functions as introduced here.

The design of the experiment results from the hypotheses about specialists' experience. Briefly, experience provides the following to physicians:

a) higher precision in the use of vague linguistics terms;
b) higher agreement with other specialists;
c) higher predictive capacity when using vague terms.

Combining scaling methods with aggregation and comparison tools of membership functions allows us to formalize the hypotheses. We have shown how formalized hypotheses can be checked for their acceptance or refusal.

Furthermore, the experiment provides information about each of the doctors and their diagnosis, their predictive capacities about the stimuli displayed, and finally, but no less important, about the vague adjectives used.

References

[1] Calcedo, B.A., Mental disorder classification at primary care, *Monografías de Psiquiatría*, IX, Extra Issue, (in Spanish) pp. 41-53, 1997.

[2] Herrán, A., Vázquez-Barquero, J.L., and Artal, J., Depression identification at primary health care, *Monografías de Psiquiatría*, IX, Extra Issue, (in Spanish) pp. 54-75, 1997.

[3] Norwich, A.M. and Turksen, I.B., The fundamental measurement of fuzziness, *Fuzzy Set and Possibility Theory*, Ronald R. Yager (Ed.), 49-60, Pergamon Press, NY, 1982.

[4] Norwich, A. and Turksen, I.B., The construction of memberships functions, *Fuzzy Set and Possibility Theory,* Ronald R. Yager (Ed.), 61-67, Pergamon Press, NY, 1982.

[5] Norwich, A. and Turksen, I.B., Meaningfulness in fuzzy set theory, *Fuzzy Set and Possibility Theory,* Ronald R. Yager (Ed.), 68-74, Pergamon Press, NY, 1982.

[6] Norwich, A. and Turksen, I.B., Stochastic fuzziness, *Approximate Reasoning in decision analysis*, M.M. Gupta and E. Sanchez (Eds.), North-Holland, Amsterdam, 13-22, 1982.

[7] Norwich, A. and Turksen, I.B., A model for the measurement of membership and the consequences of its empirical implementations, *Fuzzy sets and systems*, 12, pp. 1-25, 1984.

[8] Krantz, D.H., Luce, R.D., Suppes, P., and Tversky, A., *Foundations of Measurement*, Vol. 1, Academic Press, NY, 1971.

[9] Dunn-Rankin, P., *Scaling Methods*, Lawrence Erlabum Associates. Hillsdale, 1983.

[10] Likert, E.A., Technique for the measurement of attitudes, *Archives of Psychology* 140; 22, pp. 44-53, 1932.

[11] Miller, G.A., The magical number seven plus or minus two: some limits on our capacity for processing information, *The Psychology of Communication,* Penguin Books Inc., 1967.

[12] Bonisonne, P.P. and Decker, K.S., Selecting uncertainty calculi and granularity: an experiment in trading-off precision and complexity, *KBS Working Paper,* Gen. El. Corp., Schenectady, NY, 1985.

[13] Osgood, C.E., *Method and Theory in Experimental Psychology*, Oxford University Press, London, 1962.

[14] Verdegay, J.L. and Sancho-Royo, A., Empirical determination of membership functions for stimuli comparison, *Proceedings Fuzzy Systems Conference IEEE*, Vol III, pp. 1327-1332, 1997. (A more detailed reference is Sancho, A., Stimuli Assessment with Fuzzy Characteristics, Tesis Doctoral, Univ. de Granada, Dept. Ciencias de la Computación e Inteligencia Artificial, November 1997, in Spanish.)

[15] Fishburn, P.C., The axioms and algebra of ambiguity, *Theory and Decision*, 34, pp. 119-137, 1993.

[16] Yager, R.R., On a measure of ambiguity, *Int. J. of Intelligent Systems*, Vol. 10, pp. 1001-1019, 1995.

[17] Yager, R.R., On the measure of fuzziness and negation. Part I: membership in the unit interval, *Int. J. Intelligent Systems*, 5, pp. 221-229, 1979.

[18] Yager, R.R., On the measure of fuzziness and negation. Part II: lattices, *Inf. Control*, 44, pp. 236-280, 1980.

Index of Terms